Injury & Trauma Sourcebook

Learning Disabilities Sourcebook, 4th Edition

Leukemia Sourcebook

Liver Disorders Sourcebook

Medical Tests Sourcebook, 4th Edition

Men's Health Concerns Sourcebook, 4th Edition

Mental Health Disorders Sourcebook, 5th Edition

Mental Retardation Sourcebook

Movement Disorders Sourcebook, 2nd Edition

Multiple Sclerosis Sourcebook

Muscular Dystrophy Sourcebook

Obesity Sourcebook

Osteoporosis Sourcebook

Pain Sourcebook, 3rd Edition

Pediatric Cancer Sourcebook

Physical & Mental Issues in Aging Sourcebook

Podiatry Sourcebook, 2nd Edition

Pregnancy & Birth Sourcebook, 3rd Edition

Prostate & Urological Disorders Sourcebook

Prostate Cancer Sourcebook

Rehabilitation Sourcebook

Respiratory Disorders Sourcebook, 2nd Edition

Sexually Transmitted Diseases Sourcebook, 5th Edition

Sleep Disorders Sourcebook, 3rd Edition

Smoking Concerns Sourcebook

Sports Injuries Sourcebook, 4th Edition

Stress-Related Disorders Sourcebook, 3rd Edition

Stroke Sourcebook, 2nd Edition

Surgery Sourcebook, 2nd Edition

Thyroid Disorders Sourcebook

Transplantation Sourcebook

Traveler's Health Sourcebook

Urinary Tract & Kidney Diseases & Disorders Sourcebook, 2nd Edition

Vegetarian Sourcebook

Women's Health Concerns Sourcebook, 3rd Edition

Workplace Health & Safety Sourcebook

Worldwide Health Sourcebook

Teen Health Series

Abuse & Violence Information for Teens

Accident & Safety Information for Teens

Alcohol Information for Teens, 2nd Edition

Allergy Information for Teens

Asthma Information for Teens, 2nd Edition

Body Information for Teens

Cancer Information for Teens, 2nd Edition

Complementary & Alternative Medicine Information for Teens

Diabetes Information for Teens, 2nd Edition

Diet Information for Teens, 3rd Edition

Drug Information for Teens, 3rd Edition

Eating Disorders Information for Teens, 2nd Edition

Fitness Information for Teens, 3rd Edition

Learning Disabilities Information for Teens

Mental Health Information for Teens, 3rd Edition

Pregnancy Information for Teens, 2nd Edition

Sexual Health Information for Teens, 3rd Edition

Skin Health Information for Teens, 2nd Edition

Sleep Information for Teens

Sports Injuries Information for Teens, 3rd Edition

Stress Information for Teens

Suicide Information for Teens, 2nd Edition

Tobacco Information for Teens, 2nd Edition

Depression
SOURCEBOOK

Third Edition

Depression
SOURCEBOOK

Basic Consumer Health Information about the Symptoms, Causes, and Types of Depression, Including Major Depression, Dysthymia, Atypical Depression, Bipolar Disorder, Depression during and after Pregnancy, Premenstrual Dysphoric Disorder, Schizoaffective Disorder, and Seasonal Affective Disorder

Along with Facts about Depression and Chronic Illness, Treatment-Resistant Depression and Suicide, Mental Health Medications, Therapies, and Treatments, Tips for Improving Self-Esteem, Resilience, and Quality of Life While Living with Depression, a Glossary of Related Terms, and Resources for Additional Help and Information

Edited by
Amy L. Sutton

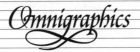

155 W. Congress, Suite 200, Detroit, MI 48226

Bibliographic Note

Because this page cannot legibly accommodate all the copyright notices, the Bibliographic Note portion of the Preface constitutes an extension of the copyright notice.

Edited by Amy L. Sutton

Health Reference Series

Karen Bellenir, *Managing Editor*
David A. Cooke, MD, FACP, *Medical Consultant*
Elizabeth Collins, *Research and Permissions Coordinator*
Cherry Edwards, *Permissions Assistant*
EdIndex, Services for Publishers, *Indexers*

* * *

Omnigraphics, Inc.

Matthew P. Barbour, *Senior Vice President*
Kevin M. Hayes, *Operations Manager*

* * *

Peter E. Ruffner, *Publisher*

Copyright © 2012 Omnigraphics, Inc.

ISBN 978-0-7808-1257-4

E-ISBN 978-0-7808-1258-1

Library of Congress Cataloging-in-Publication Data

Depression sourcebook : basic consumer health information about the symptoms, causes, and types of depression, including major depression, dysthymia, atypical depression, bipolar disorder, depression during and after pregnancy, premenstrual dysphoric disorder, schizoaffective disorder, and seasonal affective disorder; along with facts about depression and chronic illness, treatment-resistant depression and suicide, mental health medications, therapies, and treatments, tips for improving self-esteem, resilience, and quality of life while living with depression ... / edited by Amy L. Sutton. -- 3rd ed.

p. cm. -- (Health reference series)

Summary: "Provides basic consumer health information about the causes, symptoms, diagnosis, and treatment of various forms of depression, along with coping tips and strategies for building resilience and self-esteem. Includes index, glossary of related terms, and other resources"-- Provided by publisher.

Includes bibliographical references and index.

ISBN 978-0-7808-1257-4 (hardcover : alk. paper) 1. Depression, Mental--Popular works. I. Sutton, Amy L.

RC537.D4455 2012

616.85'27--dc23

2011052939

This book is printed on acid-free paper meeting the ANSI Z39.48 Standard. The infinity symbol that appears above indicates that the paper in this book meets that standard.

Printed in the United States

Table of Contents

Visit www.healthreferenceseries.com to view *A Contents Guide to the Health Reference Series*, a listing of more than 16,000 topics and the volumes in which they are covered.

Part II: Types of Depression

Part III: Who Develops Depression?

Part IV: Causes and Risk Factors for Depression

Part VI: Diagnosis and Treatment of Depression

Part VII: Strategies for Managing Depression

Part VIII: Suicide

Part IX: Additional Help and Information

Preface

About This Book

Depression, which is characterized by persistent sadness, hopelessness, trouble concentrating, fatigue, and changes in appetite and sleep habits, is one of the most disabling health problems in the world. It is also one of the most common. Approximately one in five women (20%) and one in ten men (10%) will experience it during the course of a lifetime. A variety of factors, including genetics, biology, and environment, may contribute to the development of depression, but prompt diagnosis and treatment helps those who suffer manage their symptoms and develop strategies for living with this chronic disease.

Depression Sourcebook, Third Edition offers basic information about the prevalence, symptoms, and types of depressive mood disorders, including major depression, dysthymia, atypical depression, bipolar disorder, depression during and after pregnancy, premenstrual dysphoric disorder, depression with psychosis, and seasonal affective disorder. It discusses genetic, biological, and environmental risk factors for depression and examines the impact of depression among the chronically ill, minority populations, children, adolescents, college students, men, women, and older adults. Information about depression's diagnosis and treatment—including therapy, medications, and brain stimulation techniques—is provided, along with facts about alternative and complementary therapies used to improve depression symptoms. Strategies for managing depression are also discussed, along with information about the warning signs and prevalence of suicide. The book concludes with a glossary of related terms and a directory of resources for additional help and information.

How to Use This Book

This book is divided into parts and chapters. Parts focus on broad areas of interest. Chapters are devoted to single topics within a part.

Part I: Introduction to Mental Health Disorders and Depression defines depression and discusses how brain function and chemistry play a role in the development and severity of mental health disorders. It reports on myths and facts about depression, identifies common symptoms of depression, and notes statistics and trends in mental health disorder diagnosis, treatment costs, and the number of people who receive care.

Part II: Types of Depression identifies the most common types of depression and related mental health disorders, including major depression, dysthymia, atypical depression, bipolar disorder, depression during and after pregnancy, premenstrual dysphoric disorder, seasonal affective disorder, and psychotic depression.

Part III: Who Develops Depression? provides information about gender, age, and racial disparities in the diagnosis of depression. Facts about depression in men, women, children, adolescents, college students, and seniors are discussed, along with information about mental health problems in minority populations. The chapter also provides information about the prevalence of depression in employed adults, veterans, and caregivers.

Part IV: Causes and Risk Factors for Depression highlights genetic, environmental, and situational factors that can predispose a person to developing depression. The impact of stress, trauma, unemployment, poverty, and substance use and addiction on the development of depression is also included.

Part V: Depression and Chronic Illness discusses chronic illnesses often linked to depression, such as autoimmune diseases, brain injury, cancer, diabetes, heart disease, human immunodeficiency virus (HIV), multiple sclerosis, Alzheimer disease, Parkinson disease, and stroke.

Part VI: Diagnosis and Treatment of Depression describes the process of receiving a depression diagnosis, paying for mental health care, and finding and choosing a mental health care provider. It also identifies mental health medications and therapies used to treat depression, including psychotherapy (talk therapy), cognitive-behavioral therapy, and family and group therapy. Other forms of treatment, including light therapy for seasonal affective disorder and electroconvulsive therapy, are also discussed. The part concludes with a discussion of alternative and complementary depression therapies, treatments for adolescents and children with depression, and strategies for treating severe or relapsed forms of depression.

Part VII: Strategies for Managing Depression discusses strategies for maintaining emotional wellness in people who have depression. People with depression will find information on developing resilience, avoiding depression triggers, and improving self-esteem and self-image, as well as tips on managing workplace depression, dealing with trauma, and coping with grief, bereavement, and loss. Facts about mental health support groups and strategies for helping a family member or friend with depression are also included.

Part VIII: Suicide offers information about the prevalence of suicide. It describes the warning signs of suicide and suggests next steps if you or a loved one expresses thoughts about suicide. The part concludes with information about coping with your own feelings if someone you love has died by suicide.

Part IX: Additional Help and Information provides a glossary of important terms related to depression and a directory of organizations that help people with depression and suicidal thoughts.

Bibliographic Note

This volume contains documents and excerpts from publications issued by the following U.S. government agencies: Agency for Healthcare Research and Quality (AHRQ); Centers for Disease Control and Prevention (CDC); Centers for Medicare and Medicaid Services (CMS); National Cancer Institute (NCI); National Center for Complementary and Alternative Medicine (NCCAM); National Center for Posttraumatic Stress Disorder (NCPTSD); National Diabetes Education Program (NDEP); National Health Information Center (NHIC); National Institute of Arthritis and Musculoskeletal and Skin Diseases (NIAMS); National Institute of Mental Health (NIMH); National Institute on Aging (NIA); National Institutes of Health (NIH); Office on Women's Health (OWH); Substance Abuse and Mental Health Services Administration

(SAMHSA); U.S. Department of Justice (DOJ); and the U.S. Food and Drug Administration (FDA).

In addition, this volume contains copyrighted documents from the following organizations: A.D.A.M., Inc.; AIDS InfoNet; Alzheimer's Association; American Psychiatric Association; American Psychological Association; Anxiety Disorders Association of America; BSCS; Canadian Mental Health Association; Caring, Inc.; Centre for Clinical Interventions; Family Caregiver Alliance; Fibromyalgia Network; Hazelden Foundation; Lupus Foundation of America, Inc.; Multiple Sclerosis Association of America; NAMI Los Angeles; National Alliance on Mental Illness; Nemours Foundation; Parkinson's Disease Foundation; and Psych Central.

Full citation information is provided on the first page of each chapter or section. Every effort has been made to secure all necessary rights to reprint the copyrighted material. If any omissions have been made, please contact Omnigraphics to make corrections for future editions.

Acknowledgements

Thanks go to the many organizations, agencies, and individuals who have contributed materials for this *Sourcebook* and to medical consultant Dr. David Cooke and prepress service provider Whimsy Ink. Special thanks go to managing editor Karen Bellenir and research and permissions coordinator Liz Collins for their help and support.

About the Health Reference Series

The *Health Reference Series* is designed to provide basic medical information for patients, families, caregivers, and the general public. Each volume takes a particular topic and provides comprehensive coverage. This is especially important for people who may be dealing with a newly diagnosed disease or a chronic disorder in themselves or in a family member. People looking for preventive guidance, information about disease warning signs, medical statistics, and risk factors for health problems will also find answers to their questions in the *Health Reference Series*. The *Series*, however, is not intended to serve as a tool for diagnosing illness, in prescribing treatments, or as a substitute for the physician/patient relationship. All people concerned about medical symptoms or the possibility of disease are encouraged to seek professional care from an appropriate health care provider.

A Note about Spelling and Style

Health Reference Series editors use *Stedman's Medical Dictionary* as an authority for questions related to the spelling of medical terms and the *Chicago Manual of Style* for questions related to grammatical structures, punctuation, and other editorial concerns. Consistent adherence is not always possible, however, because the individual volumes within the *Series* include many documents from a wide variety of different producers and copyright holders, and the editor's primary goal is to present material from each source as accurately as is possible following the terms specified by each document's producer. This sometimes means that information in different chapters or sections may follow other guidelines and alternate spelling authorities. For example, occasionally a copyright holder may require that eponymous terms be shown in possessive forms (Crohn's disease *vs.* Crohn disease) or that British spelling norms be retained (leukaemia *vs.* leukemia).

Locating Information within the Health Reference Series

The *Health Reference Series* contains a wealth of information about a wide variety of medical topics. Ensuring easy access to all the fact sheets, research reports, in-depth discussions, and other material contained within the individual books of the *Series* remains one of our highest priorities. As the *Series* continues to grow in size and scope, however, locating the precise information needed by a reader may become more challenging.

A *Contents Guide to the Health Reference Series* was developed to direct readers to the specific volumes that address their concerns. It presents an extensive list of diseases, treatments, and other topics of general interest compiled from the Tables of Contents and major index headings. To access *A Contents Guide to the Health Reference Series*, visit www.healthreferenceseries.com.

Medical Consultant

Medical consultation services are provided to the *Health Reference Series* editors by David A. Cooke, MD, FACP. Dr. Cooke is a graduate of Brandeis University, and he received his M.D. degree from the University of Michigan. He completed residency training at the University of Wisconsin Hospital and Clinics. He is board-certified in Internal Medicine. Dr. Cooke currently works as part of the University of Michigan Health System and practices in Ann Arbor, MI. In his free time, he enjoys writing, science fiction, and spending time with his family.

Our Advisory Board

We would like to thank the following board members for providing guidance to the development of this *Series*:

- Dr. Lynda Baker, Associate Professor of Library and Information Science, Wayne State University, Detroit, MI

- Nancy Bulgarelli, William Beaumont Hospital Library, Royal Oak, MI

- Karen Imarisio, Bloomfield Township Public Library, Bloomfield Township, MI

- Karen Morgan, Mardigian Library, University of Michigan-Dearborn, Dearborn, MI

- Rosemary Orlando, St. Clair Shores Public Library, St. Clair Shores, MI

Health Reference Series *Update Policy*

The inaugural book in the *Health Reference Series* was the first edition of *Cancer Sourcebook* published in 1989. Since then, the *Series* has been enthusiastically received by librarians and in the medical community. In order to maintain the standard of providing high-quality health information for the layperson the editorial staff at Omnigraphics felt it was necessary to implement a policy of updating volumes when warranted.

Medical researchers have been making tremendous strides, and it is the purpose of the *Health Reference Series* to stay current with the most recent advances. Each decision to update a volume is made on an individual basis. Some of the considerations include how much new information is available and the feedback we receive from people who use the books. If there is a topic you would like to see added to the update list, or an area of medical concern you feel has not been adequately addressed, please write to:

Editor
Health Reference Series
Omnigraphics, Inc.
155 W. Congress, Suite 200
Detroit, MI 48226
E-mail: editorial@omnigraphics.com

Part One

Introduction to Mental Health Disorders and Depression

Chapter 1

What Are Mental Health Disorders?

Defining Mental Illness

We can all be "sad" or "blue" at times in our lives. We have all seen movies about the madman and his crime spree, with the underlying cause of mental illness. We sometimes even make jokes about people being crazy or nuts, even though we know that we shouldn't. We have all had some exposure to mental illness, but do we really understand it or know what it is? Many of our preconceptions are incorrect. A mental illness can be defined as a health condition that changes a person's thinking, feelings, or behavior (or all three) and that causes the person distress and difficulty in functioning. As with many diseases, mental illness is severe in some cases and mild in others. Individuals who have a mental illness don't necessarily look like they are sick, especially if their illness is mild. Other individuals may show more explicit symptoms such as confusion, agitation, or withdrawal. There are many different mental illnesses, including depression, schizophrenia, attention deficit hyperactivity disorder (ADHD), autism, and obsessive-compulsive disorder. Each illness alters a person's thoughts, feelings, and/or behaviors in distinct ways.

Not all brain diseases are categorized as mental illnesses. Disorders such as epilepsy, Parkinson disease, and multiple sclerosis are brain disorders, but they are considered neurological diseases rather than mental illnesses.

Interestingly, the lines between mental illnesses and these other brain or neurological disorders is blurring somewhat. As scientists continue to investigate the brains of people who have mental illnesses, they are learning that mental illness is associated with changes in the brain's structure, chemistry, and function and that mental illness does indeed have a biological basis. This ongoing research is, in some ways, causing scientists to minimize the distinctions between mental illnesses and these other brain disorders. In this text, we will restrict our discussion of mental illness to those illnesses that are traditionally classified as mental illnesses, as listed in the previous paragraph.

Mental Illness in the Population

Many people feel that mental illness is rare, something that only happens to people with life situations very different from their own, and that it will never affect them. Studies of the epidemiology of mental illness indicate that this belief is far from accurate. In fact, the surgeon general reports that mental illnesses are so common that few U.S. families are untouched by them.

Mental Illness in Adults

Even if you or a family member has not experienced mental illness directly, it is very likely that you have known someone who has. Estimates are that at least one in four people is affected by mental illness either directly or indirectly.

Consider the following statistics to get an idea of just how widespread the effects of mental illness are in society:

- According to recent estimates, approximately 20 percent of Americans, or about one in five people over the age of 18, suffer from a diagnosable mental disorder in a given year.

- Four of the 10 leading causes of disability—major depression, bipolar disorder, schizophrenia, and obsessive-compulsive disorder—are mental illnesses.

- About 3 percent of the population have more than one mental illness at a time.

- About 5 percent of adults are affected so seriously by mental illness that it interferes with their ability to function in society. These severe and persistent mental illnesses include schizophrenia, bipolar disorder, other severe forms of depression, panic disorder, and obsessive-compulsive disorder.

- Approximately 20 percent of doctors' appointments are related to anxiety disorders such as panic attacks.

- Eight million people have depression each year.

- Two million Americans have schizophrenia disorders, and 300,000 new cases are diagnosed each year.

Mental Illness in Children and Adolescents

Mental illness is not uncommon among children and adolescents. Approximately 12 million children under the age of 18 have mental disorders. The National Mental Health Association has compiled some statistics about mental illness in children and adolescents:

- Mental health problems affect one in every five young people at any given time.

- An estimated two-thirds of all young people with mental health problems are not receiving the help they need.

- Less than one-third of the children under age 18 who have a serious mental health problem receive any mental health services.

- As many as one in every 33 children may be depressed. Depression in adolescents may be as high as one in eight.

- Suicide is the third leading cause of death for 15- to 24-year-olds and the sixth leading cause of death for 5- to 15-year-olds.

- Schizophrenia is rare in children under age 12, but it occurs in about three of every 1,000 adolescents.

- Between 118,700 and 186,600 youths in the juvenile justice system have at least one mental illness.

- Of the 100,000 teenagers in juvenile detention, an estimated 60 percent have behavioral, cognitive, or emotional problems.

Warning Signs for Mental Illness

Each mental illness has its own characteristic symptoms. However, there are some general warning signs that might alert you that someone needs professional help. Some of these signs include:

- marked personality change;

- inability to cope with problems and daily activities;

- strange or grandiose ideas;

- excessive anxieties;

- prolonged depression and apathy;

- marked changes in eating or sleeping patterns;

- thinking or talking about suicide or harming oneself;

- extreme mood swings—high or low;

- abuse of alcohol or drugs; and

- excessive anger, hostility, or violent behavior.

A person who shows any of these signs should seek help from a qualified health professional.

Diagnosing Mental Illness

Mental Health Professionals

To be diagnosed with a mental illness, a person must be evaluated by a qualified professional who has expertise in mental health. Mental health professionals include psychiatrists, psychologists, psychiatric nurses, social workers, and mental health counselors. Family doctors, internists, and pediatricians are usually qualified to diagnose common mental disorders such as depression, anxiety disorders, and ADHD. In many cases, depending on the individual and his or her symptoms, a mental health professional who is not a psychiatrist will refer the patient to a psychiatrist. A psychiatrist is a medical doctor (MD) who has received additional training in the field of mental health and mental illnesses. Psychiatrists evaluate the person's mental condition in coordination with his or her physical condition and can prescribe medication. Only psychiatrists and other MDs can prescribe medications to treat mental illness.

Mental Illnesses Are Diagnosed by Symptoms

Unlike some disease diagnoses, doctors can't do a blood test or culture some microorganisms to determine whether a person has a mental illness. Maybe scientists will develop discrete physiological tests for mental illnesses in the future; until then, however, mental health professionals will have to diagnose mental illnesses based on the symptoms that a person has. Basing a diagnosis on symptoms and not on a quantitative medical test, such as a blood chemistry test, a throat swab, X-rays, or urinalysis, is not unusual. Physicians diagnose many diseases, including migraines, Alzheimer disease, and Parkinson disease based on their symptoms alone. For other diseases, such as asthma or mononucleosis, doctors rely on analyzing symptoms to get a good idea of what the problem is and then use a physiological test to provide additional information or to confirm their diagnosis.

When a mental health professional works with a person who might have a mental illness, he or she will, along with the individual, determine what symptoms the individual has, how long the symptoms have persisted, and how his or her life is being affected. Mental health professionals often gather information through an interview during which they ask the patient about his or her symptoms, the length of time that the symptoms have occurred, and the severity of the symptoms. In many cases, the professional will also get information about the patient from family members to obtain a more comprehensive picture. A physician likely will conduct a physical exam and consult the patient's history to rule out other health problems.

Mental health professionals evaluate symptoms to make a diagnosis of mental illness. They rely on the criteria specified in the *Diagnostic and Statistical Manual of Mental Disorders (DSM-IV*; currently, the fourth edition), published by the American Psychiatric Association, to diagnose a specific mental illness.

For each mental illness, the *DSM-IV* gives a general description of the disorder and a list of typical symptoms. Mental health professionals refer to the *DSM-IV* to confirm that the symptoms a patient exhibits match those of a specific mental illness. Although the *DSM-IV* provides valuable information that helps mental health professionals diagnose mental illness, these professionals realize that it is important to observe patients over a period of time to understand the individual's mental illness and its effects on his or her life.

Chapter 2

Brain Function, Biology, and Mental Health Disorders

The term mental illness clearly indicates that there is a problem with the mind. But is it just the mind in an abstract sense, or is there a physical basis to mental illness? As scientists continue to investigate mental illnesses and their causes, they learn more and more about how the biological processes that make the brain work are changed when a person has a mental illness.

The Basics of Brain Function

Before thinking about the problems that occur in the brain when someone has a mental illness, it is helpful to think about how the brain functions normally.

The brain is an incredibly complex organ. It makes up only 2 percent of our body weight, but it consumes 20 percent of the oxygen we breathe and 20 percent of the energy we take in. It controls virtually everything we as humans experience, including movement, sensing our environment, regulating our involuntary body processes such as breathing, and controlling our emotions. Hundreds of thousands of chemical reactions occur every second in the brain; those reactions underlie the thoughts, actions, and behaviors with which we respond to environmental stimuli. In short, the brain dictates the internal processes and behaviors that allow us to survive.

How does the brain take in all this information, process it, and cause a response? The basic functional unit of the brain is the neuron. A neuron is a specialized cell that can produce different actions because of its precise connections with other neurons, sensory receptors, and muscle cells. A typical neuron has four structurally and functionally defined regions: The cell body, dendrites, axons, and the axon terminals.

The cell body is the metabolic center of the neuron. The nucleus is located in the cell body and most of the cell's protein synthesis occurs here.

A neuron usually has multiple fibers called dendrites that extend from the cell body. These processes usually branch out somewhat like tree branches and serve as the main apparatus for receiving input from other nerve cells.

The cell body also gives rise to the axon. The axon is usually much longer than the dendrites; in some cases, an axon can be up to 1 m long. The axon is the part of the neuron that is specialized to carry messages away from the cell body and to relay messages to other cells. Some large axons are surrounded by a fatty insulating material called myelin, which enables the electrical signals to travel down the axon at higher speeds.

Near its end, the axon divides into many fine branches that have specialized swellings called axon terminals or presynaptic terminals. The axon terminals end near the dendrites of another neuron. The dendrites of one neuron receive the message sent from the axon terminals of another neuron.

The site where an axon terminal ends near a receiving dendrite is called the synapse. The cell that sends out information is called the presynaptic neuron, and the cell that receives the information is called the postsynaptic neuron. It is important to note that the synapse is not a physical connection between the two neurons; there is no cytoplasmic connection between the two neurons. The intercellular space between the presynaptic and postsynaptic neurons is called the synaptic space or synaptic cleft. An average neuron forms approximately 1,000 synapses with other neurons. It has been estimated that there are more synapses in the human brain than there are stars in our galaxy. Furthermore, synaptic connections are not static. Neurons form new synapses or strengthen synaptic connections in response to life experiences. This dynamic change in neuronal connections is the basis of learning.

Neurons communicate using both electrical signals and chemical messages. Information in the form of an electrical impulse is carried away from the neuron's cell body along the axon of the presynaptic neuron toward the axon terminals. When the electrical signal reaches the presynaptic axon terminal, it cannot cross the synaptic space, or synaptic cleft. Instead, the electrical signal triggers chemical changes that can cross the synapse to affect the postsynaptic cell. When the electrical impulse reaches the presynaptic axon terminal, membranous sacs called vesicles move toward the membrane of the axon terminal. When the vesicles reach the membrane, they fuse with the membrane and release their contents into the synaptic space. The molecules contained in the vesicles are chemical compounds called neurotransmitters. Each vesicle contains many molecules of a neurotransmitter. The released neurotransmitter molecules drift across the synaptic cleft and then bind to special proteins, called receptors, on the postsynaptic neuron. A neurotransmitter molecule will bind only to a specific kind of receptor.

The binding of neurotransmitters to their receptors causes that neuron to generate an electrical impulse. The electrical impulse then moves away from the dendrite ending toward the cell body. After the neurotransmitter stimulates an electrical impulse in the postsynaptic neuron, it releases from the receptor back into the synaptic space. Specific proteins called transporters or reuptake pumps carry the neurotransmitter back into the presynaptic neuron. When the neurotransmitter molecules are back in the presynaptic axon terminal, they can be repackaged into vesicles for release the next time an electrical impulse reaches the axon terminal. Enzymes present in the synaptic space degrade neurotransmitter molecules that are not taken back up into the presynaptic neuron.

The nervous system uses a variety of neurotransmitter molecules, but each neuron specializes in the synthesis and secretion of a single type of neurotransmitter. Some of the predominant neurotransmitters in the brain include glutamate, GABA [gamma-aminobutyric acid], serotonin, dopamine, and norepinephrine. Each of these neurotransmitters has a specific distribution and function in the brain; the specifics of each are beyond the scope of this text, but a few of the names will arise in reference to particular mental illnesses.

Investigating Brain Function

Mental health professionals base their diagnosis and treatment of mental illness on the symptoms that a person exhibits. The goal for these professionals in treating a patient is to relieve the symptoms that are interfering with the person's life so that the person can function well. Research scientists, on the other hand, have a different goal.

They want to learn about the chemical or structural changes that occur in the brain when someone has a mental illness. If scientists can determine what happens in the brain, they can use that knowledge to develop better treatments or find a cure.

The techniques that scientists use to investigate the brain depend on the questions they are asking. For some questions, scientists use molecular or biochemical methods to investigate specific genes or proteins in the neurons. For other questions, scientists want to visualize changes in the brain so that they can learn more about how the activity or structure of the brain changes. Historically, scientists could examine brains only after death, but new imaging procedures enable scientists to study the brain in living animals, including humans. It is important to realize that these brain imaging techniques are not used for diagnosing mental illness. Mental illnesses are diagnosed by the set of symptoms that an individual exhibits. The imaging techniques described in the following paragraphs would not enable the mental health professional to diagnose or treat the patient more effectively. Some of the techniques are also invasive and expose patients to small amounts of radiation. Research studies using these tests are generally not conducted with children or adolescents.

One extensively used technique to study brain activity and how mental illness changes the brain is positron emission tomography (PET). PET measures the spatial distribution and movement of a radioactive chemical injected into the tissues of living subjects. Because the patient is awake, the technique can be used to investigate the relationship between behavioral and physiological effects and changes in brain activity. PET scans can detect very small (nanomolar) concentrations of tracer molecules and achieve spatial resolution of about 4 mm. In addition, computers can reconstruct images obtained from a PET scan in two or three dimensions.

PET requires the use of compounds that are labeled with positron-emitting isotopes. A positron has the same mass and spin as an electron but the opposite charge; an electron has a negative charge and a positron has a positive charge. A cyclotron accelerates protons into the nucleus of nitrogen, carbon, oxygen, or fluorine to generate these isotopes. The additional proton makes the isotope unstable. To become stable again, the proton must break down into a neutron and a positron. The unstable positron travels away from the site of generation and dissipates energy along the way. Eventually, the positron collides with an electron, leading to the emission of two gamma rays at 180 degrees from one another. The gamma rays reach a pair of detectors that record the event. Because the detectors respond only to simultaneous emissions, scientists can precisely map the location where the gamma rays were generated. The radioactive chemicals used for PET are very short lived. The half-life (the time for half of the radioactive label to disintegrate) of the commonly used radioisotopes ranges from approximately 2 minutes to less than 2 hours, depending on the specific compound. Because a PET scan requires only small amounts (a few mcg) of short-lived radioisotopes, this technique can be used safely in humans.

PET scans can answer a variety of questions about brain function, including where the neurons are most active. Scientists use different radiolabeled compounds to investigate different biological questions. For example, radiolabeled glucose can identify parts of the brain that become more active in response to a specific stimulus. Active neurons metabolize more glucose than inactive neurons. Active neurons emit more positrons, and this shows as red or yellow on PET scans compared with blue or purple in areas where the neurons are not highly active. (Different computer enhancement techniques may use a different color scheme, but the use of a spectrum with red indicating high activity and blue indicating low activity is common.) Scientists can use PET to measure changes in the activity of specific brain areas in a person who has a mental illness. Scientists can also investigate how the mentally ill brain changes after a person receives treatment.

PET imaging is not the only technique that researchers use to investigate how mental illness changes the brain. Different techniques provide different information to scientists. Another important technique is magnetic resonance imaging (MRI). Unlike PET, which reveals changes in activity level, MRI is used to look at structural changes in the brain. For example, MRI studies reveal that the ventricles, or spaces within the brain, are larger in individuals who have schizophrenia compared with those of healthy individuals.

Other techniques that scientists use to investigate function in the living brain include single photon emission computed tomography (SPECT), functional magnetic resonance imaging (fMRI), and electroencephalography (EEG). Each technique has its own advantages, and each provides different information about brain structure and function. Scientists often use more than one technique when conducting their research.

Chapter 3

Myths and Facts about Mental Health Disorders

Mental illnesses are very common. They are also widely misunderstood. People with mental illnesses are frequently stigmatized by others who think it's an uncommon condition. The truth is, mental illness can happen to anybody.

Myth: *There's no hope for people with mental illnesses.*

Fact: There are more treatments, services, and community support systems than ever before, and more are in the works. People with mental illnesses lead active, productive lives.

Myth: *I can't do anything for a person with mental illness.*

Fact: You can do a lot, starting with how you act and speak. You can create an environment that builds on people's strengths and promotes understanding. For example:

- Don't label people with words like "crazy," "wacko," or "loony" or define them by their diagnosis. Instead of saying someone is "a schizophrenic," say he or she "has schizophrenia." Don't say "a schizophrenic person," say "a person with schizophrenia." This is called "people-first" language, and it's important to make a distinction between the person and the illness.

Excerpted from "Mental Illness: Myths and Facts," by the Substance Abuse and Mental Health Services Administration (SAMHSA, www.whatadifference .samhsa.gov), 2007.

- Learn the facts about mental health and share them with others, especially if you hear something that isn't true.

- Treat people with mental illnesses with respect and dignity, just as you would anybody else.

- Respect the rights of people with mental illnesses and don't discriminate against them when it comes to housing, employment, or education. Like other people with disabilities, people with mental health problems are protected under federal and state laws.

Myth: People with mental illnesses are violent and unpredictable.

Fact: Actually, the vast majority of people with mental health conditions are no more violent than anyone else. People with mental illnesses are much more likely to be the victims of crime. You probably know someone with a mental illness and don't even realize it.

Myth: Mental illnesses don't affect me.

Fact: Mental illnesses are surprisingly common; they affect almost every family in America. Mental illnesses do not discriminate—they can affect anyone.

Myth: Mental illness is the same as mental retardation.

Fact: These are different conditions. Mental retardation is characterized by limitations in intellectual functioning and difficulties with certain daily living skills. In contrast, people with mental illnesses—health conditions that cause changes in a person's thinking, mood, and behavior—have varied intellectual functioning, just like the general population.

Myth: Mental illnesses are brought on by a weakness of character.

Fact: Mental illnesses are a product of the interaction of biological, psychological, and social factors. Social influences, like the loss of a loved one or a job, can also contribute to the development of various mental health problems.

Myth: People with mental illnesses cannot tolerate the stress of holding down a job.

Fact: All jobs are stressful to some extent. Anybody is more productive when there's a good match between the employee's needs and the working conditions, whether or not the worker has a mental health problem.

Myth: People with mental health needs, even those who have recovered, tend to be second-rate workers.

Fact: Employers who have hired people with mental illnesses report good attendance and punctuality as well as motivation, good work, and job tenure on par with or greater than other employees. Studies by the National Institute of Mental Health (NIMH) and the National Alliance on Mental Illness (NAMI) show that there are no differences in productivity when people with mental illnesses are compared to other employees.

Myth: Once people develop mental illnesses, they will never recover.

Fact: Studies show that most people with mental illnesses get better, and many recover completely. Recovery refers to the process in which people are able to live, work, learn, and participate fully in their communities. For some individuals, recovery is the ability to live a fulfilling and productive life. For others, recovery implies the reduction or complete remission of symptoms. Science has shown that hope plays an integral role in an individual's recovery.

Myth: Therapy and self-help are a waste of time. Why bother when you can just take a pill?

Fact: Treatment varies depending on the individual. A lot of people work with therapists, counselors, friends, psychologists, psychiatrists, nurses, and social workers during the recovery process. They also use self-help strategies and community supports. Often they combine these with some of the most advanced medications available.

Myth: Children don't experience mental illnesses. Their actions are just products of bad parenting.

Fact: A report from the President's New Freedom Commission on Mental Health showed that in any given year five to nine percent of children experience serious emotional disturbances. Just like adult mental illnesses, these are clinically diagnosable health conditions that are a product of the interaction of biological, psychological, and social factors.

Myth: Children misbehave or fail in school just to get attention.

Fact: Behavior problems can be symptoms of emotional, behavioral, or mental problems, rather than merely attention-seeking devices. These children can succeed in school with appropriate understanding, attention, and mental health services.

Chapter 4

Depression: Symptoms of the Most Common Mental Health Disorder

What is depression?

Everyone occasionally feels blue or sad. But these feelings are usually short-lived and pass within a couple of days. When you have depression, it interferes with daily life and causes pain for both you and those who care about you. Depression is a common but serious illness.

Many people with a depressive illness never seek treatment. But the majority, even those with the most severe depression, can get better with treatment. Medications, psychotherapies, and other methods can effectively treat people with depression.

What are the different forms of depression?

There are several forms of depressive disorders.

Major depressive disorder, or major depression, is characterized by a combination of symptoms that interfere with a person's ability to work, sleep, study, eat, and enjoy once-pleasurable activities. Major depression is disabling and prevents a person from functioning normally. Some people may experience only a single episode within their lifetime, but more often a person may have multiple episodes.

Excerpted from "Depression," by the National Institute of Mental Health (NIMH, www.nimh.nih.gov), part of the National Institutes of Health, May 6, 2011.

Dysthymic disorder, or dysthymia, is characterized by long-term (2 years or longer) symptoms that may not be severe enough to disable a person but can prevent normal functioning or feeling well. People with dysthymia may also experience one or more episodes of major depression during their lifetimes.

Minor depression is characterized by having symptoms for 2 weeks or longer that do not meet full criteria for major depression. Without treatment, people with minor depression are at high risk for developing major depressive disorder.

Some forms of depression are slightly different, or they may develop under unique circumstances. However, not everyone agrees on how to characterize and define these forms of depression. They include the following:

- Psychotic depression occurs when a person has severe depression plus some form of psychosis, such as having disturbing false beliefs or a break with reality (delusions), or hearing or seeing upsetting things that others cannot hear or see (hallucinations).

- Postpartum depression is much more serious than the baby blues that many women experience after giving birth, when hormonal and physical changes and the new responsibility of caring for a newborn can be overwhelming. It is estimated that 10 to 15 percent of women experience postpartum depression after giving birth.

- Seasonal affective disorder (SAD) is characterized by the onset of depression during the winter months, when there is less natural sunlight. The depression generally lifts during spring and summer. SAD may be effectively treated with light therapy, but nearly half of those with SAD do not get better with light therapy alone. Antidepressant medication and psychotherapy can reduce SAD symptoms, either alone or in combination with light therapy.

Bipolar disorder, also called manic-depressive illness, is not as common as major depression or dysthymia. Bipolar disorder is characterized by cycling mood changes—from extreme highs (e.g., mania) to extreme lows (e.g., depression).

What are the signs and symptoms of depression?

People with depressive illnesses do not all experience the same symptoms. The severity, frequency, and duration of symptoms vary depending on the individual and his or her particular illness.

Signs and symptoms include the following:

- Persistent sad, anxious, or "empty" feelings
- Feelings of hopelessness or pessimism
- Feelings of guilt, worthlessness, or helplessness
- Irritability and restlessness
- Loss of interest in activities or hobbies once pleasurable, including sex
- Fatigue and decreased energy
- Difficulty concentrating, remembering details, and making decisions
- Insomnia, early-morning wakefulness, or excessive sleeping
- Overeating or appetite loss
- Thoughts of suicide or suicide attempts
- Aches or pains, headaches, cramps, or digestive problems that do not ease even with treatment

What illnesses often coexist with depression?

Other illnesses may come on before depression, cause it, or be a consequence of it. But depression and other illnesses interact differently in different people. In any case, co-occurring illnesses need to be diagnosed and treated.

Anxiety disorders, such as posttraumatic stress disorder (PTSD), obsessive-compulsive disorder, panic disorder, social phobia, and generalized anxiety disorder, often accompany depression. PTSD can occur after a person experiences a terrifying event or ordeal, such as a violent assault, a natural disaster, an accident, terrorism, or military combat. People experiencing PTSD are especially prone to having coexisting depression.

In a National Institute of Mental Health (NIMH)-funded study, researchers found that more than 40 percent of people with PTSD also had depression four months after the traumatic event.

Alcohol and other substance abuse or dependence may also coexist with depression. Research shows that mood disorders and substance abuse commonly occur together.

Depression also may occur with other serious medical illnesses such as heart disease, stroke, cancer, HIV/AIDS [human immunodeficiency virus/acquired immunodeficiency syndrome], diabetes, and Parkinson disease. People who have depression along with another medical illness tend to have more severe symptoms of both depression and the medical illness, more difficulty adapting to their medical condition, and more medical costs than those who do not have coexisting depression. Treating the depression can also help improve the outcome of treating the co-occurring illness.

What causes depression?

Most likely, depression is caused by a combination of genetic, biological, environmental, and psychological factors.

Depressive illnesses are disorders of the brain. Longstanding theories about depression suggest that important neurotransmitters—chemicals that brain cells use to communicate—are out of balance in depression. But it has been difficult to prove this.

Brain-imaging technologies, such as magnetic resonance imaging (MRI), have shown that the brains of people who have depression look different than those of people without depression. The parts of the brain involved in mood, thinking, sleep, appetite, and behavior appear different. But these images do not reveal why the depression has occurred. They also cannot be used to diagnose depression.

Some types of depression tend to run in families. However, depression can occur in people without family histories of depression, too. Scientists are studying certain genes that may make some people more prone to depression. Some genetics research indicates that risk for depression results from the influence of several genes acting together with environmental or other factors. In addition, trauma, loss of a loved one, a difficult relationship, or any stressful situation may trigger a depressive episode. Other depressive episodes may occur with or without an obvious trigger.

How do women experience depression?

Depression is more common among women than among men. Biological, life cycle, hormonal, and psychosocial factors that women experience may be linked to women's higher depression rate. Researchers have shown that hormones directly affect the brain chemistry that controls emotions and mood. For example, women are especially vulnerable to developing postpartum depression after giving birth, when hormonal and physical changes and the new responsibility of caring for a newborn can be overwhelming.

Some women may also have a severe form of premenstrual syndrome (PMS) called premenstrual dysphoric disorder (PMDD). PMDD is associated with the hormonal changes that typically occur around ovulation and before menstruation begins.

During the transition into menopause, some women experience an increased risk for depression. In addition, osteoporosis—bone thinning or loss—may be associated with depression. Scientists are exploring all of these potential connections and how the cyclical rise and fall of estrogen and other hormones may affect a woman's brain chemistry.

Finally, many women face the additional stresses of work and home responsibilities, caring for children and aging parents, abuse, poverty, and relationship strains. It is still unclear, though, why some women faced with enormous challenges develop depression, while others with similar challenges do not.

How do men experience depression?

Men often experience depression differently than women. While women with depression are more likely to have feelings of sadness, worthlessness, and excessive guilt, men are more likely to be very tired, irritable, lose interest in once-pleasurable activities, and have difficulty sleeping.

Men may be more likely than women to turn to alcohol or drugs when they are depressed. They also may become frustrated, discouraged, irritable, angry, and sometimes abusive. Some men throw themselves into their work to avoid talking about their depression with family or friends, or behave recklessly. And although more women attempt suicide, many more men die by suicide in the United States.

How do older adults experience depression?

Depression is not a normal part of aging. Studies show that most seniors feel satisfied with their lives, despite having more illnesses or physical problems. However, when older adults do have depression, it may be overlooked because seniors may show different, less obvious symptoms. They may be less likely to experience or admit to feelings of sadness or grief.

Sometimes it can be difficult to distinguish grief from major depression. Grief after loss of a loved one is a normal reaction to the loss and generally does not require professional mental health treatment. However, grief that is complicated and lasts for a very long time following a loss may require treatment. Researchers continue to study the relationship between complicated grief and major depression.

Older adults also may have more medical conditions such as heart disease, stroke, or cancer, which may cause depressive symptoms. Or they may be taking medications with side effects that contribute to depression. Some older adults may experience what doctors call vascular depression, also called arteriosclerotic depression or subcortical ischemic depression. Vascular depression may result when blood vessels become less flexible and harden over time, becoming constricted. Such hardening of vessels prevents normal blood flow to the body's organs, including the brain. Those with vascular depression may have, or be at risk for, coexisting heart disease or stroke.

Although many people assume that the highest rates of suicide are among young people, older white males age 85 and older actually have the highest suicide rate in the United States. Many have a depressive illness that their doctors are not aware of, even though many of these suicide victims visit their doctors within 1 month of their deaths.

Most older adults with depression improve when they receive treatment with an antidepressant, psychotherapy, or a combination of both. Research has shown that medication alone and combination treatment are both effective in reducing depression in older adults. Psychotherapy alone also can be effective in helping older adults stay free of depression, especially among those with minor depression. Psychotherapy is particularly useful for those who are unable or unwilling to take antidepressant medication.

How do children and teens experience depression?

Children who develop depression often continue to have episodes as they enter adulthood. Children who have depression also are more likely to have other more severe illnesses in adulthood.

A child with depression may pretend to be sick, refuse to go to school, cling to a parent, or worry that a parent may die. Older children may sulk, get into trouble at school, be negative and irritable, and feel misunderstood. Because these signs may be viewed as normal mood swings typical of children as they move through developmental stages, it may be difficult to accurately diagnose a young person with depression.

Before puberty, boys and girls are equally likely to develop depression. By age 15, however, girls are twice as likely as boys to have had a major depressive episode.

Depression during the teen years comes at a time of great personal change—when boys and girls are forming an identity apart from their parents, grappling with gender issues and emerging sexuality, and making independent decisions for the first time in their lives. Depression in adolescence frequently co-occurs with other disorders such as anxiety, eating disorders, or substance abuse. It can also lead to increased risk for suicide.

An NIMH-funded clinical trial of 439 adolescents with major depression found that a combination of medication and psychotherapy was the most effective treatment option. Other NIMH-funded researchers are developing and testing ways to prevent suicide in children and adolescents.

How is depression diagnosed and treated?

Depression, even the most severe cases, can be effectively treated. The earlier that treatment can begin, the more effective it is.

The first step to getting appropriate treatment is to visit a doctor or mental health specialist. Certain medications, and some medical conditions such as viruses or a thyroid disorder, can cause the same symptoms as depression. A doctor can rule out these possibilities by doing a physical exam, interview, and lab tests. If the doctor can find no medical condition that may be causing the depression, the next step is a psychological evaluation.

The doctor may refer you to a mental health professional, who should discuss with you any family history of depression or other mental disorder, and get a complete history of your symptoms. You should discuss when your symptoms started, how long they have lasted, how severe they are, and whether they have occurred before and if so, how they were treated. The mental health professional may also ask if you are using alcohol or drugs, and if you are thinking about death or suicide.

Once diagnosed, a person with depression can be treated in several ways. The most common treatments are medication and psychotherapy.

Medication: Antidepressants primarily work on brain chemicals called neurotransmitters, especially serotonin and norepinephrine. Other antidepressants work on the neurotransmitter dopamine. Scientists have found that these particular chemicals are involved in regulating mood, but they are unsure of the exact ways that they work.

Popular newer antidepressants: Some of the newest and most popular antidepressants are called selective serotonin reuptake inhibitors (SSRIs). Fluoxetine (Prozac), sertraline (Zoloft), escitalopram (Lexapro), paroxetine (Paxil), and citalopram (Celexa) are some of the most commonly prescribed SSRIs for depression. Most are available in generic versions. Serotonin and norepinephrine reuptake inhibitors (SNRIs) are similar to SSRIs and include venlafaxine (Effexor) and duloxetine (Cymbalta).

SSRIs and SNRIs tend to have fewer side effects than older antidepressants, but they sometimes produce headaches, nausea, jitters, or insomnia when people first start to take them. These symptoms tend to fade with time. Some people also experience sexual problems with SSRIs or SNRIs, which may be helped by adjusting the dosage or switching to another medication.

One popular antidepressant that works on dopamine is bupropion (Wellbutrin). Bupropion tends to have similar side effects as SSRIs and SNRIs, but it is less likely to cause sexual side effects. However, it can increase a person's risk for seizures.

Tricyclics: Tricyclics are older antidepressants. Tricyclics are powerful, but they are not used as much today because their potential side effects are more serious. They may affect the heart in people with heart conditions. They sometimes cause dizziness, especially in older adults. They also may cause drowsiness, dry mouth, and weight gain. These side effects can usually be corrected by changing the dosage or switching to another medication. However, tricyclics may be especially dangerous if taken in overdose. Tricyclics include imipramine and nortriptyline.

MAOIs: Monoamine oxidase inhibitors (MAOIs) are the oldest class of antidepressant medications. They can be especially effective in cases of atypical depression, such as when a person experiences increased appetite and the need for more sleep rather than decreased appetite and sleep. They also may help with anxious feelings or panic and other specific symptoms.

However, people who take MAOIs must avoid certain foods and beverages (including cheese and red wine) that contain a substance called tyramine. Certain medications, including some types of birth control pills, prescription pain relievers, cold and allergy medications, and herbal supplements, also should be avoided while taking an MAOI. These substances can interact with MAOIs to cause dangerous increases in blood pressure. The development of a new MAOI skin patch may help reduce these risks. If you are taking an MAOI, your doctor should give you a complete list of foods, medicines, and substances to avoid.

MAOIs can also react with SSRIs to produce a serious condition called "serotonin syndrome," which can cause confusion, hallucinations, increased sweating, muscle stiffness, seizures, changes in blood pressure or heart rhythm, and other potentially life-threatening conditions. MAOIs should not be taken with SSRIs.

How should I take medication?

All antidepressants must be taken for at least 4 to 6 weeks before they have a full effect. You should continue to take the medication, even if you are feeling better, to prevent the depression from returning.

Medication should be stopped only under a doctor's supervision. Some medications need to be gradually stopped to give the body time to adjust. Although antidepressants are not habit-forming or addictive, suddenly ending an antidepressant can cause withdrawal symptoms or lead to a relapse of the depression. Some individuals, such as those with chronic or recurrent depression, may need to stay on the medication indefinitely.

In addition, if one medication does not work, you should consider trying another. NIMH-funded research has shown that people who did not get well after taking a first medication increased their chances of beating the depression after they switched to a different medication or added another medication to their existing one.

Sometimes stimulants, antianxiety medications, or other medications are used together with an antidepressant, especially if a person has a coexisting illness. However, neither antianxiety medications nor stimulants are effective against depression when taken alone, and both should be taken only under a doctor's close supervision.

Report any unusual side effects to a doctor immediately.

Psychotherapy: Several types of psychotherapy—or talk therapy—can help people with depression.

Two main types of psychotherapies—cognitive-behavioral therapy (CBT) and interpersonal therapy (IPT)—are effective in treating depression. CBT helps people with depression restructure negative thought patterns. Doing so helps people interpret their environment and interactions with others in a positive and realistic way. It may also help you recognize things that may be contributing to the depression and help you change behaviors that may be making the depression worse. IPT helps people understand and work through troubled relationships that may cause their depression or make it worse.

For mild to moderate depression, psychotherapy may be the best option. However, for severe depression or for certain people, psychotherapy may not be enough.

For teens, a combination of medication and psychotherapy may be the most effective approach to treating major depression and reducing the chances of it coming back. Another study looking at depression treatment among older adults found that people who responded to initial treatment of medication and IPT were less likely to have recurring depression if they continued their combination treatment for at least 2 years.

Electroconvulsive therapy and other brain stimulation therapies: For cases in which medication and/or psychotherapy does not help relieve a person's treatment-resistant depression, electroconvulsive therapy (ECT) may be useful. ECT, formerly known as shock therapy, once had a bad reputation. But in recent years, it has greatly improved and can provide relief for people with severe depression who have not been able to feel better with other treatments.

Before ECT begins, a patient is put under brief anesthesia and given a muscle relaxant. He or she sleeps through the treatment and does not consciously feel the electrical impulses. Within one hour after the treatment session, which takes only a few minutes, the patient is awake and alert.

A person typically will undergo ECT several times a week, and often will need to take an antidepressant or other medication along with the ECT treatments.

Although some people will need only a few courses of ECT, others may need maintenance ECT—usually once a week at first, then gradually decreasing to monthly treatments. Ongoing NIMH-supported ECT research is aimed at developing personalized maintenance ECT schedules.

ECT may cause some side effects, including confusion, disorientation, and memory loss. Usually these side effects are short-term, but sometimes they can linger.

Newer methods of administering the treatment have reduced the memory loss and other cognitive difficulties associated with ECT. Research has found that after one year of ECT treatments, most patients showed no adverse cognitive effects.

Nevertheless, patients always provide informed consent before receiving ECT, ensuring that they understand the potential benefits and risks of the treatment.

Other more recently introduced types of brain stimulation therapies used to treat severe depression include vagus nerve stimulation (VNS), and repetitive transcranial magnetic stimulation (rTMS). These methods are not yet commonly used, but research has suggested that they show promise.

How can I help a loved one who is depressed?

If you know someone who is depressed, it affects you, too. The most important thing you can do is help your friend or relative get a diagnosis and treatment.

You may need to make an appointment and go with him or her to see the doctor. Encourage your loved one to stay in treatment, or to seek different treatment if no improvement occurs after six to eight weeks.

To help your friend or relative, try the following:

- Offer emotional support, understanding, patience, and encouragement.

- Talk to him or her, and listen carefully.

- Never dismiss feelings, but point out realities and offer hope.

- Never ignore comments about suicide, and report them to your loved one's therapist or doctor.

- Invite your loved one out for walks, outings, and other activities. Keep trying if he or she declines, but don't push him or her to take on too much too soon.

- Provide assistance in getting to the doctor's appointments.

- Remind your loved one that with time and treatment, the depression will lift.

How can I help myself if I am depressed?

If you have depression, you may feel exhausted, helpless, and hopeless. It may be extremely difficult to take any action to help yourself. But as you begin to recognize your depression and begin treatment, you will start to feel better.

To help yourself, try the following:

- Do not wait too long to get evaluated or treated. There is research showing the longer one waits, the greater the impairment can be down the road. Try to see a professional as soon as possible.

- Try to be active and exercise. Go to a movie, a ball game, or another event or activity that you once enjoyed.

- Set realistic goals for yourself.

- Break up large tasks into small ones, set some priorities, and do what you can as you can.

- Try to spend time with other people and confide in a trusted friend or relative. Try not to isolate yourself, and let others help you.

- Expect your mood to improve gradually, not immediately. Do not expect to suddenly snap out of your depression. Often during treatment for depression, sleep and appetite will begin to improve before your depressed mood lifts.

- Postpone important decisions, such as getting married or divorced or changing jobs, until you feel better. Discuss decisions with others who know you well and have a more objective view of your situation.

- Remember that positive thinking will replace negative thoughts as your depression responds to treatment.

- Continue to educate yourself about depression.

Where can I go for help?

If you are unsure where to go for help, ask your family doctor. Others who can help include the following:

- Mental health specialists, such as psychiatrists, psychologists, social workers, or mental health counselors

- Health maintenance organizations

- Community mental health centers

- Hospital psychiatry departments and outpatient clinics

- Mental health programs at universities or medical schools

- State hospital outpatient clinics

- Family services, social agencies, or clergy

- Peer support groups

- Private clinics and facilities

- Employee assistance programs

- Local medical and/or psychiatric societies

You can also check the phone book under "mental health," "health," "social services," "hotlines," or "physicians" for phone numbers and addresses. An emergency room doctor also can provide temporary help and can tell you where and how to get further help.

What if I or someone I know is in crisis?

If you are thinking about harming yourself, or know someone who is, tell someone who can help immediately and do the following:

- Do not leave your friend or relative alone, and do not isolate yourself.

- Call your doctor.

- Call 911 or go to a hospital emergency room to get immediate help, or ask a friend or family member to help you do these things.

- Call the toll-free, 24-hour hotline of the National Suicide Prevention Lifeline at 800-273-TALK (800-273-8255); TTY: 800-799-4TTY (4889) to talk to a trained counselor.

Chapter 5

Statistics on Depression and Related Mental Health Disorders

Chapter Contents

Section 5.1

Mental Health Disorders by the Numbers

"Mental Illness: Facts and Numbers," © 2011 NAMI, the National Alliance on Mental Illness, www.nami.org. Reprinted with permission.

- One in four adults—approximately 57.7 million Americans—experience a mental health disorder in a given year. One in 17 lives with a serious mental illness such as schizophrenia, major depression, or bipolar disorder[1] and about one in 10 children live with a serious mental or emotional disorder.[2]

- About 2.4 million Americans, or 1.1 percent of the adult population, lives with schizophrenia.[1]

- Bipolar disorder affects 5.7 million American adults, approximately 2.6 percent of the adult population per year.[1]

- Major depressive disorder affects 6.7 percent of adults, or about 14.8 million American adults.[1] According to the 2004 *World Health Report*, this is the leading cause of disability in the United States and Canada in ages between 15–44.[3]

- Anxiety disorders, including panic disorder, obsessive-compulsive disorder (OCD), posttraumatic stress disorder (PTSD), generalized anxiety disorder, and phobias, affect about 18.7 percent of adults, an estimated 40 million individuals. Anxiety disorders frequently co-occur with depression or addiction disorders.[1]

- An estimated 5.2 million adults have co-occurring mental health and addiction disorders.[4] Of adults using homeless services, 31 percent reported having combination of these conditions.[5]

- One-half of all lifetime cases of mental illness begin by age 14, three-quarters by age 24.[6] Despite effective treatments, there are long delays—sometimes decades—between the first onset of symptoms and when people seek and receive treatment.[7]

- Fewer than one-third of adults and one-half of children with a diagnosable mental disorder receive mental health services in a given year.[2]

- Racial and ethnic minorities are less likely to have access to mental health services and often receive a poorer quality of care.[8]

- In the United States, the annual economic, indirect cost of mental illness is estimated to be $79 billion. Most of that amount—approximately $63 billion—reflects the loss of productivity as a result of illnesses.[2]

- Individuals living with serious mental illness face an increased risk of having chronic medical conditions.[9] Adults living with serious mental illness die 25 years earlier than other Americans, largely due to treatable medical conditions.[10]

- Suicide is the eleventh-leading cause of death in the United States and the third-leading cause of death for people ages 10–24 years. More than 90 percent of those who die by suicide have a diagnosable mental disorder.[11]

- In July 2007, a nationwide report indicated that male veterans are twice as likely to die by suicide as compared with their civilian peers in the general United States population.[12]

- Twenty-four percent of state prisoners and 21 percent of local jail prisoners have a recent history of a mental health disorder.[13]

- Seventy percent of youth in juvenile justice systems have at least one mental disorder with at least 20 percent experiencing significant functional impairment from a serious mental illness.[14]

- Over 50 percent of students with a mental disorder age 14 and older drop out of high school—the highest dropout rate of any disability group.[15]

References

1. "NIMH: The numbers count—Mental disorders in America." National Institute of Health. Available at www.nimh.nih.gov/publicat/numbers.cfm.

2. U.S. Department of Health and Human Services. *Mental Health: A Report of the Surgeon General.* Rockville, MD, U.S. Department of Health and Human Services, Substance Abuse and Mental Health Services Administration, Center for Mental Health Services, 1999, pp. 408–409, 411.

3. "NIMH: The numbers count—Mental disorders in America." National Institute of Health. Available at www.nimh.nih.gov/ publicat/numbers.cfm. [Citing 2004 *World Health Report* Annex Table 3 Burden of disease in DALYs by cause, sex and mortality stratum in WHO regions, estimates for 2002. Geneva: World Health Organization].

4. Substance Abuse and Mental Health Services Administration. (2007, February). National Outcome Measures (NOMs) for Co-occurring Disorders. [Citing 2005 data from the National Survey on Drug Use and Health (NSDUH)].

5. Burt, M. (2001). "What will it take to end homelessness?" Urban Institute: Washington, DC, p. 3. Available at www.urban.org/ UploadedPDF/end_homelessness.pdf.

6. Kessler, R., Berglund, P., Demler, O., Jin, R., Merikangas, & Walters, E., Lifetime prevalence and age-of-onset distributions of *DSM-IV* disorders in the National Co-morbidity Survey Replication (NCSR). *General Psychiatry*, 62, June 2005, 593–602.

7. Wang, P., Berglund, P., et al. Failure and delay in initial treatment contact after first onset of mental disorders in the National Co-morbidity Survey Replication (NCS-R). *General Psychiatry*, 62, June 2005, 603–613.

8. New Freedom Commission on Mental Health, Achieving the Promise: Transforming Mental Health Care in America. Final Report. United States Department of Health and Human Services: Rockville, MD, 2003, pp. 49–50.

9. Colton, C.W. & Manderscheid, R.W., (2006, April). Congruencies in increased mortality rates, years of potential life lost, and causes of death among public mental health clients in eight States. *Preventing Chronic Disease: Public Health Research, Practice and Policy*, 3(2), 1–14. Available at www.pubmedcentral.nih.gov/article render.fcgi?tool=pubmed&pubmedid=16539783.

10. Manderscheid, R., Druss, B., & Freeman, E. (2007, August 15). Data to manage the mortality crisis: Recommendations to the Substance Abuse and Mental Health Services Administration, Washington, DC.

11. National Institute of Mental Health. Suicide in the U.S.: Statistics and prevention. Available at www.nimh.nih.gov/publicat/ harmsway.cfm.

12. Kaplan, M.S., Huguet, N., McFarland, B., & Newsom, J.T. (2007). Suicide among male veterans: A perspective population-based study. *Journal of Epidemiol Community Health*, 61(7), 619–624.

13. Glaze, L.E. & James, D.J. (2006, September). Mental Health Problems of Prison and Jail Inmates. US Department of Justice, Office of Justice Programs, Bureau of Justice Statistics: Washington, DC.

14. Skowyra, K.R. & Cocozza, J.J. (2007) Blueprint for change. National Center for Mental Health and Juvenile Justice; Policy Research Associates, Inc. The Office of Juvenile Justice and Delinquency Prevention. Available at http://www.ncmhjj.com/Blueprint/default.shtml.

15. U.S. Department of Education. Twenty-third annual report to Congress on the implementation of the Individuals with Disabilities Act. Washington, DC, 2006.

Section 5.2

One in Ten U.S. Adults Report Depression

Excerpted from "An Estimated 1 in 10 U.S. Adults Report Depression," by the Centers for Disease Control and Prevention (CDC, www.cdc.gov), March 31, 2011.

Depression is a mental illness that can be costly and debilitating to sufferers. Depression can adversely affect the course and outcome of common chronic conditions, such as arthritis, asthma, cardiovascular disease, cancer, diabetes, and obesity. Depression also can result in increased work absenteeism, short-term disability, and decreased productivity.

Current Depression in U.S. Adults

Current depression was defined as meeting criteria for either major depression or "other depression" (fewer symptoms than major depression, but still meet criteria for a depressive disorder according to the *Diagnostic and Statistical Manual of Mental Disorders, 4th edition,* could be classified as nonspecified depression or minor depression or dysthymia) during the two weeks preceding the survey.

Estimates indicate that, among 235,067 adults (in 45 states, the District of Columbia [DC], Puerto Rico, and the U.S. Virgin Islands), 9.1% met the criteria for current depression (significant symptoms for at least 2 weeks before the survey), including 4.1% who met the criteria for major depression. In this study, increased prevalence of depression was found in southeastern states, where a greater prevalence of chronic conditions associated with depression has been observed (e.g., obesity and stroke). By state, age-standardized estimates for current depression ranged from 4.8% in North Dakota to 15.0% in Puerto Rico.

Who Tends to Be Most Depressed?

This study found the following groups to be more likely to meet criteria for major depression:

- Persons 45–64 years of age
- Women

- Blacks, Hispanics, non-Hispanic persons of other races or multiple races
- Persons with less than a high school education
- Those previously married
- Individuals unable to work or unemployed
- Persons without health insurance coverage

Similar patterns were found among persons with "other depression" with the two following exceptions: Adults aged 18–24 years were most likely to report "other depression" as were Hispanics (instead of other non-Hispanics).

Section 5.3

Just over Half of Americans Diagnosed with Major Depression Receive Care

From the National Institute of Mental Health (NIMH, www.nimh.nih .gov), part of the National Institutes of Health, January 4, 2010.

Overall, only about half of Americans diagnosed with major depression in a given year receive treatment for it, and even fewer—about one fifth—receive treatment consistent with current practice guidelines, according to data from nationally representative surveys supported by the National Institute of Mental Health (NIMH). Among the ethnic/racial groups surveyed, African Americans and Mexican Americans had the lowest rates of use of depression care; all groups reported higher use of past-year psychotherapy vs. medication for depression.

Background

Depression is a leading cause of disability in the United States. Past research has found that many people with depression never received treatment, and that the percentage of those receiving treatment varies with ethnicity and race. In order to provide comprehensive and up-to-date information on depression care, with a particular emphasis on minority groups, NIMH's Collaborative Psychiatric Epidemiology Surveys initiative (CPES) has combined data from three nationally representative studies, including the National Survey of American Life, the National Comorbidity Survey-Replication, and the National Latino and Asian American Study.

This Study

Scientists at Wayne State University, Detroit, MI; the University of Michigan, Ann Arbor; the University of California, Los Angeles; and the Harvard School of Public Health, Boston, MA, carried out the current study, which reports on data from CPES collected between February 2001 and November 2003 from 15,762 residents 18 years and older. The size of the sample makes it possible to examine health care use in ethnic/racial groups with a new level of detail, distinguishing between groups often surveyed as one population. The investigators were able to break out types of care used, and to assess to what extent the care used was consistent with the American Psychiatric Association (APA) Practice Guidelines for the Treatment of Patients with Major Depressive Disorder. Finally, they examined how factors enabling healthcare access—insurance, education, and household income—influenced rates of care.

A central finding was that overall, 51 percent of all those in the study who met criteria for major depression during the prior year received some kind of treatment for it, with only 21 percent receiving care that was consistent with the APA Guidelines.

Other key study findings addressed disparities, types and quality of care received, and factors that enable access to healthcare.

- Prevalence and severity of major depression was similar among the five studied ethnic/racial groups—Mexican Americans, Puerto Ricans, Caribbean Blacks, African Americans, and non-Latino Whites. However, African Americans and Mexican Americans were least likely to receive any care or care consistent with practice guidelines. Compared with non-Latino Whites for example, of whom 54 percent with depression received care, 40 percent of African Americans and 34 percent of Mexican Americans did. The rate of care for Puerto Ricans was close to that of Whites, 50 percent.

- Across these population groups, psychotherapy was used more frequently than medications (pharmacotherapy). Overall, 34 percent received pharmacotherapy; 45 percent psychotherapy. Psychotherapy was more likely to be consistent with APA guidelines than pharmacotherapy, suggesting that adherence—the extent to which patients completed the recommended therapy—was greater for psychotherapy than pharmacotherapy. The contrast between the rates of Guideline-consistent psychotherapy and pharmacotherapy use was greatest among Caribbean Blacks, African Americans, and Mexican Americans.

- Puerto Ricans had rates of treatment use, and treatment that was consistent with care guidelines, that were similar to, or higher than, non-Latino Whites.

- Differences in factors enabling healthcare access appeared to contribute substantially to disparities in mental healthcare use, particularly for Mexican Americans. When differences in these enabling factors were controlled for statistically—so in effect, the population groups being compared had the same rates of enabling factors—the degree of disparities in use of care by Mexican Americans was reduced. For Caribbean Blacks and African Americans, statistical control of enabling factors reduced disparities in psychotherapy use, but not use of pharmacotherapy.

- Health insurance coverage was associated with a greater likelihood of depression care, but not guideline consistent care. The pattern with education was reversed: education was associated with a greater likelihood of care that was consistent with the APA Guidelines, but not with greater use of care in general.

Significance

This study, with its large sample size and emphasis on minority groups, provides a more nuanced and detailed picture of the care received for major depression among different ethnic/racial groups and of factors that contribute to disparities. Lead author Hector González at Wayne State University said that Mexican-Americans make up over two-thirds of Latinos in the United States. "We found in our study that there are some really distinctive differences in mental healthcare use between Mexican Americans and other Latino subgroups that have not been previously reported." Estimates suggest that Latinos will make up close to one-third of the U.S. population by mid-century; the study findings suggest that Mexican Americans should be a focus of efforts to reduce health disparities to ensure the nation's health in coming decades.

All groups were more likely to have received psychotherapy than pharmacotherapy. Caribbean Blacks and African Americans were particularly unlikely to receive pharmacotherapy consistent with APA guidelines; enabling factors such as education, health insurance, and income did not explain the lower rates of medication use. The authors note possible reasons for this, including research indicating that perceived discrimination can shape health care seeking. They speculate that the non-immigrant status of Puerto Ricans—and with that, greater predominance of English language use within this group—may be factors in their relatively high rates of health care use.

Findings from this study will inform future research on adherence to various depression therapies, and the factors that shape differences in care among racial/ethnic groups. "Future studies," say the authors, "should explore the extent to which patients' subjective experiences of racial bias may affect their access and utilization of mental healthcare."

Reference

González, H.M., Vega, W.A., Williams, D.R., Tarraf, W., West, B.T., and Neighbors, H.W. *Archives of General Psychiatry* 2010;67(1):37–46.

Section 5.4

The Cost of Treating Mental Health Disorders

Excerpted from "Statistical Brief 303: Anxiety and Mood Disorders: Use and Expenditures for Adults 18 and Older, U.S. Civilian Noninstitutionalized Population, 2007," by Anita Soni, PhD, part of the Medical Expenditure Panel Survey (www.meps.ahrq.gov), by the Agency for Healthcare Research and Quality (www.ahrq.gov), December 2010.

This text presents estimates on the use of and expenditures for ambulatory care and prescribed medications to treat anxiety and mood disorders among adults 18 and older in the U.S. civilian noninstitutionalized population.

Anxiety and mood disorders often occur together and are two of the main reasons individuals seek treatment for mental health problems.

The estimates are based on the Household Component of the Medical Expenditure Panel Survey (MEPS-HC). Average annual estimates are shown by type of service and source of payment. All differences between estimates noted in the text are statistically significant at the 0.05 level or better.

Findings

Number of Treated Cases of Anxiety and Mood Disorders, by Sex

In 2007, 26.8 million U.S. adults ages 18 and older adults reported receiving treatment for anxiety and mood disorders. More females received treatment for anxiety and mood disorders than males (18.0 million versus 8.8 million).

Total and Mean Health Care Expenditures on Anxiety and Mood Disorders, by Type of Service

Even though expenditures for treatment of anxiety and mood disorders accounted for less than 5 (4.3) percent of expenditures on treatment of all conditions for adults ages 18 and older, a total of $36.8 billion was spent on treatment of anxiety and mood disorders. Half of expenditures for anxiety and mood disorders were spent on prescription medications ($18.4 billion) compared to about one-fourth on ambulatory visits ($8.7 billion).

Average expenditures for the treatment of anxiety and mood disorders for those with an anxiety or mood disorder related expense were $1,374 in 2007. The mean expense per adult for those with a prescription medicine expense was $763 and $646 per adult for those with an expense related to ambulatory care visits.

Distribution of Average Annual Health Care Expenditures for Anxiety and Mood Disorders, by Source of Payment and Type of Service

A little less than one third (30.5 percent) of the expenditures for the treatment of anxiety and mood disorders for adults in 2007 were paid by private insurance, with Medicare paying one fourth (25.0 percent), and out-of-pocket payments accounting for about one fifth (19.5 percent). One fourth of the expenses for ambulatory visits and prescription medicines were paid out of pocket. A little over one third of the expenditures for prescription medications and ambulatory care was paid by private insurance (36.3 percent and 34.6 percent, respectively).

About MEPS-HC

MEPS-HC is a nationally representative longitudinal survey that collects detailed information on health care utilization and expenditures, health insurance, and health status, as well as a wide variety of social, demographic, and economic characteristics for the U.S. civilian noninstitutionalized population. It is cosponsored by the Agency for Healthcare Research and Quality and the National Center for Health Statistics. For more information about MEPS, call the MEPS information coordinator at the Agency for Healthcare Research and Quality (301) 427-1656 or visit the MEPS website at www.meps.ahrq.gov.

Part Two

Types of Depression

Chapter 6

Major Depression

Introduction

Like diabetes and heart disease, major depression is a serious medical illness that is quite common. Psychological, biological, environmental, and genetic factors contribute to its development.

For many years, people living with depression and their families were blamed and experienced societal prejudice as a result of their illness, partly because their illness was so poorly understood. During the last few decades, however, scientific research has greatly expanded our understanding and firmly established that mental illnesses like major depression are biologically based brain diseases.

Major depression affects about 5–8 percent of the United States' adult population in any 12-month period which means that, based on the last census, approximately 15 million Americans will have an episode of major depression this year. Depression occurs twice as frequently in women as in men for reasons that are not fully understood. More than one-half of those who experience a single episode of depression will continue to have episodes that occur as frequently as once or even twice a year. Without treatment, the frequency as well as the severity of symptoms of depressive illness tend to increase over time.

Major depression is also known as clinical depression, major depressive illness, major affective disorder, and unipolar mood disorder. It involves some combination of the following symptoms: Depressed mood (sadness), poor concentration, sleep disturbances, fatigue, appetite disturbances, excessive guilt, and even suicidal thoughts. Thus, left untreated, depression can lead to serious impairment in daily functioning and even suicide, which is the eleventh-leading cause of death in the United States. Devastating as this disease may be, it is treatable. The availability of effective treatments and a better understanding of the biological basis for depression may lessen the barriers that can prevent early detection, accurate diagnosis, and the decision to seek medical treatment.

This text is intended to answer your questions about depression and give you valuable, accurate information about this illness and how it is treated. Unfortunately, major depression often goes unrecognized and untreated. You may need this information because you suspect you may have depression or you may want to become knowledgeable because a family member or friend has the disorder.

Major depression is only one form of depressive illness. Bipolar disorder is a less-common form of depression characterized by symptoms such as mood swings, loss of sleep, extreme "highs," increased energy and activity, increased risk-taking and poor judgments, feelings of great pleasure or irritability, aggressiveness and racing, disconnected thoughts as well as "low" periods very similar to those experienced by individuals with depressive illness.

Having a physician make the right distinction between unipolar depression and bipolar depression is critical since treatments for these two depressive disorders differ. On the one hand, antidepressant treatment (the cornerstone of treatment of unipolar depression) can in some cases activate manic symptoms or even worsen depressive symptoms, including suicidal thinking, in people living with bipolar depression. On the other hand, standard treatments for bipolar disorder (lithium, mood stabilizers, antipsychotics) do not appear to be effective in treating unipolar depression and may simply burden people suffering from unipolar depression with side effects.

What Is Major Depression?

Major depression is a mood state that goes well beyond temporarily feeling sad or blue. It is a serious medical illness that affects one's thoughts, feelings, behavior, mood, and physical health.

Major depression can occur at any age, even in rare cases starting as young as preschool. Some individuals may only have one episode of depression in a lifetime, but more often people have recurrent episodes. More than one-half of those who experience a first episode of depression will have at least one other episode in their lives. Some people may have several episodes in the course of a year, and others may have ongoing symptoms. If untreated, episodes commonly last anywhere from a few months to many years.

The outward behavior of the person with depression often does not attract attention. The behavior of the depressed individual, although quite worrisome to family members and friends and even to him- or herself, rarely disrupts the lives of others to the extent that some other serious mental illnesses do.

However, major depression is disruptive in other ways, such as causing people to withdraw from their relationships, from their work, and from the very fabric of society. In fact, major depression ranks as the largest cause of disability in the developed world and the fourth-largest cause of disability in the developing world. To make matters worse, researchers believe that more than one half of people who succeed in committing suicide were suffering from depression at the time.

The normal human emotion we sometimes call "depression" is a common response to a loss, failure, or disappointment. Major depression is different. It is a serious emotional and biological disease that—with a correct diagnosis—can be treated effectively. Major depression may require long-term treatment to keep symptoms from returning just like any other chronic medical illness. For some, biological depression is a life-long condition in which periods of wellness alternate with recurrences of illness.

The use of alcohol, a central nervous system depressant, can be a serious complication for depressed individuals who use it to try to change moods. All alcohol should be avoided during treatment for depression for several reasons. First, after its initial anti-anxiety effect, alcohol produces increased feelings of depression. Regular alcohol alone can cause a depressed mood that lasts for weeks, even after the use of alcohol stops. Second, in combination with many antidepressants, alcohol can make drug side effects much worse, even dangerously so, and may make antidepressants less effective. Third, alcohol reduces inhibitions, which increases the risk of suicide or suicidal gestures.

Getting an accurate diagnosis is important. First, rule out other possible medical conditions that mimic depression—such as hypothyroidism (underactive thyroid), substance abuse, infectious processes, anemia, and neurological disorders.

What Are the Symptoms?

The onset of the first episode of major depression may not be obvious if it is brief or mild. Unrecognized or left untreated, however, it may recur with greater seriousness or progress to a syndrome with the following symptoms: A profoundly sad or irritable mood lasting at least two weeks accompanied by pronounced changes in sleep, appetite, energy, ability to concentrate, and remember, a lack of interest in usual activities and a decreased ability to experience pleasure. Frequently, there are feelings of hopelessness, worthlessness, sadness, emptiness, or guilt. Very depressed persons cannot respond to positive events in their lives. A depressive episode may develop gradually or affect a person quite suddenly and it frequently is unrelated to current events in the person's life.

The symptoms of clinical depression characteristically represent a significant change in how a person functions. Often, when all of those symptoms co-exist at a severe level for a long time, individuals become so discouraged and hopeless that death seems preferable to life. These feelings can lead to passive suicidal wishes, suicidal plans, and even attempted and completed suicide.

Changes in sleep: The changes in sleep can go in either direction. Some depressed individuals have difficulty falling asleep, wake throughout the night, and awaken an hour to several hours earlier than desired in the morning. Other individuals experiencing depression will sleep more than the usual amount. In most cases, individuals awaken without feeling rested.

Changes in appetite: Many people in a clinical depression experience a decrease in appetite and weight loss that can often be considerable. Others will experience an increased desire to eat and will gain weight. Most of these people will report that the food they are eating does not actually appeal to them.

Impaired concentration and decision making: The inability to concentrate and make decisions experienced by depressed individuals can be a frightening aspect of the disorder. In the midst of a severe depression, individuals may find that they cannot follow the thread of a simple newspaper article or the story line of a half-hour comedy on television. Major decision making is often impossible. This leads depressed individuals to feel as though they are literally losing their minds.

Loss of energy: Equally distressing to depressed persons is the loss of energy and profound fatigue experienced by both those who sleep more and those who sleep less during an episode. Mental speed and activity are usually reduced, as is the ability to perform normal daily routines. Ideas are fewer and responses to the environment are painfully slowed.

Loss of interest: Depressed people feel sad and lose interest in usual activities. They lose the capacity to experience pleasure. For instance, eating and sex are often no longer enjoyable. Former regular activities seem boring or unrewarding and the ability to feel and offer love may be diminished or lost.

Low self-esteem: During periods of depression, individuals often dwell on memories of losses or failures and they feel excessive guilt and helplessness. Negative thoughts such as "I am not worth much" or "the world is a terrible place" may take over.

Feelings of hopelessness or guilt: The symptoms of depression often come together to produce a strong feeling of hopelessness, a belief that nothing will ever improve. Periods of depression can lead to the wish to die or thoughts of suicide.

Movement changes: People who are depressed may literally look slowed down and physically depleted or, alternatively, activated and agitated. For example, a depressed person may awaken very early in the morning and pace the floor for hours.

Depression may be as disabling (in terms of time spent in bed and loss of work productivity) as other chronic illnesses, such as hypertension and diabetes. It has been estimated that the annual cost of depressive illness in the United States is $80 billion due to lost productivity and illness care.

Who Develops Major Depression?

All age groups and all racial, ethnic, and socioeconomic groups can experience depression. An estimated 15 million American adults are affected by major depression in a given year. Only about one third of those with major depression receive some form of treatment.

Youth: Many symptoms of depression in children and adolescents are similar to those in other age groups but there are some differences. Grade-school children are more likely to complain of aches and pains than they are to report feeling hopeless or sad. Depressed teens may "act out" by showing anger or irritability, becoming aggressive, abusing drugs or alcohol, doing poorly in school, or running away. In contrast to outward appearances when acting out, an adolescent's own experience of depression is of feeling isolated, empty, and hopeless. Suicide is the third-leading cause of death among children ages 15–19, following accidents and homicides. Therefore, it is essential for young people with severe symptoms or symptoms lasting for several weeks to be evaluated by doctors. Even though the use of antidepressant medication in children may sometimes be controversial, some observe that depression is itself lethal for many and lack of treatment is also a serious concern.

Adults age 65 and over: An estimated 10 percent of American adults age 65 and older have a diagnosable depressive disorder, including major depression, dysthymia (a mild form of depression), and adjustment disorder with depressed mood. Experts believe that depression is under-treated in older adults because it can be difficult to recognize. Certain problems associated with aging, such as backaches, headaches, joint pain, or stomach problems, are often not recognized as signs of depression. Medical illnesses common in the elderly, such as Parkinson's disease, dementia, and heart disease, often have symptoms that overlap with those of a depression syndrome, and physicians and families may not recognize the concurrent presence of major depression. Contrary to popular belief, depression is not a normal part of aging. It can be successfully treated when recognized and diagnosed by a physician. Treatment is especially important in this population, due to a higher risk of associated suicide.

What Causes Major Depression?

The general scientific understanding is that depression does not have a single cause; it arises from multiple factors that may need to occur simultaneously. A person's life experience, genetic inheritance, age, sex, brain chemistry imbalance, hormone changes, substance use, and other illnesses all play significant roles in the development of a depression. It also may occur that there is no observable trigger leading to the illness; depression may occur spontaneously and be unassociated with any life crisis, physical illness, or other currently known risks.

Mood disorders and suicides tend to run in families. In the case of complete genetic inheritance, such as with identical twins, it appears that only about 30 percent of the time when one twin develops depression will the other twin ever do so as well. We know that a biologically inherited tendency to develop depression is associated with a younger age of depression onset, and that new onset depression occurring after age 60 is less likely to be due to a genetic predisposition. Life factors and events seem to influence whether an inherited, genetic tendency to develop depression will ever lead to an episode of major depression.

Social variables like marital status, financial standing, and place of residence have some relationship to the likelihood of developing depression but conclusions are not easily reached as to which causes the other. For instance, though depression is more common in people who are homeless, it may be that the depression strongly influences why any given person becomes homeless. We also know that long-lasting stressors like unemployment or a difficult marriage play a more significant role in developing depression than sudden stressors like an argument or receiving bad news.

Traumatic experiences may not only contribute to one's general state of stress, but also seem to alter how the brain functions for years to come. Early-life traumatic experiences have been shown to cause long-term changes in how the brain responds to future fears and stresses. This may be what accounts for the greater lifetime incidence of major depression in people who have a history of significant childhood trauma.

Other proposed genetic pathways in the development of depression include changes observed in regional brain functioning. For instance, imaging studies have shown consistently that the left, front portion of the brain becomes less active during depression. Also, brain patterns during sleep change in a characteristic way during depression. Depression is also associated with changes in how the pituitary gland and hypothalamus respond to hormone stimulation.

Other factors that have been linked to depression include abnormalities in neurotransmitter levels or function (particularly of serotonin, norepinephrine, and dopamine), a history of sleep disturbances, medical illness, chronic pain, anxiety, attention deficit hyperactivity disorder, alcoholism, or drug abuse. Our current understanding is that major depression can have many causes and can develop from a variety of genetic pathways.

How Is Major Depression Treated?

Of all the mental illnesses, major depression is among the most responsive to treatment. Although major depression can be a devastating illness, it is highly treatable. Most people diagnosed with serious depression can be effectively treated and can return to their routine daily activities and experience relief from their feelings of depression. Many types of treatment are available; the type chosen depends on the individual and the severity and patterns of the illness. There are three well-established types of treatment for depression: Medications, psychotherapy, and electroconvulsive therapy (ECT). A new treatment called transcranial magnetic stimulation (TMS) has recently been cleared by the FDA [U.S. Food and Drug Administration] for individuals who have not done well on one trial of an antidepressant. For some people who have a seasonal component to their depression, light therapy may be useful. These treatments may be used alone or in combination.

Medications

It often takes 2 to 4 weeks for antidepressants to start having an effect, and 6 to 12 weeks for antidepressants to have their full effect. In some cases, patients may have to try various doses and different antidepressants before finding the one or the combination that is most effective. Friends and relatives will usually notice an improvement on medication before the depressed person him- or herself will notice any changes. Antidepressant medications are not habit-forming; however, they should not be stopped abruptly as withdrawal symptoms (muscle aches, stomach upset, headaches) may occur.

Below is a list of options:

- **Selective serotonin reuptake inhibitors (SSRIs)** act specifically on the neurotransmitter serotonin. They are the most common agents prescribed for depression worldwide. These agents block the reuptake of serotonin from the synapse to the nerve, which increases levels of serotonin. SSRIs include fluoxetine (Prozac), sertraline (Zoloft), paroxetine (Paxil), citalopram (Celexa), escitalopram (Lexapro), and fluvoxamine (Luvox).

- **Serotonin and norepinephrine reuptake inhibitors (SNRIs)** are the second-most popular antidepressants worldwide. These agents block the reuptake of both serotonin and norepinephrine from the synapse into the nerve which increases the amounts of these chemicals. SNRIs include venlafaxine (Effexor), desvenlafaxine (Pristiq), and duloxetine (Cymbalta).

- **Bupropion (Wellbutrin)** is a popular antidepressant medication classified as a norepinephrine-dopamine reuptake inhibitor (NDRI). It acts by blocking the reuptake of dopamine and norepinephrine and increases these neurotransmitters in the brain. It also helps with smoking cessation strategies.

- **Mirtazapine (Remeron)** works differently from the compounds discussed above. Mirtazapine targets specific serotonin and norepinephrine receptors in the brain, thus indirectly increasing the activity of several brain circuits.

- **Aripiprazole (Abilify)** is an atypical antipsychotic that was approved by the FDA in 2007, and is used to augment depression when used along with antidepressants.

- **Tricyclic antidepressants (TCAs)** are older agents rarely used today as first-line treatment. They work similarly to the SNRIs, but have other properties that often result in higher rates of side effects, as compared to almost all other antidepressants. They are sometimes used in cases where other antidepressants have not worked. TCAs include amitriptyline (Elavil, Limbitrol), desipramine (Norpramin), doxepin (Sinequan), imipramine (Tofranil), nortriptyline (Pamelor, Aventyl), and protriptyline (Vivactil). TCAs may be helpful with chronic pain as well.

- **Monoamine oxidase inhibitors (MAOIs)** are less commonly used today. MAOIs work by inactivating enzymes in the brain which catabolize (break down) serotonin, norepinephrine, and dopamine from the synapse, thus increasing the levels of these chemicals in the brain. MAOIs can sometimes be effective for people who do not respond to other medications or who have "atypical" (abnormal) depression with marked anxiety, excessive sleeping, irritability, hypochondria, or phobic characteristics. They have important food and medication interactions, which requires strict adherence to a particular diet. MAOIs include phenelzine (Nardil), isocarboxazid (Marplan) tranylcypromine sulfate (Parnate), and selegiline patch (Emsam). Selegiline (Emsam) is a patch approved by the FDA in 2006. This delivery system reduces the risk of the dietary concerns noted in the preceding text.

The FDA periodically approves medications. For a current list, visit www.fda.gov.

Side Effects

Different medications produce different side effects, and people differ in the type and severity of side effects they experience. About 50 percent of people who take antidepressant medications experience some side effects, particularly during the first weeks of treatment. Side effects that are particularly bothersome can often be treated by changing the dose of the medication, switching to a different medication, or treating the side effects directly with additional medications. Rarely, serious side effects such as fainting, heart problems, or seizure may occur, but they are almost always treatable.

SSRIs and SNRIs, the most commonly prescribed treatments for depression, have similar side effect profiles. Common side effects with SSRIs and SNRIs include nausea, dry mouth, headaches, nervousness, insomnia, daytime sleepiness, diarrhea, constipation, rash, agitation, mild to modest weight gain, or sexual side effects such as problems with arousal or satisfaction. SSRIs and SNRIs should never be combined with MAOIs; combination of the two can result in serious health problems and may even be lethal. Effexor and Cymbalta should be used with some caution in those with high blood pressure or cardiovascular disorders. Effexor and Cymbalta are generally not recommended for young children.

Bupropion (Wellbutrin) generally causes fewer side effects than most other antidepressants (particularly nausea, sexual side effects, weight gain, and fatigue or sleepiness). Its side effects include restlessness, insomnia, headache or a worsening of pre-existing migraine tendencies, tremor, dry mouth, agitation, rapid heartbeat, dizziness, nausea, constipation, menstrual complaints, and rash. For some people, Wellbutrin can cause significant anxiety symptoms.

Of note: Although antidepressants generally reduce suicidal thoughts along with other symptoms of depression, in the vast majority of children who benefit from them, children starting an antidepressant medication should be monitored frequently for the emergence or worsening of suicidal thoughts due to the association, in some studies, of increased suicidality in a small minority of patients on antidepressant medication. The FDA public health advisory on this issue is available at www.fda.gov.

Medications often effectively control the symptoms of depression but people with this disorder must learn to recognize their individual patterns of illness and learn ways to cope with them.

Taking medication prescribed by a doctor is just one way to manage major depression. Psychotherapy is another way to help manage depression and research demonstrates that a combination of medication and psychotherapy is often the most effective treatment. Education, peer, and mutual support endeavors are also useful in supporting recovery.

Psychotherapy

There are several types of psychotherapy that have been shown to be effective for depression, including cognitive behavioral therapy (CBT) and interpersonal therapy (IPT). In general, these two types of therapies are short-term; treatments usually last only 10–20 weeks. Research has shown that mild to moderate depression can often be treated successfully with either medication or psychotherapy alone. However, severe depression appears more likely to respond to a combination of these two treatments.

- **Cognitive-behavioral therapy (CBT)** helps to change the negative thinking and behavior associated with depression while teaching people how to unlearn the behavioral patterns that contribute to their illness. The goal of this therapy is to recognize negative thoughts or mindsets (e.g., "I can't do anything right") and replace them with positive thoughts (e.g., "I can do this correctly"), leading to more effective, beneficial behavior. It is also noted that simply changing one's behavior can lead to an improvement in thoughts and mood. This might be as simple as leaving the house and taking a 15-minute walk every day.

- **Interpersonal therapy (IPT)** focuses on improving personal relationships that may contribute to a person's depression. The therapist teaches people to evaluate their interactions with others and to become aware of self-isolation and difficulties getting along with, relating to or understanding others.

- **Psychodynamic psychotherapy** is often more available than CBT and IPT in many communities, but researchers in depression recommend it less often due to a relative lack of data indicating that it works for this condition. This type of therapy is based on discovering one's unconscious desires and greater self-awareness.

Other forms of psychosocial treatments may help people and their families manage major depression more effectively. These treatments include psychoeducation, family psychoeducation, and self-help and support groups.

- Psychoeducation involves teaching a person about his or her illness, how to treat it, and how to recognize signs of relapse so that he or she can get necessary treatment before the illness worsens or occurs again.

- Family psychoeducation helps to reduce distress, confusion, and anxieties within the family and can help the person recover.

- Self-help and support groups for people and families dealing with mental illnesses are becoming more widely available. In this venue, people rely on their lived experience to share frustrations and successes, referrals to qualified specialists and community resources, and information about what works best when trying to recover. They also share friendship and hope for themselves, their loved ones, and others in the group.

Electroconvulsive Therapy (ECT)

ECT is a highly effective treatment for severe depression episodes. When medication or psychotherapy are not effective or if treatments are too slow to relieve severe symptoms such as psychosis or thoughts of suicide or if a person cannot take antidepressants, ECT may be considered. ECT can be combined with antidepressants for some individuals. Memory problems can follow ECT treatments, so a careful risk-benefit assessment needs to be made for this important and effective intervention.

Transcranial Magnetic Stimulation (TMS)

In October of 2008, the FDA cleared the use of TMS for major depression. Early returns indicate it to be a low-risk intervention that may help a person who has not responded to one antidepressant trial. It is neither as effective nor as risky as ECT. More will be learned about this new treatment over time.

How Successful Are Treatments for a Person with Major Depression?

How well treatment works depends on the type of depression, its severity, how long it has been going on, and the medical and psychological interventions offered. A multicenter trial funded by the National Institute of Mental Health (NIMH) called STAR*D (www.nimh.nih. gov/healthinformation/stard.cfm) is currently offering new information on treatment outcomes in real-world settings. This is a study to watch, going forward.

The development over the past 25 years of antidepressants and mood-stabilizing drugs has revolutionized the treatment of clinical depression, particularly for those with more serious or recurrent forms of the disorder. Biological treatments are effective overall, and most people with biological depression get significant relief from medications—whether the depression is mild or severe, recent or long-term. Left untreated, however, depression can become more serious or go on indefinitely. Treatment is important because it works and continued treatment after getting well can prevent recurrences. More than one-half of people who experience a first episode of depression will have at least one other episode in their lives. After two episodes, the chances of having a third episode are even greater.

The STAR*D study noted above has already shown that it can take up to six to eight weeks to get a good response to treatment and that people should keep trying different strategies. For instance, one-third of people who did not get better with a first treatment got all symptoms reduced (into remission) with the addition of a second medicine. Another one-quarter improved to remission after switching to another antidepressant. This study helps to support the idea that staying with the battle against depression is essential.

Although most people who live with depression can be treated successfully as outpatients, severe episodes and episodes accompanied by suicidal thinking may require brief hospitalization for careful evaluation, protection, and initiation of treatment. In combined treatments, medications are used to treat the symptoms of depression, while psychotherapy is used to help alleviate the problems depression causes in daily living. Psychotherapy is particularly important to undertake for anyone experiencing suicidal thoughts or profound psychosocial impairment.

What About Side Effects?

Different medications produce different side effects, and people differ in the type and severity of side effects they experience. About 50 percent of people who take antidepressant medications experience some side effects, particularly during the first weeks of treatment. Side effects that are particularly bothersome can often be treated by changing the dose of the medication, switching to a different medication, or treating the side effects directly with additional medications. Rarely, serious side effects such as fainting, heart problems, or seizure may occur but they are almost always treatable.

SSRIs and SNRIs, the most commonly prescribed treatments for depression, have similar side-effect profiles. Common side effects with SSRIs and SNRIs include nausea, dry mouth, headaches, nervousness, insomnia, daytime sleepiness, diarrhea, constipation, rash, agitation, mild to modest weight gain, or sexual side effects such as problems with arousal or satisfaction. SSRIs and SNRIs should never be combined with MAOIs; combination of the two can result in serious health problems and may even be fatal. Effexor and Cymbalta should be used with some caution in those with high blood pressure or cardiovascular disorder. Effexor and Cymbalta are generally not recommended for young children.

Bupropion (Wellbutrin) generally causes fewer side effects than most other antidepressants (particularly nausea, sexual side effects, weight gain, and fatigue or sleepiness). Its side effects include restlessness, insomnia, headache, or a worsening of pre-existing migraine tendencies, tremor, dry mouth, agitation, rapid heartbeat, dizziness, nausea, constipation, menstrual complaints, and rash. For some people, Wellbutrin causes significant anxiety symptoms and for others it is a very effective treatment for anxiety. However, Wellbutrin has been shown to increase the likelihood of having a seizure in those prone to this occurrence at doses above 450mg per day and should never be taken at doses above the recommended maximum of 450mg per day. Wellbutrin is not recommended in patients with a history of an eating disorder, head injury, or seizure disorder.

Mirtazapine (Remeron) is used less often than other, newer antidepressants (SSRIs, SNRIs, bupropion) because it is associated with more weight gain, sedation, and sleepiness. However, it appears to be less likely to result in insomnia, sexual side effects, and nausea than the SSRIs and SNRIs. Other side effects include headaches, dry mouth, and constipation. Remeron is not recommended for those with hepatic or renal dysfunction, a history of mania, or seizure disorder.

Tricyclic antidepressants (TCAs) generally have more side effects than all other antidepressants, including headaches, sleepiness and drowsiness, significant weight gain, nervousness, dry mouth, constipation, bladder problems, sexual problems, blurred vision, dizziness, drowsiness, skin rash, and heart conduction changes.

Monoamine oxidase inhibitors (MAOIs) are less commonly used. While their side effect profile is not as burdensome as the TCAs', the MAOIs are generally less safe than other antidepressants. People taking oral MAOIs may have to be careful about their diet, including restricting foods like alcohol or cheese as they contain high amounts of tyramine, which can cause severe high blood pressure in combination with a MAOI.

Other, less serious side effects may also occur with MAOIs including weight gain, constipation, dry mouth, dizziness, headache, drowsiness, insomnia, and sexual side effects, such as problems with arousal or satisfaction. MAOIs should generally not be combined with other antidepressant medications and, due to multiple other medication interactions, every treating physician should be notified that a consumer is taking this medication.

Specific body chemistry, age, the type and dosage of medication taken, other medications being taken (including nonprescription medications and supplements), and other medical conditions can all contribute to the side effects an individual may experience. Therefore, it is important always to discuss medications, medical conditions, and side effects with your health care provider.

What Type of Help Does a Person with Major Depression Need?

Above all, people with major depression need accurate diagnosis and early treatment. Family, friends, and coworkers should encourage a depressed person to seek expert evaluation. Those who are ill also need understanding, compassion, patience, and respect.

Insurance plans often make primary care physicians a required entry point for a consumer to receive psychiatric treatment, and different primary care physicians vary in their comfort levels with managing major depression. For instance, some primary care physicians will feel comfortable initiating medications while others prefer to refer to a specialist. Individuals living with mental illness and their families should not feel afraid to seek expert advice early in the course of a depressive illness if they feel things are not improving. It is recognized that the longer a person remains depressed, the harder successful treatment becomes. It is important that every depressed patient be thoroughly examined for possible physical illnesses, as there are some occasions when depression is being caused by another medical problem.

Experts in the treatment of depression include psychiatrists, psychologists, psychiatric social workers, psychiatric nurses, some mental health counselors, and persons living with mental illness and families themselves. A psychiatrist is a medical doctor who specializes in mental disorders and, in most states, is the only one of the mental health professionals who can prescribe medication. A clinical psychologist conducts psychotherapy and works with individuals, couples, and families to resolve problems associated with depression. Psychiatric or clinical social workers are trained in counseling, psychotherapy, and client-centered advocacy, including information, referral, and direct intervention with government and civic agencies. Mental health counselors provide professional counseling services that may include psychotherapy and they have a professional goal of promoting healthy, satisfying lifestyles. Peer education and support can promote recovery. Attention to lifestyle, including diet, regular aerobic exercise, and smoking cessation can result in better health, including mental health.

How Can Family and Friends Help?

Talking through feelings may help the depressed person recognize that he or she needs professional help, so friends and family should be willing to listen. They should be willing to find out more about depression, to learn the symptoms, and to help with the treatment.

People living with depression often must be encouraged to seek help. If they are severely depressed, they may need help finding a health care professional and may depend on being brought in by someone else for their diagnosis and treatment. Once treatment has begun, they may need help managing their medications, recognizing side effects, and observing changes in symptoms. Do not ignore remarks about suicide or death. Report them to the health care provider.

If a person does not want his or her health care professional to speak with family or friends about the details of an illness, the health care professional is bound to honor the person's wishes except in case of emergency. However, friends and family members are not restricted from offering information to the health care professional by telephone or in writing. This is particularly important to do when there is concern for the safety of the person living with depression, such as suicide threats.

Friends and family members who understand major depression are in the best position to help the person living with depression. They understand that the illness affects functioning, personality, attitude, and perspective as well as what to expect during acute stages of depression and over the long term. They also understand that their own lives will be disrupted as well.

Because depression often means a loss of self-esteem or self-confidence, friends and family should try to increase the person's feeling of self-worth by maintaining as normal a relationship as possible, talking through unwarranted negative thinking (such as examining the evidence against the idea of being worthless), encouraging efforts to improve, and acknowledging that the person is suffering from an illness. Care and respect are important ways to help someone who is having difficulty at work, home, or school. Pointing out the effectiveness of treatments may be useful when feelings of hopelessness become intense. In doing all of this, however, it is important to acknowledge that the depressed person's lack of confidence or feelings of hopelessness seem reasonable to him or her at the time and that things will look different when the illness begins to improve.

Chapter 7

Dysthymia:
Chronic Depression

Dysthymia is a chronic type of depression in which a person's moods are regularly low. However, symptoms are not as severe as with major depression.

Causes

The exact cause of dysthymia is unknown. It tends to run in families. Dysthymia occurs more often in women than in men and affects up to 5% of the general population.

Many people with dysthymia have a long-term medical problem or another mental health disorder, such as anxiety, alcohol abuse, or drug addiction. About half of people with dysthymia will also have an episode of major depression at some point in their lives.

Dysthymia in the elderly is often caused by:

- difficulty caring for themselves;
- mental decline;
- isolation;
- medical illnesses.

Symptoms

The main symptom of dysthymia is a low, dark, or sad mood on most days for at least two years. In children and adolescents, the mood can be irritable instead of depressed and may last for at least one year.

In addition, two or more of the following symptoms will be present almost all of the time that the person has dysthymia:

"Dysthymia," © 2011, A.D.A.M., Inc. Reprinted with permission.

- Feelings of hopelessness
- Too little or too much sleep
- Low energy or fatigue
- Low self-esteem
- Poor appetite or overeating
- Poor concentration

People with dysthymia will often take a negative or discouraging view of themselves, their future, other people, and life events. Problems often seem more difficult to solve.

Exams and Tests

Your health care provider will take a history of your mood and other mental health symptoms. The health care provider may also check your blood and urine to rule out medical causes of depression.

Treatment

Treatment for dysthymia includes antidepressant drug therapy, along with some type of talk therapy.

Medications often do not work as well for dysthymia as they do for major depression. It also may take longer after starting medication for you to feel better.

The following medications are used to treat dysthymia:

- Selective serotonin reuptake inhibitors (SSRIs) are the drugs most commonly used for dysthymia. They include fluoxetine (Prozac), sertraline (Zoloft), paroxetine (Paxil), fluvoxamine (Luvox), citalopram (Celexa), and escitalopram (Lexapro).

- Other antidepressants used to treat dysthymia include serotonin norepinephrine reuptake inhibitors (SNRIs), bupropion (Wellbutrin), tricyclic antidepressants, and monoamine oxidase inhibitors (MAOIs).

People with dysthymia often benefit from some type of talk therapy. Talk therapy is a good place to talk about feelings and thoughts, and most importantly, to learn ways to deal with them. Types of talk therapy include:

- Cognitive behavioral therapy (CBT) teaches depressed people ways of correcting negative thoughts. People can learn to be more aware of their symptoms, learn what seems to make depression worse, and learn problem-solving skills.

- Insight-oriented or psychodynamic psychotherapy can help someone with depression understand the psychological factors that may be behind their depressive behaviors, thoughts, and feelings.

Joining a support group of people who are experiencing problems like yours can also help. Ask your therapist or health care provider for a recommendation.

Outlook (Prognosis)

Dysthymia is a chronic condition that lasts many years. Though some people completely recover, others continue to have some symptoms, even with treatment.

Although it is not as severe as major depression, dysthymia symptoms can affect a person's ability to function in their family, and at work.

Dysthymia also increases the risk for suicide.

Possible Complications

If it is not treated, dysthymia can turn into a major depressive episode. This is known as double depression.

When to Contact a Medical Professional

Call for an appointment with your health care provider if:

- you regularly feel depressed or low; or

- your symptoms are getting worse.

Call for help immediately if you or someone you know develops these symptoms, which are signs of a suicide risk:

- Giving away belongings, or talking about going away and the need to get affairs in order

- Performing self-destructive behaviors, such as injuring themselves

- Suddenly changing behaviors, especially being calm after a period of anxiety

- Talking about death or suicide, or even stating the desire to harm themselves

- Withdrawing from friends or being unwilling to go out anywhere

Chapter 8

Atypical Depression

The existence of a subgroup of atypical depressed patients—distinguishable in terms of symptoms, drug response, and possibly even underlying neurobiology—suggests that depression is less a disease than a description, encompassing a variety of subtypes.

Twenty-five years ago a depressed patient told researchers at Columbia University College of Physicians and Surgeons, "You know those people who run around the park with lead weights? I feel like that all the time. I feel so heavy and leaden [that] I can't get out of a chair."

The statement graphically portrayed a symptom peculiar to a subset of depressed patients first described by English psychiatrists a generation earlier as atypical. The Columbia researchers, seeking to define the group more rigorously, incorporated that symptom—which they called leaden paralysis—into the criteria that currently serve as the basis for a diagnosis of depression with atypical features.

That diagnosis depends on the presence of mood reactivity—depressed mood that can brighten readily at a positive turn of events—in conjunction with any two of the following: hypersomnia, hyperphagia, leaden paralysis, and interpersonal rejection sensitivity.

But while experts agree that the definition roughly describes a subgroup of people who are different from those with classic melancholic

"Atypical Depression: What's in a Name?" Psychiatric News, Volume 38, Number 20, October 17, 2003. Copyright 2003 American Psychiatric Association, reproduced with permission of The American Psychiatric Association via Copyright Clearance Center. Reviewed by David A. Cooke, MD, FACP, November 19, 2011.

depression, much about the description, including the centrality of mood reactivity, is debated.

Even researchers involved in developing the original Columbia University criteria agree that the diagnosis requires refinement.

"There is something out there that we can call atypical depression, but the problem is that the *DSM* [*Diagnostic and Statistical Manual of Mental Disorders*] criteria are too broad," said Jonathan Stewart, MD, a professor of clinical psychiatry at Columbia and a research psychiatrist at the New York State Psychiatric Institute.

"It's clear to me that even though it captures most of the people who have the disorder—whatever it is—it probably captures a lot who have something else."

Not Like Melancholic Depression

As Stewart recounted, almost 50 years ago the English psychiatrists West and Dally first described a subset of patients who were depressed but whose clinical symptoms differed from those of classic melancholic depression. Moreover, while this group did not respond to tricyclic antidepressants, it did respond to monoamine oxidase inhibitors (MAOIs).

Stewart said the Columbia research in the 1980s confirmed the latter, identifying a group of depressed patients who preferentially responded to the MAOI phenelzine sulfate. The treatment studies also validated criteria for atypical depression that originated with published observations by the English group and by the American Donald F. Klein, MD, with reactivity of mood as the basic distinguishing characteristic.

"If you are depressed and something nice happens, you feel better for a while," Stewart explained. "In contrast, the quintessential melancholic is an emotional rock. The melancholic is not going to have any reaction at all."

Stewart and colleagues also found the opposite to be true of the patients with atypical depression—that they had an extreme reaction to negative events, particularly interpersonal rejection that others might just brush off. In contrast to the insomnia and loss of appetite usually seen in patients with melancholic depression, the patients with atypical depression were prone to overeating and oversleeping.

Since the development of the Columbia criteria, however, the uncertainty about how exactly to characterize these patients has become apparent, with some researchers and clinicians emphasizing some aspects over others.

"The original criteria were adopted on the basis of nonresponse to tricyclic antidepressants, not on the basis of a biological or genetic finding," said Linda Carpenter, MD, chief of the mood disorders program at Butler Hospital in Providence, Rhode Island, and an assistant professor of psychiatry at Brown University School of Medicine. In this way, she said, people with atypical depression are a subgroup that has been defined by researchers—and the definition is still in the making. Carpenter added that the picture is complicated by the fact that patients with bipolar disorder, anxious depression, and personality disorders share some of the features of atypical depression.

So, even a reasonable estimate of prevalence is elusive, depending on what criteria are used to identify the atypical patient.

"The term atypical depression makes it sound like some rare thing," said Frederick E. Miller, MD, PhD, chair of the department of psychiatry at Evanston Northwestern Healthcare in Evanston, Illinois.

"Of the patients I see, it's a common minority, depending on how much you stress the requirements in the *DSM* criteria. But it is not uncommon to see someone whose chief complaint is lethargy, who says [he or she] can sleep a thousand hours, but who also doesn't eat a lot.

"Are we making rational distinctions?" Miller wonders. "Or are we just sort of splitting certain symptoms that are part of a more general condition?"

Reverse Vegetative Symptoms Give Clue

A recent analysis of depressed patients with atypical features emphasizing the reverse vegetative symptoms—overeating and oversleeping—suggest that those two symptoms alone might serve as important markers of atypical depression for primary care physicians who might not otherwise look for the disorder.

The study, appearing in the September [2003] *Archives of General Psychiatry*, used the two symptoms to identify 836 patients with major depression, 304 of whom had atypical features and 532 who did not, in the National Comorbidity Survey.

Study author Louis S. Matza, PhD, told *Psychiatric News* that the analysis suggests that the simpler criteria emphasizing overeating and oversleeping could be readily used by primary care physicians to identify depressed patients who are liable to have a different clinical course and possibly a different response to treatment.

He noted that the study found that the patients who fit the criteria had an earlier onset of illness. They also reported higher rates of depressive symptoms, suicidal thoughts and attempts, psychiatric comorbidity, drug dependence, and a history of paternal depression, childhood neglect, and sexual abuse.

Matza is with MEDTAP International of Bethesda, Maryland. MEDTAP is a research organization specializing in health outcomes research.

Stewart, a co-author of the study, noted that the earlier age of onset found among the patients identified by the NCS is "exactly what we see in patients with atypical depression as diagnosed according to the full *DSM-IV* criteria."

Experts React

Experts who reviewed the study for Psychiatric News found compelling the use of the reverse vegetative symptoms to identify atypical depression in such a large national sample.

Carpenter agreed that hypersomnia and hyperphagia are prominent. "A person with atypical depression is usually slowed down, as opposed to agitated and moving around a lot," she said. "They will tell you they are oversleeping and overeating—that is sort of a classic characteristic. If you had to say what jumps out when you see these patients, that would be it."

But she and others expressed surprise, and some skepticism, about the finding of an increased-risk profile for suicide and comorbid psychiatric disorders among people with atypical depression.

"There have been plenty of typically melancholic depressed patients who are significantly ill," said Mark Frye, MD, director of the bipolar research program at the University of California, Los Angeles. "The idea that [atypical patients] have more drug use is remarkable as well. I am not sure I have seen that. It makes me think that many of these patients are covert bipolars."

Miller, too, expressed surprise at the finding and—underscoring the complicated picture of atypical depression—wondered whether the increased risk found among the sample could reflect the confluence of personality disorders.

All the clinicians interviewed by Psychiatric News agreed that reverse vegetative symptoms cannot be used as criteria to start patients on MAOIs as a first-line treatment.

"Why force someone into following an MAOI regimen with its side-effect problems until you have demonstrated that less problematic treatments are not going to work?," Stewart asked.

Distinct Biological Disorder?

Stewart told *Psychiatric News* that he and colleagues have refined their definition of atypical depression, focusing on early onset and chronic course as critical features.

"If you sort the patients who meet the criteria [for atypical depression] into those who have early-onset chronic illness and those who have later-onset or nonchronic illness, those two groups look entirely different," he said.

Moreover, the "true" atypical patients with early onset and chronic course differ from both late-onset nonchronic patients and from patients with classic melancholic depression on cortisol testing and auditory perceptual processing, as well as on their response to tricyclic antidepressants.

"The patients with melancholic depression and late-onset atypical depression lie on the same side of normal controls on cortisol testing and perceptual processing, while these early-onset chronic patients lie on the opposite side of normal controls," Stewart said. "This demonstrates to me that they have biologically different disorders. It argues against the notion of depression as a continuum and in favor of the idea that these categorical distinctions make some sense, that they are biologically distinct disorders."

More generally, experts said, the stubborn existence of a subgroup of atypical depressed patients—distinguishable in terms of symptoms, drug response, and possibly even underlying neurobiology—points to the possibility that depression itself is less a disease than a description, encompassing a variety of subtypes.

"As we learn more about the biology of depression—not just the phenomenology, but the biological markers—we will be able to lump less and split more," Carpenter said. "The nosology will reflect more subtypes as we have greater understanding of the biological, genetic, and psychosocial contributions."

An abstract of the study, "Depression With Atypical Features in the National Comorbidity Survey: Classification, Description, and Consequences," is posted on the Web at http://archpsyc.ama-assn.org/cgi/content/abstract/60/8/817?.

Chapter 9

Bipolar Disorder (Manic-Depressive Illness)

Bipolar Disorder

What is bipolar disorder?

Bipolar disorder, also known as manic-depressive illness, is a brain disorder that causes unusual shifts in mood, energy, activity levels, and the ability to carry out day-to-day tasks. Symptoms of bipolar disorder are severe. They are different from the normal ups and downs that everyone goes through from time to time. Bipolar disorder symptoms can result in damaged relationships, poor job or school performance, and even suicide. But bipolar disorder can be treated, and people with this illness can lead full and productive lives.

Bipolar disorder often develops in a person's late teens or early adult years. At least half of all cases start before age 25. Some people have their first symptoms during childhood, while others may develop symptoms late in life.

Bipolar disorder is not easy to spot when it starts. The symptoms may seem like separate problems, not recognized as parts of a larger problem. Some people suffer for years before they are properly diagnosed and treated. Like diabetes or heart disease, bipolar disorder

This chapter contains text from "Bipolar Disorder," by the National Institute of Mental Health (NIMH, www.nimh.nih.gov), part of the National Institutes of Health, 2008; "Same Genes Suspected in Both Depression and Bipolar Illness," by the NIMH, January 28, 2010; and "Symptoms of Bipolar Disorder May Go Undiagnosed in Some Adults with Major Depression," by the NIMH, August 16, 2010.

is a long-term illness that must be carefully managed throughout a person's life.

What are the symptoms of bipolar disorder?

People with bipolar disorder experience unusually intense emotional states that occur in distinct periods called mood episodes. An overly joyful or overexcited state is called a manic episode, and an extremely sad or hopeless state is called a depressive episode. Sometimes, a mood episode includes symptoms of both mania and depression. This is called a mixed state. People with bipolar disorder also may be explosive and irritable during a mood episode.

Extreme changes in energy, activity, sleep, and behavior go along with these changes in mood. It is possible for someone with bipolar disorder to experience a long-lasting period of unstable moods rather than discrete episodes of depression or mania.

A person may be having an episode of bipolar disorder if he or she has a number of manic or depressive symptoms for most of the day, nearly every day, for at least one or two weeks. Sometimes symptoms are so severe that the person cannot function normally at work, school, or home.

Symptoms of mania or a manic episode include the following:

- Mood changes:
    - A long period of feeling high, or an overly happy or outgoing mood
    - Extremely irritable mood, agitation, feeling jumpy or wired

- Behavioral changes:
    - Talking very fast, jumping from one idea to another, having racing thoughts
    - Being easily distracted
    - Increasing goal-directed activities, such as taking on new projects
    - Being restless
    - Sleeping little
    - Having an unrealistic belief in one's abilities
    - Behaving impulsively and taking part in a lot of pleasurable, high-risk behaviors, such as spending sprees, impulsive sex, and impulsive business investments

Symptoms of depression or a depressive episode include the following:

- Mood changes:
  - A long period of feeling worried or empty
  - Loss of interest in activities once enjoyed, including sex
- Behavioral changes:
  - Feeling tired or slowed down
  - Having problems concentrating, remembering, and making decisions
  - Being restless or irritable
  - Changing eating, sleeping, or other habits
  - Thinking of death or suicide, or attempting suicide

In addition to mania and depression, bipolar disorder can cause a range of moods. One side of the scale includes severe depression, moderate depression, and mild low mood. Moderate depression may cause less extreme symptoms, and mild low mood is called dysthymia when it is chronic or long-term. In the middle of the scale is normal or balanced mood. At the other end of the scale are hypomania and severe mania. Some people with bipolar disorder experience hypomania. During hypomanic episodes, a person may have increased energy and activity levels that are not as severe as typical mania, or he or she may have episodes that last less than a week and do not require emergency care. A person having a hypomanic episode may feel very good, be highly productive, and function well. This person may not feel that anything is wrong even as family and friends recognize the mood swings as possible bipolar disorder. Without proper treatment, however, people with hypomania may develop severe mania or depression.

During a mixed state, symptoms often include agitation, trouble sleeping, major changes in appetite, and suicidal thinking. People in a mixed state may feel very sad or hopeless while feeling extremely energized.

Sometimes, a person with severe episodes of mania or depression has psychotic symptoms too, such as hallucinations or delusions. The psychotic symptoms tend to reflect the person's extreme mood. For example, psychotic symptoms for a person having a manic episode may include believing he or she is famous, has a lot of money, or has special powers. In the same way, a person having a depressive episode may believe he or she is ruined and penniless, or has committed a crime. As a result, people with bipolar disorder who have psychotic symptoms are sometimes wrongly diagnosed as having schizophrenia, another severe mental illness that is linked with hallucinations and delusions.

People with bipolar disorder may also have behavioral problems. They may abuse alcohol or substances, have relationship problems, or perform poorly in school or at work. At first, it's not easy to recognize these problems as signs of a major mental illness.

How does bipolar disorder affect someone over time?

Bipolar disorder usually lasts a lifetime. Episodes of mania and depression typically come back over time. Between episodes, many people with bipolar disorder are free of symptoms, but some people may have lingering symptoms.

Doctors usually diagnose mental disorders using guidelines from the *Diagnostic and Statistical Manual of Mental Disorders,* or *DSM*. According to the *DSM*, there are four basic types of bipolar disorder:

* Bipolar I disorder is mainly defined by manic or mixed episodes that last at least seven days, or by manic symptoms that are so severe that the person needs immediate hospital care. Usually, the person also has depressive episodes, typically lasting at least two weeks. The symptoms of mania or depression must be a major change from the person's normal behavior.

* Bipolar II disorder is defined by a pattern of depressive episodes shifting back and forth with hypomanic episodes, but no full-blown manic or mixed episodes.

* Bipolar disorder not otherwise specified (BP-NOS) is diagnosed when a person has symptoms of the illness that do not meet diagnostic criteria for either bipolar I or II. The symptoms may not last long enough, or the person may have too few symptoms, to be diagnosed with bipolar I or II. However, the symptoms are clearly out of the person's normal range of behavior.

* Cyclothymic disorder, or cyclothymia, is a mild form of bipolar disorder. People who have cyclothymia have episodes of hypomania that shift back and forth with mild depression for at least two years. However, the symptoms do not meet the diagnostic requirements for any other type of bipolar disorder.

Some people may be diagnosed with rapid-cycling bipolar disorder. This is when a person has four or more episodes of major depression, mania, hypomania, or mixed symptoms within a year. Some people experience more than one episode in a week, or even within one day. Rapid cycling seems to be more common in people who have severe bipolar disorder and may be more common in people who have their first episode at a younger age. One study found that people with rapid cycling had their first episode about four years earlier, during mid to late teen years, than people without rapid cycling bipolar disorder. Rapid cycling affects more women than men.

Bipolar disorder tends to worsen if it is not treated. Over time, a person may suffer more frequent and more severe episodes than when the illness first appeared. Also, delays in getting the correct diagnosis and treatment make a person more likely to experience personal, social, and work-related problems.

Proper diagnosis and treatment helps people with bipolar disorder lead healthy and productive lives. In most cases, treatment can help reduce the frequency and severity of episodes.

What illnesses often co-exist with bipolar disorder?

Substance abuse is very common among people with bipolar disorder, but the reasons for this link are unclear. Some people with bipolar disorder may try to treat their symptoms with alcohol or drugs. However, substance abuse may trigger or prolong bipolar symptoms, and the behavioral control problems associated with mania can result in a person drinking too much.

Anxiety disorders, such as posttraumatic stress disorder (PTSD) and social phobia, also co-occur often among people with bipolar disorder. Bipolar disorder also co-occurs with attention deficit hyperactivity disorder (ADHD), which has some symptoms that overlap with bipolar disorder, such as restlessness and being easily distracted.

People with bipolar disorder are also at higher risk for thyroid disease, migraine headaches, heart disease, diabetes, obesity, and other physical illnesses. These illnesses may cause symptoms of mania or depression. They may also result from treatment for bipolar disorder.

Other illnesses can make it hard to diagnose and treat bipolar disorder. People with bipolar disorder should monitor their physical and mental health. If a symptom does not get better with treatment, they should tell their doctor.

What are the risk factors for bipolar disorder?

Scientists are learning about the possible causes of bipolar disorder. Most scientists agree that there is no single cause. Rather, many factors likely act together to produce the illness or increase risk.

Genetics: Bipolar disorder tends to run in families, so researchers are looking for genes that may increase a person's chance of developing the illness. Genes are the "building blocks" of heredity. They help control how the body and brain work and grow. Genes are contained inside a person's cells that are passed down from parents to children.

Children with a parent or sibling who has bipolar disorder are four to six times more likely to develop the illness, compared with children who do not have a family history of bipolar disorder. However, most children with a family history of bipolar disorder will not develop the illness.

Genetic research on bipolar disorder is being helped by advances in technology. This type of research is now much quicker and more far-reaching than in the past. One example is the launch of the Bipolar Disorder Phenome Database, funded in part by NIMH. Using the database, scientists will be able to link visible signs of the disorder with the genes that may influence them. So far, researchers using this database found that most people with bipolar disorder had:

- missed work because of their illness;

- other illnesses at the same time, especially alcohol and/or substance abuse and panic disorders;

- been treated or hospitalized for bipolar disorder.

The researchers also identified certain traits that appeared to run in families, including:

- history of psychiatric hospitalization;

- co-occurring obsessive-compulsive disorder (OCD);

- age at first manic episode;

- number and frequency of manic episodes.

Scientists continue to study these traits, which may help them find the genes that cause bipolar disorder some day. But genes are not the only risk factor for bipolar disorder. Studies of identical twins have shown that the twin of a person with bipolar illness does not always develop the disorder. This is important because identical twins share all of the same genes. The study results suggest factors besides genes are also at work. Rather, it is likely that many different genes and a person's environment are involved. However, scientists do not yet fully understand how these factors interact to cause bipolar disorder.

Brain structure and functioning: Brain-imaging studies are helping scientists learn what happens in the brain of a person with bipolar disorder. Newer brain-imaging tools, such as functional magnetic resonance imaging (fMRI) and positron emission tomography (PET), allow researchers to take pictures of the living brain at work. These tools help scientists study the brain's structure and activity.

Some imaging studies show how the brains of people with bipolar disorder may differ from the brains of healthy people or people with other mental disorders. For example, one study using MRI found that the pattern of brain development in children with bipolar disorder was similar to that in children with multi-dimensional impairment, a disorder that causes symptoms that overlap somewhat with bipolar disorder and schizophrenia. This suggests that the common pattern of brain development may be linked to general risk for unstable moods.

Learning more about these differences, along with information gained from genetic studies, helps scientists better understand bipolar disorder. Someday scientists may be able to predict which types of treatment will work most effectively. They may even find ways to prevent bipolar disorder.

How is bipolar disorder diagnosed?

The first step in getting a proper diagnosis is to talk to a doctor, who may conduct a physical examination, an interview, and lab tests. Bipolar disorder cannot currently be identified through a blood test or a brain scan, but these tests can help rule out other contributing factors, such as a stroke or brain tumor. If the problems are not caused by other illnesses, the doctor may conduct a mental health evaluation. The doctor may also provide a referral to a trained mental health professional, such as a psychiatrist, who is experienced in diagnosing and treating bipolar disorder.

The doctor or mental health professional should conduct a complete diagnostic evaluation. He or she should discuss any family history of bipolar disorder or other mental illnesses and get a complete history of symptoms. The doctor or mental health professionals should also talk to the person's close relatives or spouse and note how they describe the person's symptoms and family medical history.

People with bipolar disorder are more likely to seek help when they are depressed than when experiencing mania or hypomania. Therefore, a careful medical history is needed to assure that bipolar disorder is not mistakenly diagnosed as major depressive disorder, which is also called unipolar depression. Unlike people with bipolar disorder, people who have unipolar depression do not experience mania. Whenever possible, previous records and input from family and friends should also be included in the medical history.

How is bipolar disorder treated?

To date, there is no cure for bipolar disorder. But proper treatment helps most people with bipolar disorder gain better control of their mood swings and related symptoms. This is also true for people with the most severe forms of the illness.

Because bipolar disorder is a lifelong and recurrent illness, people with the disorder need long-term treatment to maintain control of bipolar symptoms. An effective maintenance treatment plan includes medication and psychotherapy for preventing relapse and reducing symptom severity.

Medications: Bipolar disorder can be diagnosed and medications prescribed by people with an MD (doctor of medicine). Usually, bipolar medications are prescribed by a psychiatrist. In some states, clinical psychologists, psychiatric nurse practitioners, and advanced psychiatric nurse specialists can also prescribe medications. Check with your state's licensing agency to find out more.

Not everyone responds to medications in the same way. Several different medications may need to be tried before the best course of treatment is found. Keeping a chart of daily mood symptoms, treatments, sleep patterns, and life events can help the doctor track and treat the illness most effectively. Sometimes this is called a daily life chart. If a person's symptoms change or if side effects become serious, the doctor may switch or add medications.

Mood stabilizing medications are usually the first choice to treat bipolar disorder. In general, people with bipolar disorder continue treatment with mood stabilizers for years. Except for lithium, many of these medications are anticonvulsants. Anticonvulsant medications are usually used to treat seizures, but they also help control moods. These medications are commonly used as mood stabilizers in bipolar disorder:

Lithium (sometimes known as Eskalith or Lithobid) was the first mood-stabilizing medication approved by the U.S. Food and Drug Administration (FDA) in the 1970s for treatment of mania. It is often very effective in controlling symptoms of mania and preventing the recurrence of manic and depressive episodes.

Valproic acid or divalproex sodium (Depakote), approved by the FDA [U.S. Food and Drug Administration] in 1995 for treating mania, is a popular alternative to lithium for bipolar disorder. It is generally as effective as lithium for treating bipolar disorder.

More recently, the anticonvulsant lamotrigine (Lamictal) received FDA approval for maintenance treatment of bipolar disorder.

Other anticonvulsant medications, including gabapentin (Neurontin), topiramate (Topamax), and oxcarbazepine (Trileptal) are sometimes prescribed. No large studies have shown that these medications are more effective than mood stabilizers.

Valproic acid, lamotrigine, and other anticonvulsant medications have an FDA warning. The warning states that their use may increase the risk of suicidal thoughts and behaviors. People taking anticonvulsant medications for bipolar or other illnesses should be closely monitored for new or worsening symptoms of depression, suicidal thoughts or behavior, or any unusual changes in mood or behavior. People taking these medications should not make any changes without talking to their health care professional.

Atypical antipsychotic medications are sometimes used to treat symptoms of bipolar disorder. Often, these medications are taken with other medications. Atypical antipsychotic medications are called "atypical" to set them apart from earlier medications, which are called "conventional" or "first-generation" antipsychotics.

Olanzapine (Zyprexa), when given with an antidepressant medication, may help relieve symptoms of severe mania or psychosis. Olanzapine is also available in an injectable form, which quickly treats agitation associated with a manic or mixed episode. Olanzapine can be used for maintenance treatment of bipolar disorder as well, even when a person does not have psychotic symptoms. However, some studies show that people taking olanzapine may gain weight and have other side effects that can increase their risk for diabetes and heart disease. These side effects are more likely in people taking olanzapine when compared with people prescribed other atypical antipsychotics.

Aripiprazole (Abilify), like olanzapine, is approved for treatment of a manic or mixed episode. Aripiprazole is also used for maintenance treatment after a severe or sudden episode. As with olanzapine, aripiprazole also can be injected for urgent treatment of symptoms of manic or mixed episodes of bipolar disorder.

Quetiapine (Seroquel) relieves the symptoms of severe and sudden manic episodes. In that way, quetiapine is like almost all antipsychotics. In 2006, it became the first atypical antipsychotic to also receive FDA approval for the treatment of bipolar depressive episodes.

Risperidone (Risperdal) and ziprasidone (Geodon) are other atypical antipsychotics that may also be prescribed for controlling manic or mixed episodes.

Antidepressant medications are sometimes used to treat symptoms of depression in bipolar disorder. People with bipolar disorder who take antidepressants often take a mood stabilizer, too. Doctors usually require this because taking only an antidepressant can increase a person's risk of switching to mania or hypomania, or of developing rapid cycling symptoms. To prevent this switch, doctors who prescribe antidepressants for treating bipolar disorder also usually require the person to take a mood-stabilizing medication at the same time.

Recently, a large-scale, NIMH-funded study showed that for many people, adding an antidepressant to a mood stabilizer is no more effective in treating the depression than using only a mood stabilizer.

Fluoxetine (Prozac), paroxetine (Paxil), sertraline (Zoloft), and bupropion (Wellbutrin) are examples of antidepressants that may be prescribed to treat symptoms of bipolar depression.

Some medications are better at treating one type of bipolar symptoms than another. For example, lamotrigine (Lamictal) seems to be helpful in controlling depressive symptoms of bipolar disorder.

What are the side effects of these medications?

Before starting a new medication, people with bipolar disorder should talk to their doctor about the possible risks and benefits.

The psychiatrist prescribing the medication or pharmacist can also answer questions about side effects. Over the last decade, treatments have improved, and some medications now have fewer or more tolerable side effects than earlier treatments. However, everyone responds differently to medications. In some cases, side effects may not appear until a person has taken a medication for some time.

If the person with bipolar disorder develops any severe side effects from a medication, he or she should talk to the doctor who prescribed it as soon as possible. The doctor may change the dose or prescribe a different medication.

People being treated for bipolar disorder should not stop taking a medication without talking to a doctor first. Suddenly stopping a medication may lead to "rebound," or worsening of bipolar disorder symptoms. Other uncomfortable or potentially dangerous withdrawal effects are also possible.

Is psychotherapy effective for treating bipolar disorder?

In addition to medication, psychotherapy, or talk therapy, can be an effective treatment for bipolar disorder. It can provide support, education, and guidance to people with bipolar disorder and their families. Some psychotherapy treatments used to treat bipolar disorder include the following:

- Cognitive behavioral therapy (CBT) helps people with bipolar disorder learn to change harmful or negative thought patterns and behaviors.

- Family-focused therapy includes family members. It helps enhance family coping strategies, such as recognizing new episodes early and helping their loved one. This therapy also improves communication and problem-solving.

- Interpersonal and social rhythm therapy helps people with bipolar disorder improve their relationships with others and manage their daily routines.

- Regular daily routines and sleep schedules may help protect against manic episodes.

- Psychoeducation teaches people with bipolar disorder about the illness and its treatment. This treatment helps people recognize signs of relapse so they can seek treatment early, before a full-blown episode occurs. Usually done in a group, psychoeducation may also be helpful for family members and caregivers.

A licensed psychologist, social worker, or counselor typically provides these therapies. This mental health professional often works with the psychiatrist to track progress. The number, frequency, and type of sessions should be based on the treatment needs of each person. As with medication, following the doctor's instructions for any psychotherapy will provide the greatest benefit.

Recently, NIMH funded a clinical trial called the Systematic Treatment Enhancement Program for Bipolar Disorder (STEP-BD). This was the largest treatment study ever conducted for bipolar disorder. In a study on psychotherapies, STEP-BD researchers compared people in two groups. The first group was treated with collaborative care (three sessions of psychoeducation over six weeks). The second group was treated with medication and intensive psychotherapy (30 sessions over 9 months of CBT, interpersonal and social rhythm therapy, or family-focused therapy). Researchers found that the second group had fewer relapses, lower hospitalization rates, and were better able to stick with their treatment plans. They were also more likely to get well faster and stay well longer.

What about other treatments?

Electroconvulsive therapy (ECT): For cases in which medication and/or psychotherapy does not work, electroconvulsive therapy (ECT) may be useful. ECT, formerly known as shock therapy, once had a bad reputation. But in recent years, it has greatly improved and can provide relief for people with severe bipolar disorder who have not been able to feel better with other treatments.

Before ECT is administered, a patient takes a muscle relaxant and is put under brief anesthesia. He or she does not consciously feel the electrical impulse administered in ECT. On average, ECT treatments last from 30–90 seconds.

People who have ECT usually recover after 5–15 minutes and are able to go home the same day.

Sometimes ECT is used for bipolar symptoms when other medical conditions, including pregnancy, make the use of medications too risky. ECT is a highly effective treatment for severely depressive, manic, or mixed episodes, but is generally not a first-line treatment.

ECT may cause some short-term side effects, including confusion, disorientation, and memory loss. But these side effects typically clear soon after treatment. People with bipolar disorder should discuss possible benefits and risks of ECT with an experienced doctor.

Sleep medications: People with bipolar disorder who have trouble sleeping usually sleep better after getting treatment for bipolar disorder. However, if sleeplessness does not improve, the doctor may suggest a change in medications. If the problems still continue, the doctor may prescribe sedatives or other sleep medications.

People with bipolar disorder should tell their doctor about all prescription drugs, over-the-counter medications, or supplements they are taking. Certain medications and supplements taken together may cause unwanted or dangerous effects.

What can people with bipolar disorder expect from treatment?

Bipolar disorder has no cure, but can be effectively treated over the long term. It is best controlled when treatment is continuous, rather than on and off. In the STEP-BD study, a little more than half of the people treated for bipolar disorder recovered over one year's time. For this study, recovery meant having two or fewer symptoms of the disorder for at least eight weeks.

However, even with proper treatment, mood changes can occur. In the STEP-BD study, almost half of those who recovered still had lingering symptoms. These people experienced a relapse or recurrence that was usually a return to a depressive state. If a person had a mental illness in addition to bipolar disorder, he or she was more likely to experience a relapse. Scientists are unsure, however, how these other illnesses or lingering symptoms increase the chance of relapse. For some people, combining psychotherapy with medication may help to prevent or delay relapse.

Treatment may be more effective when people work closely with a doctor and talk openly about their concerns and choices. Keeping track of mood changes and symptoms with a daily life chart can help a doctor assess a person's response to treatments. Sometimes the doctor needs to change a treatment plan to make sure symptoms are controlled most effectively. A psychiatrist should guide any changes in type or dose of medication.

How can I help a friend or relative who has bipolar disorder?

If you know someone who has bipolar disorder, it affects you, too. The first and most important thing you can do is help him or her get the right diagnosis and treatment. You may need to make the appointment and go with him or her to see the doctor. Encourage your loved one to stay in treatment.

To help a friend or relative, you can do the following:

- Offer emotional support, understanding, patience, and encouragement.
- Learn about bipolar disorder so you can understand what your friend or relative is experiencing.
- Talk to your friend or relative and listen carefully.
- Listen to feelings your friend or relative expresses—be understanding about situations that may trigger bipolar symptoms.
- Invite your friend or relative out for positive distractions, such as walks, outings, and other activities.
- Remind your friend or relative that, with time and treatment, he or she can get better.
- Never ignore comments about your friend or relative harming himself or herself. Always report such comments to his or her therapist or doctor.

Same Genes Suspected in Both Depression and Bipolar Illness

Researchers, for the first time, have pinpointed a genetic hotspot that confers risk for both bipolar disorder and depression.

People with either of these mood disorders were significantly more likely to have risk versions of genes at this site than healthy controls. One of the genes, which codes for part of a cell's machinery that tells genes when to turn on and off, was also found to be over-expressed in the executive hub of bipolar patients' brains, making it a prime suspect. The results add to mounting evidence that major mental disorders overlap at the molecular level.

"People who carry the risk versions may differ in some dimension of brain development that may increase risk for mood disorders later in life," explained Francis McMahon, MD, of the NIMH Mood and Anxiety Disorders Program, who led the study.

McMahon and an international team of investigators, supported, in part by NIMH, reported on the findings of their genome-wide meta-analysis online January 17, 2010 in the journal *Nature Genetics*.

Background

Major mood disorders affect 20 percent of the population and are among the leading causes of disability worldwide. It's long been known that bipolar disorder and unipolar depression often run together in the same families, hinting at some shared lineage. Yet, until now, no common genes or chromosomal locations had been identified.

McMahon and colleagues analyzed data from five different genome-wide association studies (GWAS) totaling more than 13,600 people, and confirmed their results in three additional independent samples totaling 4,677 people.

Findings of This Study

Genetic variations on Chromosome 3 were significantly associated with both mood disorders. The suspect gene, called PBRM1, codes for a protein critical for chromatin remodeling, a key process in regulating gene expression. A neighboring gene is involved in the proliferation of brain stem cells.

The researchers pinpointed a "protective" version of the PBRM1 gene that is carried by 41 percent of healthy controls, but only 38 percent of people with bipolar and unipolar depression. The risk version was found in 62 percent of mood disorder cases and 59 percent of controls. The researchers also showed that PBRM1 is expressed more in the prefrontal cortex of people with bipolar disorder than in controls.

Significance

Since mood disorders likely involve altered gene expression during brain development and in response to stress, PBRM1's profile makes it a good potential candidate gene. This first genetic evidence of unipolar/bipolar overlap is also the first significant genome-wide association with any psychiatric illness in the Chromosome 3p region.

However, the findings underscore limitations of the GWAS approach, which looks for connections to gene versions that are common in the population. Having one copy of this risk variant increases vulnerability for developing a mood disorder by a modest 15 percent. Why do some people with this variant—and presumably other, yet to be discovered, shared risk genes—develop bipolar disorder while others develop unipolar depression or remain healthy? Environmental influences and epigenetic factors may be involved, suggest the researchers, who note that "genetic association findings so far seem to account for little of the inherited risk for mood disorders."

"Our results support the growing view that there aren't common genes with large effects that confer increased risk for mood disorders," said McMahon. "If there were, in this largest sample to date, we would have found them. The disorders likely involve many genes with small effects—and different genes in different families—complicating the search. Rarer genes with large effects may also exist."

What's Next?

Ultimately, findings such as these may lead to identification of common biological pathways that may play a role in both unipolar and bipolar illness and suggest strategies for better treatment, said McMahon. The results add to other evidence of overlap that is spurring a new NIMH initiative to make sense of research findings that don't fit neatly into current diagnostic categories.

Reference

Meta-analysis of genome-wide association data identifies a risk locus for major mood disorders on 3p21.1.the Bipolar Disorder Genome Study (BiGS) Consortium, McMahon FJ, Akula N, Schulze TG, Muglia P, Tozzi F, Detera-Wadleigh SD, Steele CJ, Breuer R, Strohmaier J, Wendland JR, Mattheisen M, Mühleisen TW, Maier W, Nöthen MM, Cichon S, Farmer A, Vincent JB, Holsboer F, Preisig M, Rietschel M. *Nat Genet.* 2010 Jan 17 (epub ahead of print).

Symptoms of Bipolar Disorder May Go Undiagnosed in Some Adults with Major Depression

Nearly 40 percent of people with major depression may also have subthreshold hypomania, a form of mania that does not fully meet current diagnostic criteria for bipolar disorder, according to an NIMH-funded study. The study was published online ahead of print August 15, 2010, in the *American Journal of Psychiatry*.

Background

Mania is a symptom of bipolar disorder. According to the *Diagnostic and Statistical Manual for Mental Disorders (DSM-IV)*, it is generally defined as a discrete period of increased energy, activity, euphoria, or irritability that leads to marked impairment in one's daily life. The *DSM-IV* states that a manic episode lasts for one week or more, and may sometimes require hospitalization.

Hypomania is defined as a milder form of mania that lasts for four days at a time, but does not interfere with one's daily activities. The majority of people diagnosed with bipolar disorder experience repeated episodes of hypomania rather than mania.

For this study, Kathleen Merikangas, PhD, of NIMH, and colleagues aimed to characterize the full spectrum of mania by identifying hypomanic episodes that last less than four days among those diagnosed with major depression. They described this type of hypomania as subthreshold hypomania. Merikangas and colleagues used data from 5,692 respondents of the National Comorbidity Survey Replication (NCS-R), a nationally representative survey of American adults ages 18 and older.

Results of the Study

The researchers found that nearly 40 percent of those identified as having major depression also had symptoms of subthreshold hypomania. Compared to those with major depression alone, those with depression plus subthreshold hypomania tended to be younger at age of onset and to have had more coexisting health problems, more episodes of depression and more suicide attempts. They also found that among those with subthreshold hypomania, a family history of mania was just as common as it was among people with bipolar disorder.

Significance

According to the researchers, the findings indicate that many adults with major depression may in fact have mild but clinically significant symptoms of bipolar disorder. In addition, because many with subthreshold hypomania had a family history of mania, the researchers suggest that subthreshold hypomania may be predictive of future hypomania or mania. Previous research has indicated that young people with subthreshold hypomania symptoms are more likely to develop bipolar disorder over time, compared to those without subthreshold hypomania, said the authors.

What's Next?

The researchers suggest that depression and mania may be defined as dimensions, rather than as discrete diagnostic categories. Clinicians should be aware that patients who report repeated episodes of subthreshold hypomania may have a risk of developing mania, the researcher concluded.

Reference

Angst J, Cui L, Swendsen J, Rothen S, Cravchik A, Kessler R, Merikangas K. Major depressive disorder with sub-threshold bipolarity in the National Comorbidity Survey Replication. *American Journal of Psychiatry*. Online ahead of print August 15, 2010.

Chapter 10

Depression during and after Pregnancy

What is depression?

Depression is more than just feeling blue or down in the dumps for a few days. It's a serious illness that involves the brain. With depression, sad, anxious, or empty feelings don't go away and interfere with day-to-day life and routines. These feelings can be mild to severe. The good news is that most people with depression get better with treatment.

How common is depression during and after pregnancy?

Depression is a common problem during and after pregnancy. About 13 percent of pregnant women and new mothers have depression.

How do I know if I have depression?

When you are pregnant or after you have a baby, you may be depressed and not know it. Some normal changes during and after pregnancy can cause symptoms similar to those of depression. But if you have any of the following symptoms of depression for more than two weeks, call your doctor:

- Feeling restless or moody
- Feeling sad, hopeless, and overwhelmed

From "Frequently Asked Questions: Depression during and after Pregnancy," by the Office on Women's Health (www.womenshealth.gov), part of the U.S. Department of Health and Human Services, March 6, 2009.

- Crying a lot
- Having no energy or motivation
- Eating too little or too much
- Sleeping too little or too much
- Having trouble focusing or making decisions
- Having memory problems
- Feeling worthless and guilty
- Losing interest or pleasure in activities you used to enjoy
- Withdrawing from friends and family
- Having headaches, aches and pains, or stomach problems that don't go away

Your doctor can figure out if your symptoms are caused by depression or something else.

What causes depression? What about postpartum depression?

There is no single cause. Rather, depression likely results from a combination of factors:

- Depression is a mental illness that tends to run in families. Women with a family history of depression are more likely to have depression.
- Changes in brain chemistry or structure are believed to play a big role in depression.
- Stressful life events, such as death of a loved one, caring for an aging family member, abuse, and poverty, can trigger depression.
- Hormonal factors unique to women may contribute to depression in some women. We know that hormones directly affect the brain chemistry that controls emotions and mood. We also know that women are at greater risk of depression at certain times in their lives, such as puberty, during and after pregnancy, and during perimenopause. Some women also have depressive symptoms right before their period.

Depression after childbirth is called postpartum depression. Hormonal changes may trigger symptoms of postpartum depression. When you are pregnant, levels of the female hormones estrogen and progesterone increase greatly. In the first 24 hours after childbirth, hormone levels quickly return to normal. Researchers think the big change in hormone levels may lead to depression. This is much like the way smaller hormone changes can affect a woman's moods before she gets her period.

Levels of thyroid hormones may also drop after giving birth. The thyroid is a small gland in the neck that helps regulate how your body uses and stores energy from food. Low levels of thyroid hormones can cause symptoms of depression. A simple blood test can tell if this condition is causing your symptoms. If so, your doctor can prescribe thyroid medicine.

Other factors may play a role in postpartum depression. You may feel the following:

- Tired after delivery

- Tired from a lack of sleep or broken sleep

- Overwhelmed with a new baby

- Doubts about your ability to be a good mother

- Stress from changes in work and home routines

- An unrealistic need to be a perfect mom

- Loss of who you were before having the baby

- Less attractive

- A lack of free time

Are some women more at risk for depression during and after pregnancy?

Certain factors may increase your risk of depression during and after pregnancy:

- A personal history of depression or another mental illness

- A family history of depression or another mental illness

- A lack of support from family and friends

- Anxiety or negative feelings about the pregnancy

- Problems with a previous pregnancy or birth

- Marriage or money problems

- Stressful life events

- Young age

- Substance abuse

Women who are depressed during pregnancy have a greater risk of depression after giving birth.

What is the difference between baby blues, postpartum depression, and postpartum psychosis?

Many women have the baby blues in the days after childbirth. If you have the baby blues, you may experience these symptoms:

- Have mood swings

- Feel sad, anxious, or overwhelmed

- Have crying spells

- Lose your appetite

- Have trouble sleeping

The baby blues most often go away within a few days or a week. The symptoms are not severe and do not need treatment.

The symptoms of postpartum depression last longer and are more severe.

Postpartum depression can begin anytime within the first year after childbirth. If you have postpartum depression, you may have any of the symptoms of depression listed in the preceding text. Symptoms may also include the following:

- Thoughts of hurting the baby

- Thoughts of hurting yourself

- Not having any interest in the baby

Postpartum depression needs to be treated by a doctor.

Postpartum psychosis is rare. It occurs in about one to four out of every 1,000 births. It usually begins in the first two weeks after childbirth. Women who have bipolar disorder or another mental health problem called schizoaffective disorder have a higher risk for postpartum psychosis. Symptoms may include the following:

- Seeing things that aren't there

- Feeling confused

- Having rapid mood swings

- Trying to hurt yourself or your baby

What should I do if I have symptoms of depression during or after pregnancy?

Call your doctor if the following occur:

- Your baby blues don't go away after two weeks
- Symptoms of depression get more and more intense
- Symptoms of depression begin any time after delivery, even many months later
- It is hard for you to perform tasks at work or at home
- You cannot care for yourself or your baby
- You have thoughts of harming yourself or your baby

Your doctor can ask you questions to test for depression. Your doctor can also refer you to a mental health professional who specializes in treating depression.

Some women don't tell anyone about their symptoms. They feel embarrassed, ashamed, or guilty about feeling depressed when they are supposed to be happy. They worry they will be viewed as unfit parents.

Any woman may become depressed during pregnancy or after having a baby. It doesn't mean you are a bad or "not together" mom. You and your baby don't have to suffer. There is help.

Here are some other helpful tips:

- Rest as much as you can. Sleep when the baby is sleeping.
- Don't try to do too much or try to be perfect.
- Ask your partner, family, and friends for help.
- Make time to go out, visit friends, or spend time alone with your partner.
- Discuss your feelings with your partner, family, and friends.
- Talk with other mothers so you can learn from their experiences.
- Join a support group. Ask your doctor about groups in your area.
- Don't make any major life changes during pregnancy or right after giving birth. Major changes can cause unneeded stress. Sometimes big changes can't be avoided. When that happens, try to arrange support and help in your new situation ahead of time.

How is depression treated?

The two common types of treatment for depression are the following:

- **Talk therapy:** This involves talking to a therapist, psychologist, or social worker to learn to change how depression makes you think, feel, and act.

- **Medicine:** Your doctor can prescribe an antidepressant medicine. These medicines can help relieve symptoms of depression.

These treatment methods can be used alone or together. If you are depressed, your depression can affect your baby. Getting treatment is important for you and your baby. Talk with your doctor about the benefits and risks of taking medicine to treat depression when you are pregnant or breastfeeding.

What can happen if depression is not treated?

Untreated depression can hurt you and your baby. Some women with depression have a hard time caring for themselves during pregnancy. They may do the following:

- Eat poorly
- Not gain enough weight
- Have trouble sleeping
- Miss prenatal visits
- Not follow medical instructions
- Use harmful substances, like tobacco, alcohol, or illegal drugs

Depression during pregnancy can raise the risk of the following:

- Problems during pregnancy or delivery
- Having a low-birth-weight baby
- Premature birth

Untreated postpartum depression can affect your ability to parent. You may lack energy, have trouble focusing, feel moody, or not be able to meet your child's needs. As a result, you may feel guilty and lose confidence in yourself as a mother. These feelings can make your depression worse.

Researchers believe postpartum depression in a mother can affect her baby. It can cause the baby to have the following:

- Delays in language development

- Problems with mother-child bonding

- Behavior problems

- Increased crying

It helps if your partner or another caregiver can help meet the baby's needs while you are depressed.

All children deserve the chance to have a healthy mom. And all moms deserve the chance to enjoy their life and their children. If you are feeling depressed during pregnancy or after having a baby, don't suffer alone. Please tell a loved one and call your doctor right away.

Chapter 11

Premenstrual Dysphoric Disorder

Premenstrual dysphoric disorder (PMDD) is a condition in which a woman has severe depression symptoms, irritability, and tension before menstruation. The symptoms of PMDD are more severe than those seen with premenstrual syndrome (PMS).

PMS refers to a wide range of physical or emotional symptoms that typically occur about 5 to 11 days before a woman starts her monthly menstrual cycle. The symptoms usually stop when or shortly after her period begins.

Causes

The causes of PMS and PMDD have not been found.

Hormone changes that occur during a woman's menstrual cycle appear to play a role.

PMDD affects between 3% and 8% of women during the years when they are having menstrual periods.

Many women with this condition have:

- anxiety;
- major depression;
- seasonal affective disorder (SAD).

Other factors that may play a role include:

- alcohol abuse;

"Premenstrual Dysphoric Disorder," © 2011, A.D.A.M., Inc. Reprinted with permission.

- being overweight;

- drinking large amounts of caffeine;

- having a mother with a history of the disorder;

- lack of exercise.

Symptoms

The symptoms of PMDD are similar to those of PMS. However, they are generally more severe and debilitating and include at least one mood-related symptom. Symptoms occur during the week just before menstrual bleeding and usually improve within a few days after the period starts.

Five or more of the following symptoms must be present to diagnose PMDD, including one mood-related symptom:

- Disinterest in daily activities and relationships

- Fatigue or low energy

- Feeling of sadness or hopelessness, possible suicidal thoughts

- Feelings of tension or anxiety

- Feeling out of control

- Food cravings or binge eating

- Mood swings marked by periods of teariness

- Panic attack

- Persistent irritability or anger that affects other people

- Physical symptoms, such as bloating, breast tenderness, headaches, and joint or muscle pain

- Problems sleeping

- Trouble concentrating

Exams and Tests

No physical examination or lab tests can diagnose PMDD. A complete history, physical examination (including a pelvic exam), and psychiatric evaluation should be done to rule out other conditions.

Keeping a calendar or diary of symptoms can help women identify the most troublesome symptoms and the times when they are likely to occur. This information may help the health care provider diagnose PMDD and determine the best treatment.

Treatment

A healthy lifestyle is the first step to managing PMDD.

- Eat a balanced diet (with more whole grains, vegetables, fruit, and little or no salt, sugar, alcohol, and caffeine).

- Get regular aerobic exercise throughout the month to reduce the severity of PMS symptoms.

- Try changing your sleep habits before taking drugs for insomnia.

Keep a diary or calendar to record:

- the type of symptoms you are having;

- how severe they are;

- how long they last.

Antidepressants may be helpful.

The first option is usually an antidepressant known as a selective serotonin-reuptake inhibitor (SSRI). You can take SSRIs in the second part of your cycle up until your period starts, or for the whole month. Ask your doctor.

Cognitive behavioral therapy (CBT) may be used either with or instead of antidepressants. During CBT, you have about 10 visits with a mental health professional over several weeks.

Other treatments that may help include:

- Birth control pills may decrease or increase PMS symptoms, including depression.

- Diuretics may be useful for women who gain a lot of weight from fluid retention.

- Nutritional supplements—such as vitamin B6, calcium, and magnesium—may be recommended.

- Other medicines (such as Depo-Lupron) suppress the ovaries and ovulation.

- Pain relievers such as aspirin or ibuprofen may be prescribed for headache, backache, menstrual cramping, and breast tenderness.

Outlook (Prognosis)

After proper diagnosis and treatment, most women with PMDD find that their symptoms go away or drop to tolerable levels.

Possible Complications

PMDD symptoms may be severe enough to interfere with a woman's daily life. Women with depression may have worse symptoms during the second half of their cycle and may need changes in their medication.

As many as 10% of women who report PMS symptoms, especially those with PMDD, have had suicidal thoughts. Suicide in women with depression is much more likely to occur during the second half of the menstrual cycle.

PMDD may be associated with eating disorders and smoking.

When to Contact a Medical Professional

Call 911 or a local crisis line immediately if you are having suicidal thoughts.

Call for an appointment with your health care provider if:

- symptoms do not improve with self-treatment;
- symptoms interfere with your daily life.

Chapter 12

Psychotic Depression

Chapter Contents

Section 12.1

Major Depression with Psychotic Features

"Major depression with psychotic features,"
© 2011, A.D.A.M., Inc. Reprinted with permission.

Major depression with psychotic features is a mental disorder in which a person has depression along with loss of touch with reality (psychosis).

Causes

The cause is unknown. A family or personal history of depression or psychotic illness makes you more likely to develop this condition.

Symptoms

People with psychotic depression have symptoms of depression and psychosis.

Psychosis is a loss of contact with reality. It usually includes:

- **Delusions:** False beliefs about what is taking place or who one is

- **Hallucinations:** Seeing or hearing things that aren't there

The types of delusions and hallucinations are often related to your depressed feelings. For example, some patients may hear voices criticizing them, or telling them that they don't deserve to live. The person may develop false beliefs about their body, for example, that they have cancer.

Exams and Tests

Your health care provider will perform a physical exam and ask questions about your medical history and symptoms. Your answers and certain questionnaires can help your doctor diagnose this condition and determine how severe it may be.

Blood and urine tests and possibly a brain scan may be done to rule out other medical conditions with similar symptoms.

Treatment

Psychotic depression requires immediate medical care and treatment. Treatment usually involves antidepressant and antipsychotic medication. You may only need antipsychotic medication for a short period of time.

Electroconvulsive therapy can help treat depression with psychotic symptoms. However, medication is usually tried first.

Outlook (Prognosis)

This is a serious condition that requires immediate treatment and close monitoring by a doctor. You may need to take medication for a long time to prevent the depression from coming back. Depression symptoms are more likely to return than the psychotic symptoms.

Possible Complications

The risk of suicide is much higher in people with depression with psychotic symptoms than in those without psychosis. You may need to stay in the hospital if you have thoughts of suicide. The safety of others must also be considered.

When to Contact a Medical Professional

If you have thoughts of suicide or harming yourself or others, immediate call your local emergency number (such as 911) or go to the hospital emergency room.

You may also call a suicide hotline from anywhere in the United States, 24 hours a day, 7 days a week: 800-SUICIDE or 800-999-9999.

Call your doctor right away if:

- you hear voices that are not there;

- you have frequent crying spells with little or no reason;

- your depression is disrupting work, school, or family life;

- you think that your current medications are not working or are causing side effects. Never change or stop any medications without consulting your doctor.

Section 12.2

Schizoaffective Disorder

What is schizoaffective disorder?

Some psychiatric disorders are very difficult to diagnose accurately.
One of the most confusing conditions is schizoaffective disorder.

This relatively rare disorder is defined as the presence of psychotic
symptoms in the absence of mood changes for at least two weeks in
a patient who has a mood disorder. The diagnosis is used when an
individual does not fit diagnostic standards for either schizophrenia
or affective (mood) disorders such as depression and bipolar disorder
(manic depression).

Some people may have symptoms of both a depressive disorder
and schizophrenia at the same time, or they may have symptoms of
schizophrenia without mood symptoms.

Many individuals with schizoaffective disorder are originally diagnosed with manic depression. If the person experiences delusions or
hallucinations that go away in less than two weeks when the mood is
normal, bipolar disorder may be the proper diagnosis. Someone who
experiences psychosis for three or four weeks while in a manic phase
does not have schizoaffective disorder.

However, if delusions or hallucinations continue after the mood has
stabilized and are accompanied by other symptoms of schizophrenia
such as catatonia, paranoia, bizarre behavior, or thought disorders,
a diagnosis of schizoaffective disorder may be appropriate. Accurate
diagnosis is easier once the acute psychotic episode is under control.

Distinguishing between bipolar disorder and schizophrenia can
be particularly difficult in an adolescent, since at that age psychotic
features are especially common during manic periods.

Because schizoaffective disorder is so complicated, misdiagnosis
is common. Some people may be misdiagnosed as having schizophrenia. Others may be misdiagnosed as having bipolar disorder. And
those diagnosed as having schizoaffective disorder may actually have

schizophrenia with prominent mood symptoms. Or they may have a mood disorder with symptoms similar to those of schizophrenia.

What is the treatment for this disorder?

Psychiatrists often treat this disorder with an antipsychotic medication and lithium, or with carbamazepine (an anticonvulsant medication) and lithium.

As a practical matter, differentiating between schizophrenia, bipolar disorder, and schizoaffective disorder is not absolutely critical, since antipsychotic medication is recommended for all three. If a mood problem is suspected, lithium or an antidepressant should be added.

What is the prognosis for those with this disorder?

The prognosis for individuals diagnosed with schizoaffective disorder is generally better than for those diagnosed with schizophrenia, but not quite as good for those diagnosed with a mood disorder. (Schizophrenia is a chronic brain disorder interfering with a person's ability to think clearly, manage emotions, make decisions, and relate to others. Persons with schizophrenia may experience hallucinations and delusions. Mood disorders, including depression and bipolar disorder, are chronic illnesses in which the person's mood may return to normal between depressive or manic episodes.) Those with schizoaffective disorder generally respond to lithium better than those with schizophrenia, but not as well as those with mood disorders.

More research is needed to fully understand this illness and why it resists conventional treatment. New medications may be developed to treat this disorder more effectively.

Further Information

Overcoming Depression by Dimitri F. Papolos, MD, and Janice Papolos

Manic Depressive Illness by Frederick K. Goodwin, MD, and Kay Redfield Jamison, PhD

Chapter 13

Seasonal Affective Disorder (SAD)

Weather often affects people's moods. Sunlight breaking through clouds can lift our spirits, while a dull, rainy day may make us feel a little gloomy. While noticeable, these shifts in mood generally do not affect our ability to cope with daily life. Some people, however, are vulnerable to a type of depression that follows a seasonal pattern. For them, the shortening days of late autumn are the beginning of a type of clinical depression that can last until spring. This condition is called Seasonal Affective Disorder, or SAD.

A mild form of SAD, often referred to as the winter blues, causes discomfort, but is not incapacitating. However, the term winter blues can be misleading; some people have a rarer form of SAD which is summer depression. This condition usually begins in late spring or early summer.

Awareness of this mental condition has existed for more than 150 years, but it was only recognized as a disorder in the early 1980s. Many people with SAD may not be aware that it exists or that help is available. SAD can be a debilitating condition, preventing sufferers from functioning normally. It may affect their personal and professional lives, and seriously limit their potential. It is important to learn about the symptoms, and to know that there is treatment to help people with SAD live a productive life year-round.

What Causes SAD?

Research into the causes of SAD is ongoing. As yet, there is no confirmed cause. However, SAD is thought to be related to seasonal variations in light. A biological internal clock in the brain regulates our circadian (daily) rhythms. This biological clock responds to changes in season, partly because of the differences in the length of the day. For many thousands of years, the cycle of human life revolved around the daily cycle of light and dark. We were alert when the sun shone; we slept when our world was in darkness. The relatively recent introduction of electricity has relieved us of the need to be active mostly in the daylight hours. But our biological clocks may still be telling our bodies to sleep as the days shorten. This puts us out of step with our daily schedules, which no longer change according to the seasons. Other research shows that neurotransmitters, chemical messengers in the brain that help regulate sleep, mood, and appetite, may be disturbed in SAD.

What Are the Symptoms?

SAD can be difficult to diagnose, since many of the symptoms are similar to those of other types of depression or bipolar disorder. Even physical conditions, such as thyroid problems, can look like depression. Generally, symptoms that recur for at least two consecutive winters, without any other explanation for the changes in mood and behavior, indicate the presence of SAD. They may include:

- change in appetite, in particular a craving for sweet or starchy foods;
- weight gain;
- decreased energy;
- fatigue;
- tendency to oversleep;
- difficulty concentrating;
- irritability;
- avoidance of social situations;
- feelings of anxiety and despair.

The symptoms of SAD generally disappear when spring arrives. For some people, this happens suddenly with a short time of heightened activity. For others, the effects of SAD gradually dissipate.

Symptoms of summer depression may include:

- poor appetite;
- weight loss;
- trouble sleeping.

Who Is at Risk?

Research in Ontario suggests that between 2% and 3% of the general population may have SAD. Another 15% have a less severe experience described as the winter blues. SAD may affect some children and teenagers, but it tends to begin in people over the age of 20. The risk of SAD decreases with age. The condition is more common in women than in men.

Recent studies suggest that SAD is more common in northern countries, where the winter day is shorter.

Deprivation from natural sources of light is also of particular concern for shift workers and urban dwellers who may experience reduced levels of exposure to daylight in their work environments. People with SAD find that spending time in a southerly location brings them relief from their symptoms.

How Is SAD Treated?

If you feel depressed for long periods during autumn and winter, if your sleep and appetite patterns change dramatically and you find yourself thinking about suicide, you should seek professional help, for example, from your family doctor. There is effective treatment for SAD. Even people with severe symptoms can get rapid relief once they begin treatment.

People with mild symptoms can benefit from spending more time outdoors during the day and by arranging their environments so that they receive maximum sunlight. Trim tree branches that block light, for example, and keep curtains open during the day. Move furniture so that you sit near a window. Installing skylights and adding lamps can also help.

Exercise relieves stress, builds energy and increases your mental and physical well-being. Build physical activity into your lifestyle before SAD symptoms take hold. If you exercise indoors, position yourself near a window. Make a habit of taking a daily noon-hour walk. The activity and increased exposure to natural light can raise your spirits.

A winter vacation in a sunny destination can also temporarily relieve SAD symptoms, although symptoms usually recur after return home. At home, work at resisting the carbohydrate and sleep cravings that come with SAD.

Many people with SAD respond well to exposure to bright, artificial light. Light therapy involves sitting beside a special fluorescent light box for several minutes day. A health care professional should be consulted before beginning light therapy.

For people who are more severely affected by SAD, antidepressant medications are safe and effective in relieving symptoms. Counseling and therapy, especially short-term treatments such as cognitive-behavioral therapy, may also be helpful for winter depression.

Increasing your exposure to light and monitoring your diet, sleep patterns, and exercise levels are important first steps. For those who are severely affected, devising a treatment plan with a health care professional consisting of light therapy, medication, and cognitive-behavioral therapy may also be needed.

Where to Go for More Information

For further information about seasonal affective disorder, contact a community organization like the Canadian Mental Health Association to find out about support and resources in your community.

Part Three

Who Develops Depression?

Chapter 14

Men, Women, and Depression

Chapter Contents

Section 14.1

The Gender Gap in Depression

Betty can't get to sleep; Tashita can't wake up. Nothing interests Mei Wu; Carmen cries when she's home alone; and Lucy is convinced her life's not worth living. They're among the millions of women worldwide trying to cope with the symptoms of clinical depression.

Welcome to the blues sisterhood.

Rate Twice That of Males

Over the course of their lifetimes, 20 percent of all women are likely to find themselves in these women's shoes, note Subahash C. Bhatia, MD, and Shashi K. Bhatia, MD—a husband-and-wife team of professors at Creighton University School of Medicine in Omaha and University of Nebraska College of Medicine.

Writing in the July 1999 issue of *American Family Physician*, the Bhatias—both of them experienced psychiatrists—point out that although the diagnostic criteria for depression is identical for both sexes, females experience the condition twice as often as males. The National Mental Health Association in Alexandria, Virginia, notes approximately 12 million women in the United States alone experience clinical depression each year.

A Global Disease Burden

Dr. Myrna Weissman of Columbia University's New York State Psychiatric Institute and her colleagues reported a similar prevalence of depressive illnesses in women in the United States, Canada, Germany, and New Zealand. Across the four nations, Weissman's team identified double the rates of major depression and its milder form—known as dysthymia—in females compared to their male counterparts.

At the beginning of the 1990s, the World Health Organization named depression as the leading cause of "disease burden," a measure of both illness and death, in women around the globe. But although medical science has taken giant steps forward in understanding the genetic and environmental bases of many common physical and mental ills, Bhatia and Bhatia say the exact reason for the wide gender gap in depression remains unknown.

The quest for an answer has researchers pursuing an interesting and ever-lengthening list of possibilities.

Depressing Combinations

Like other experts in women's mental health, the Bhatias believe the higher prevalence of depression in women is probably due to a combination of gender-related differences in cognitive styles, certain biological factors, and a higher incidence of social, psychological, and economic stresses in females. They list the following specific risk factors for women:

- Family history of mood disorders
- Personal past history of mood disorders in early reproductive years
- Loss of a parent before the age of 10
- Childhood history of physical or sexual abuse
- Use of an oral contraceptive, particularly one with a high progesterone content
- Use of gonadotropin stimulants for treatment of infertility
- Persistent psychosocial stressors (for example, job loss, family illness, poverty)
- Loss of a social support system or the threat of such a loss (for example, through a death, move, divorce)

Other researchers have delved more deeply into genetics and female biology to determine how these factors may relate to one another and which—if any—explain why so many more women than men get depressed.

An Inherited Trait?

Stress obviously plays a role in depression, but do women experience different stressors than men, or do they simply respond to the same stressors in a different fashion?

Researchers at the Medical College of Virginia looked for clues about how females react to environmental stressors in a study of more than 1,000 twin sisters, about half of whom had a family history of depression. According to the study's director, Kenneth S. Kendler, MD, a professor of psychiatry at MCV, recent exposure to a stressful event increased the risk of depression for the twins without a family history of the disorder only six percent. For twins who had such a family history, however, the risk was more than doubled, to 14 percent.

This suggests that women with a family history of depression may have inherited a tendency toward becoming depressed themselves, Kendler and his colleagues concluded. But, as the National Institute on Mental Health (NIMH) points out, not every woman with a family history develops the illness, while others with no such family history do.

Hormonal Factors

Hormones have attracted considerable attention as a likely cause for the huge differences between rates of depression in women and men. After all, women's hormone-related reproductive events—including menstruation, pregnancy, the postpartum period, infertility, and menopause—often are associated with mood fluctuations, including depression.

But in a National Institute of Health booklet, "Depression: What Every Woman Should Know," U.S. government experts acknowledge that although female hormones do affect emotions and moods, the specific biological mechanism linking hormones such as estrogen to depression has yet to be identified.

The National Institutes of Health (NIH) further notes that some types of female depression, such as those that happen during the postpartum period or at the onset of menopause, more often occur in women who have had previous depressive episodes, even though they may not have been diagnosed or treated earlier. Other reproductive events—such as pregnancy and abortion—do not seem to result in a higher incidence of clinical depression. This knowledge has prompted study of the relationship between female hormones and depression from a different angle.

Estrogen May Set the Stage

Ellen Leibenluft, MD, Chief of the Unit on Rapid Cycling Bipolar Disorder at the National Institute of Mental Health, explained in a June 1998 Scientific American article that "[I]t now appears that estrogen might set the stage for depression indirectly by priming the body's stress response. During stressful times, adrenal glands—which set on top of the kidneys and are controlled by the pituitary gland in the brain—secrete levels of a hormone called cortisol. Cortisol increases the activity of the body's metabolic and immune systems, among others. In the normal course of events, stress increases cortisol secretion, but these elevated levels have a negative feedback effect on the pituitary, so that cortisol levels gradually return to normal."

"Evidence is emerging that estrogen might not only increase cortisol secretion, but also decrease cortisol's ability to shut down its own secretion," she added. "The result might be a stress response that is not only more pronounced but longer-lasting in women than in men."

Such research is expected to provide part—but probably not all—of the explanation for the gender gap in depressive conditions.

Small Pieces, Complex Puzzle

According to Leibenluft, figuring out why depression is more common among women than men is difficult work and progress is necessarily slow. But, she added, "What is coming into focus is that certain environmental factors— including stress, seasonal changes, and social rank— may produce different physiological changes in females than they do in males. These findings are small pieces in what is proving to be an incredibly complex puzzle."

Additional Depression Resources Online

Need more information about women and depression? These websites and organizations may be helpful to you:

National Institute of Mental Health (NIMH)
Science Writing, Press, and Dissemination Branch
6001 Executive Boulevard, Room 8184, MSC 9663
Bethesda, MD 20892-9663
Toll-Free: 866-615-6464
Toll-Free TTY: 866-415-8051
Phone: 301-443-4513
TTY: 301-443-8431
Fax: 301-443-4279
Website: www.nimh.nih.gov
E-mail: nimhinfo@nih.gov

National Foundation for Depressive Illness, Inc.
PO Box 2257
New York, NY 10116
Toll-Free: 800-248-4344
Website: www.depression.org

National Depressive and Manic-Depressive Association
730 N. Franklin Street, Suite 501
Chicago, IL 60610-3526
Toll-Free: 800-826-3632
Phone: 312-642-0049
Website: www.ndmda.org

Mental Health America
2000 North Beauregard Street, 6th Floor
Alexandria, VA 22311
Toll-Free: 800-969-6642
Toll-Free Crisis Line: 800-273-TALK (800-273-8255)
Phone: 703-684-7722
Fax: 703-684-5968
Website: www.nmha.org
E-mail: webmaster@mentalhealthamerica.net

Section 14.2

Men and Depression

From "Men and Depression," by the National Institute of
Mental Health (NIMH, www.nimh.nih.gov), part of the
National Institutes of Health, September 23, 2010.

Are you tired and irritable all the time? Have you lost interest in
your work, family, or hobbies? Are you having trouble sleeping and
feeling angry or aggressive, sad, or worthless? Have you been feeling
like this for weeks or months? If so, you may have depression.

What is depression?

Everyone feels sad or irritable sometimes, or has trouble sleeping
occasionally. But these feelings and troubles usually pass after a couple
of days. When a man has depression, he has trouble with daily life and
loses interest in anything for weeks at a time.

Both men and women get depression. But men can experience it
differently than women. Men may be more likely to feel very tired
and irritable, and lose interest in their work, family, or hobbies. They
may be more likely to have difficulty sleeping than women who have
depression. And although women with depression are more likely to
attempt suicide, men are more likely to die by suicide.

Many men do not recognize, acknowledge, or seek help for their
depression. They may be reluctant to talk about how they are feeling. But depression is a real and treatable illness. It can affect any
man at any age. With the right treatment, most men with depression can get better and gain back their interest in work, family,
and hobbies.

What are the different forms of depression?

The most common types of depression are the following:

- Major depression: Major depression involves severe symptoms
  that interfere with a man's ability to work, sleep, study, eat, and
  enjoy most aspects of life. An episode of major depression may

121

occur only once in a person's lifetime. But more often, a person can have several episodes.

- Dysthymic disorder, or dysthymia: This disorder involves depressive symptoms that last a long time (two years or longer) but are less severe than those of major depression.

- Minor depression: Minor depression is similar to major depression and dysthymia, but symptoms are less severe and may not last as long.

What are the signs and symptoms of depression in men?

Different people have different symptoms. Some symptoms of depression include:

- Feeling sad or empty

- Feeling hopeless, irritable, anxious, or angry

- Loss of interest in work, family, or once-pleasurable activities, including sex

- Feeling very tired

- Not being able to concentrate or remember details

- Not being able to sleep or sleeping too much

- Overeating or not wanting to eat at all

- Thoughts of suicide or suicide attempts

- Aches or pains, headaches, cramps, or digestive problems

- Inability to meet the responsibilities of work, caring for family, or other important activities

What causes depression in men?

Several factors may contribute to depression in men.

- **Genes:** Men with a family history of depression may be more likely to develop it than those whose family members do not have the illness.

- **Brain chemistry and hormones:** The brains of people with depression look different on scans than those of people without the illness. Also, the hormones that control emotions and mood can affect brain chemistry.

- **Stress:** Loss of a loved one, a difficult relationship, or any stressful situation may trigger depression in some men.

Most of the time, it is likely a combination of these factors.

How is depression treated?

The first step to getting the right treatment is to visit a doctor or mental health professional. He or she can do an exam or lab tests to rule out other conditions that may have the same symptoms as depression. He or she can also tell if certain medications you are taking may be affecting your mood.

The doctor needs to get a complete history of symptoms. Tell the doctor when the symptoms started, how long they have lasted, how bad they are, whether they have occurred before, and if so, how they were treated. Tell the doctor if there is a history of depression in your family.

Medication: Medications called antidepressants can work well to treat depression. But they can take several weeks to work. Antidepressants can have side effects including the following:

- Headache
- Nausea or feeling sick to your stomach
- Difficulty sleeping and nervousness
- Agitation or restlessness
- Sexual problems

Most side effects lessen over time. Talk to your doctor about any side effects you may have.

It's important to know that although antidepressants can be safe and effective for many people, they may present serious risks to some, especially children, teens, and young adults. A black box—the most serious type of warning that a prescription drug can have—has been added to the labels of antidepressant medications. These labels warn people that antidepressants may cause some people to have suicidal thoughts or make suicide attempts, especially those who become agitated when they first start taking the medication and before it begins to work. Anyone taking antidepressants should be monitored closely, especially when they first start taking them.

For most people, though, the risks of untreated depression far outweigh those of antidepressant medications when they are used under a doctor's supervision. Careful monitoring by a professional will also minimize any potential risks.

Therapy: Several types of therapy can help treat depression. Some therapies are just as effective as medications for certain types of depression. Therapy helps by teaching new ways of thinking and behaving, and changing habits that may be contributing to the depression. Therapy can also help men understand and work through difficult situations or relationships that may be causing their depression or making it worse.

How can I help a loved one who is depressed?

If you know someone who has depression, first help him find a doctor or mental health professional and make an appointment.

- Offer him support, understanding, patience, and encouragement.

- Talk to him, and listen carefully.

- Never ignore comments about suicide, and report them to his therapist or doctor.

- Invite him out for walks, outings and other activities. If he says no, keep trying, but don't push him to take on too much too soon.

- Encourage him to report any concerns about medications to his health care provider.

- Ensure that he gets to his doctor's appointments.

- Remind him that with time and treatment, the depression will lift.

How can I help myself if I am depressed?

As you continue treatment, gradually you will start to feel better. Remember that if you are taking an antidepressant, it may take several weeks for it to start working. Try to do things that you used to enjoy before you had depression. Go easy on yourself. Other things that may help include the following:

- See a professional as soon as possible. Research shows that getting treatment sooner rather than later can relieve symptoms quicker and reduce the length of time treatment is needed.

- Break up large tasks into small ones, and do what you can as you can. Don't try to do too many things at once.

- Spend time with other people and talk to a friend or relative about your feelings.

- Do not make important decisions until you feel better. Discuss decisions with others who know you well.

Section 14.3

Women and Depression

From "Women and Depression: Discovering Hope," by the National
Institute on Mental Health (NIMH, www.nimh.nih.gov), part of the
National Institutes of Health, August 31, 2010.

Causes of Depression in Women

Scientists are examining many potential causes for and contributing factors to women's increased risk for depression. It is likely that genetic, biological, chemical, hormonal, environmental, psychological, and social factors all intersect to contribute to depression.

Genetics

If a woman has a family history of depression, she may be more at risk of developing the illness. However, this is not a hard and fast rule. Depression can occur in women without family histories of depression, and women from families with a history of depression may not develop depression themselves.

Genetics research indicates that the risk for developing depression likely involves the combination of multiple genes with environmental or other factors.

Chemicals and Hormones

Brain chemistry appears to be a significant factor in depressive disorders. Modern brain-imaging technologies, such as magnetic resonance imaging (MRI), have shown that the brains of people suffering from depression look different than those of people without depression. The parts of the brain responsible for regulating mood, thinking, sleep, appetite, and behavior don't appear to be functioning normally. In addition, important neurotransmitters—chemicals that brain cells use to communicate—appear to be out of balance. But these images do not reveal why the depression has occurred.

Scientists are also studying the influence of female hormones, which change throughout life. Researchers have shown that hormones directly affect the brain chemistry that controls emotions and mood. Specific times during a woman's life are of particular interest, including puberty; the times before menstrual periods; before, during, and just after pregnancy (postpartum); and just prior to and during menopause (perimenopause).

Premenstrual Dysphoric Disorder

Some women may be susceptible to a severe form of premenstrual syndrome called premenstrual dysphoric disorder (PMDD). Women affected by PMDD typically experience depression, anxiety, irritability, and mood swings the week before menstruation, in such a way that interferes with their normal functioning. Women with debilitating PMDD do not necessarily have unusual hormone changes, but they do have different responses to these changes. They may also have a history of other mood disorders and differences in brain chemistry that cause them to be more sensitive to menstruation-related hormone changes. Scientists are exploring how the cyclical rise and fall of estrogen and other hormones may affect the brain chemistry that is associated with depressive illness.

Postpartum Depression

Women are particularly vulnerable to depression after giving birth, when hormonal and physical changes and the new responsibility of caring for a newborn can be overwhelming. Many new mothers experience a brief episode of mild mood changes known as the baby blues, but some will suffer from postpartum depression, a much more serious condition that requires active treatment and emotional support for the new mother. One study found that postpartum women are at an increased risk for several mental disorders, including depression, for several months after childbirth.

Some studies suggest that women who experience postpartum depression often have had prior depressive episodes. Some experience it during their pregnancies, but it often goes undetected. Research suggests that visits to the doctor may be good opportunities for screening for depression both during pregnancy and in the postpartum period.

Menopause

Hormonal changes increase during the transition between premenopause to menopause. While some women may transition into menopause without any problems with mood, others experience an increased risk for depression. This seems to occur even among women without a history of depression. However, depression becomes less common for women during the post-menopause period.

Stress

Stressful life events such as trauma, loss of a loved one, a difficult relationship or any stressful situation—whether welcome or unwelcome—often occur before a depressive episode. Additional work and home responsibilities, caring for children and aging parents, abuse, and poverty also may trigger a depressive episode. Evidence suggests that women respond differently than men to these events, making them more prone to depression. In fact, research indicates that women respond in such a way that prolongs their feelings of stress more so than men, increasing the risk for depression. However, it is unclear why some women faced with enormous challenges develop depression, and some with similar challenges do not.

Illnesses Often Coexist with Depression in Women

Depression often coexists with other illnesses that may precede the depression, follow it, cause it, be a consequence of it, or a combination of these. It is likely that the interplay between depression and other illnesses differs for every person and situation. Regardless, these other coexisting illnesses need to be diagnosed and treated.

Depression often coexists with eating disorders such as anorexia nervosa, bulimia nervosa, and others, especially among women. Anxiety disorders, such as posttraumatic stress disorder (PTSD), obsessive-compulsive disorder, panic disorder, social phobia, and generalized anxiety disorder, also sometimes accompany depression. Women are more prone than men to having a coexisting anxiety disorder. Women suffering from PTSD, which can result after a person endures a terrifying ordeal or event, are especially prone to having depression.

Although more common among men than women, alcohol and substance abuse or dependence may occur at the same time as depression. Research has indicated that among both sexes, the coexistence of mood disorders and substance abuse is common among the U.S. population.

Depression also often coexists with other serious medical illnesses such as heart disease, stroke, cancer, HIV/AIDS [human immunodeficiency virus/acquired immunodeficiency syndrome], diabetes, Parkinson disease, thyroid problems, and multiple sclerosis, and may even make symptoms of the illness worse. Studies have shown that both women and men who have depression in addition to a serious medical illness tend to have more severe symptoms of both illnesses. They also have more difficulty adapting to their medical condition, and more medical costs than those who do not have coexisting depression.

Research has shown that treating the depression along with the coexisting illness will help ease both conditions.

Depression Affects Adolescent Girls

Before adolescence, girls and boys experience depression at about the same frequency. By adolescence, however, girls become more likely to experience depression than boys.

Research points to several possible reasons for this imbalance. The biological and hormonal changes that occur during puberty likely contribute to the sharp increase in rates of depression among adolescent girls. In addition, research has suggested that girls are more likely than boys to continue feeling bad after experiencing difficult situations or events, suggesting they are more prone to depression. Another study found that girls tended to doubt themselves, doubt their problem-solving abilities, and view their problems as unsolvable more so than boys. The girls with these views were more likely to have depressive symptoms as well. Girls also tended to need a higher degree of approval and success to feel secure than boys.

Finally, girls may undergo more hardships, such as poverty, poor education, childhood sexual abuse, and other traumas than boys. One study found that more than 70 percent of depressed girls experienced a difficult or stressful life event prior to a depressive episode, as compared with only 14 percent of boys.

Depression Affects Older Women

As with other age groups, more older women than older men experience depression, but rates decrease among women after menopause. Evidence suggests that depression in post-menopausal women generally occurs in women with prior histories of depression. In any case, depression is not a normal part of aging.

The death of a spouse or loved one, moving from work into retirement, or dealing with a chronic illness can leave women and men alike feeling sad or distressed.

After a period of adjustment, many older women can regain their emotional balance, but others do not and may develop depression. When older women do suffer from depression, it may be overlooked because older adults may be less willing to discuss feelings of sadness or grief, or they may have less obvious symptoms of depression. As a result, their doctors may be less likely to suspect or spot it.

For older adults who experience depression for the first time later in life, other factors, such as changes in the brain or body, may be at play. For example, older adults may suffer from restricted blood flow, a condition called ischemia. Over time, blood vessels become less flexible. They may harden and prevent blood from flowing normally to the body's organs, including the brain. If this occurs, an older adult with no family or personal history of depression may develop what some doctors call vascular depression. Those with vascular depression also may be at risk for a coexisting cardiovascular illness, such as heart disease or a stroke.

Antidepressant Medications and Pregnancy

At one time, doctors assumed that pregnancy was accompanied by a natural feeling of well-being, and that depression during pregnancy was rare, or never occurred at all. However, recent studies have shown that women can have depression while pregnant, especially if they have a prior history of the illness. In fact, a majority of women with a history of depression will likely relapse during pregnancy if they stop taking their antidepressant medication either prior to conception or early in the pregnancy, putting both mother and baby at risk.

However, antidepressant medications do pass across the placental barrier, potentially exposing the developing fetus to the medication. Some research suggests the use of SSRIs [selective serotonin reuptake inhibitors] during pregnancy is associated with miscarriage and/or birth defects, but other studies do not support this. Some studies have indicated that fetuses exposed to SSRIs during the third trimester may be born with "withdrawal" symptoms such as breathing problems, jitteriness, irritability, difficulty feeding, or hypoglycemia. In 2004, the U.S. Food and Drug Administration (FDA) issued a warning against the use of SSRIs in the late third trimester, suggesting that clinicians gradually taper expectant mothers off SSRIs in the third trimester to avoid any ill effects on the baby.

Although some studies suggest that exposure to SSRIs in pregnancy may have adverse effects on the infant, generally they are mild and short-lived, and no deaths have been reported. On the flip side, women who stop taking their antidepressant medication during pregnancy increase their risk for developing depression again and may put both themselves and their infant at risk.

In light of these mixed results, women and their doctors need to consider the potential risks and benefits to both mother and fetus of taking an antidepressant during pregnancy, and make decisions based on individual needs and circumstances. In some cases, a woman and her doctor may decide to taper her antidepressant dose during the last month of pregnancy to minimize the newborn's withdrawal symptoms, and after delivery, return to a full dose during the vulnerable postpartum period.

Antidepressant Medications and Breastfeeding

Antidepressants are excreted in breast milk, usually in very small amounts. The amount an infant receives is usually so small that it does not register in blood tests. Few problems are seen among infants nursing from mothers who are taking antidepressants. However, as with antidepressant use during pregnancy, both the risks and benefits to the mother and infant should be taken into account when deciding whether to take an antidepressant while breastfeeding.

Chapter 15

Depression in Children and Adolescents

Chapter Contents

Section 15.1

Understanding Depression in Children

Depression is the most common mental health problem in the United States. Each year it affects 17 million people of all age groups, races, and economic backgrounds.

As many as one in every 33 children may have depression; in teens, that number may be as high as one in eight.

So it's wise for parents and caregivers to learn about depression and how to help if your child, or a child you know, seems depressed.

About Depression

Depression isn't just bad moods and occasional melancholy. It's not just feeling down or sad, either. These feelings are normal in kids, especially during the teen years. Even when major disappointments and setbacks make people feel sad and angry, the negative feelings usually lessen with time.

But when a depressive state, or mood, lingers for a long time—weeks, months, or even longer—and limits a person's ability to function normally, it can be diagnosed as depression.

Types of depression include: major depression, dysthymia, adjustment disorder with depressed mood, seasonal affective disorder, and bipolar disorder or manic depression. All of these can affect kids and teenagers.

Major depression is a serious condition characterized by a persistent sad mood, feelings of worthlessness or guilt, and the inability to feel pleasure or happiness. Major depression typically interferes with day-to-day functioning like eating and sleeping. A child with major depression feels depressed almost every day. In kids, depression can appear as "bad moods" or irritability that persists for a long time, even if a child doesn't acknowledge being sad.

Dysthymia may be diagnosed if sadness or irritability is not as severe but continues for a year or longer. Kids with dysthymia often feel "down in the dumps." They can have low self-esteem, feel hopeless, and even have problems sleeping and eating. Unlike major depression, dysthymia does not severely interfere with day-to-day functioning but the "down mood" is a pervasive part of the child's world. However, at least 10% of those with dysthymic disorder go on to develop major depression.

Bipolar disorder, another type of mood disturbance, is characterized by episodes of low-energy depression (sadness and hopelessness) and high-energy mania (irritability and explosive temper). Bipolar disorder may affect as many as 1% to 2% of kids. More than 2 million adults have bipolar disorder, which often develops in the late teen years and early adulthood. Research in kids is not comprehensive, but experts believe that kids and teens with bipolar disorder can experience a number of problems, including attention deficit disorders, oppositional behavior disorders, anxiety, and irritability in addition to changes in mood from depression to mania.

Causes of Depression

Depression usually isn't caused by one event or reason, but is usually the result of several factors. Causes vary from person to person.

Depression can be caused by lowered levels of neurotransmitters (chemicals that carry signals through the nervous system) in the brain, which limits a person's ability to feel good. Genetics are likely involved as depression can run in families, so someone with a close relative who has depression may be more likely to experience it.

Significant life events such as the death of a loved one, a divorce, a move to a new area, and even a breakup with a girlfriend or boyfriend can bring on symptoms of depression. Stress also can be a factor, and because the teen years can be a time of emotional and social turmoil, things that are difficult for anyone to handle can be devastating to a teen.

Also, chronic illness can contribute to depression, as can the side effects of certain medicines or infections.

Diagnosing Depression

Kids with depression have described themselves as feeling hopeless about everything or feeling that nothing is worth the effort. They honestly believe that they are "no good," that their world is a difficult place, and that they're helpless to do anything about it.

But for an accurate diagnosis of major depression to be made, a detailed clinical evaluation must be done by a medical or mental health professional (such as a psychologist or psychiatrist). To meet criteria for a diagnosis, five or more of these symptoms must be present for longer than two weeks:

- A feeling of being down in the dumps or really sad for no reason
- A lack of energy, feeling unable to do the simplest task
- An inability to enjoy the things that used to bring pleasure
- A lack of desire to be with friends or family members
- Feelings of irritability, anger, or anxiety (irritability is especially common in kids and teens)
- An inability to concentrate
- A marked weight gain or loss (or failure to gain weight as expected), and too little or too much interest in eating
- A significant change in sleep habits, such as trouble falling asleep or getting up
- Feelings of guilt or worthlessness
- Aches and pains even though nothing is physically wrong
- A lack of caring about what happens in the future
- Frequent thoughts about death or suicide

For a diagnosis of dysthymia, someone must experience two or more of these symptoms almost all the time for at least a year:

- Feelings of hopelessness
- Low self-esteem
- Sleeping too much or being unable to sleep
- Extreme fatigue
- Difficulty concentrating
- Lack of appetite or overeating

Kids and teens who are depressed are more likely to use alcohol and drugs than those who aren't depressed. Because these can momentarily allow a person to forget about the depression, they seem like easy fixes. But they can make someone with depression feel even worse.

Recognizing Depression

If you think your child has symptoms of depression, it's important to take action. Talk with your child and your doctor or others who know your child well. Many parents dismiss their concerns, thinking they'll go away, or avoid acting because they may feel guilty or prefer to solve family problems privately.

For a long time, it was commonly believed that children did not get depressed and that teenagers all went through a period of "storm and stress," so many kids and teens went untreated for depression. Now more is known about childhood depression and experts say it's important to get kids help as soon as a problem is noticed.

Parents often feel responsible for things going on with their kids, but parents don't cause depression. However, it is true that parental separation, illness, death, or other separation can cause short-term problems for kids, and sometimes can trigger a problem with longer term depression. This means that if your family is going through something stressful it's usually helpful to turn to a counselor, therapist, or other expert for support during this time.

It's also important to remind your child that you're there for support. Say this over and over again—kids with depression need to hear it a lot because sometimes they feel unworthy of love and attention.

Remember, kids who are depressed may see the world very negatively because their experiences are shaped by their depression. They might act like they don't want help or might not even know what they are really experiencing.

If You Suspect a Problem

The good news is that professionals can help. Depression can be successfully treated in more than 80% of the people who become depressed. But if it goes untreated, it can be deadly—it is a major risk factor for suicidal behavior.

Depression can be treated with psychotherapy, medicine, or a combination of therapy and medicine. A psychiatrist can prescribe medicine, and although it may take a few tries to find the right drug, most people who follow their prescribed regimen eventually begin to feel better.

Psychotherapy focuses on the causes of the depression and works to help change negative thoughts and find ways to allow someone to feel better. Cognitive behavioral therapy has been shown to be very effective in treating depression, as well as anxious feelings that may come with it. Depression can be caused by and maintained with negative thinking, and this type of therapy, when given by a trained professional, can be extremely effective in helping fight it.

Getting Help for Your Child

Your first consultation should be with your child's pediatrician, who probably will perform a complete examination to rule out physical illness. If depression is suspected, the doctor may refer you to a psychiatrist (a medical doctor who can make a diagnosis, offer treatment, and prescribe medicine), psychologist (a health professional who can diagnose and treat depression but is unable to write prescriptions), or licensed clinical social worker (a person who has a degree in social work and is qualified to treat childhood depression).

When it comes to managing your child's depression, all of these health professionals can help. The important thing is that your child feels comfortable with the person. If it's not a good fit, find another.

Your child's teacher, guidance counselor, or school psychologist also may be able to help. These professionals have the welfare of your child at heart and all information shared with them during therapy is kept confidential.

Treating Depression

Don't put off your child's treatment. Early detection and diagnosis are key in treating kids with depression.

A child or adolescent psychiatrist or psychologist can perform a complete evaluation and start a treatment plan that may include counseling, medicine, or both. The counselor may prescribe some sort of group counseling where the family works with the child in therapy sessions.

Depending on your child's age and maturity, it may be beneficial for him or her to participate in treatment decisions.

What Can I Do to Help?

Most parents think that it's their job to ensure the happiness of their kids. When your child's depressed, you may feel guilty because you can't cheer him or her up. You also may think that your child is suffering because of something you did or didn't do. This isn't true. If you're struggling with guilt, frustration, or anger, consider counseling for yourself. In the long run, this can only help both you and your child.

Other ways to help:

- Make sure your child takes any prescribed medicines and encourage healthy eating too, as this may help improve mood and outlook.

- Make sure your child stays active. Physical activity has been shown to help alleviate the symptoms of depression. Incorporate physical activities, such as bike rides or walks, into your family's routine.

- Remind your child that you're there, that you love and care about your child and want to hear what he or she has to say, even if it isn't pleasant. Although these things may be difficult for your child to believe, it's important for you to say them.

- Accept the situation and never tell your child to "snap out of it."

- Remind yourself that it isn't laziness causing your child's inability to get out of bed, complete chores, or do homework. He or she simply doesn't have the desire or the energy. However, you can still praise and reward your child for making extra effort.

- Watch for warning signs, and make sure the prescribed treatment is followed, whether it's medication, therapy, or both. Call the doctor if you see signs that your child may be thinking about self-harm. If your child talks about suicide, to you or anyone else, or shows warning signs such as giving belongings away and being preoccupied with death, call your doctor or a mental health professional immediately.

Depression can be frightening and frustrating for your child, you, and your entire family. With the proper treatment and your help, though, your child can start to feel better and go on to enjoy the teen and adult years.

Section 15.2

Depression and High School Students

From "Depression and High School Students," by the National
Institute of Mental Health (NIMH, www.nimh.nih.gov), part of
the National Institutes of Health, June 14, 2011.

Depression can occur during adolescence, a time of great personal
change. You may be facing changes in where you go to school, your
friends, your after-school activities, as well as in relationships with
your family members. You may have different feelings about the type
of person you want to be, your future plans, and may be making decisions for the first time in your life.

Many students don't know where to go for mental health treatment
or believe that treatment won't help. Others don't get help because
they think depression symptoms are just part of the typical stresses
of school or being a teen. Some students worry what other people will
think if they seek mental health care.

This text addresses common questions about depression and how
it can affect high school students.

What is depression?

Depression is a common but serious mental illness typically marked
by sad or anxious feelings. Most students occasionally feel sad or anxious, but these emotions usually pass quickly—within a couple of days.
Untreated depression lasts for a long time and interferes with your
day-to-day activities.

What are the symptoms of depression?

Different people experience different symptoms of depression. If
you are depressed, you may feel the following:

- Sad
- Anxious
- Empty
- Hopeless

- Guilty
- Worthless
- Helpless
- Irritable
- Restless

You may also experience one or more of the following symptoms:

- Loss of interest in activities you used to enjoy
- Lack of energy
- Problems concentrating, remembering information, or making decisions
- Problems falling sleep, staying asleep, or sleeping too much
- Loss of appetite or eating too much
- Thoughts of suicide or suicide attempts
- Aches, pains, headaches, cramps, or digestive problems that do not go away

Depression in adolescence frequently co-occurs with other disorders such as anxiety, disruptive behavior, eating disorders, or substance abuse. It can also lead to increased risk for suicide.

Are there different types of depression?

Yes. The most common depressive disorders are the following:

- **Major depressive disorder, also called major depression:** The symptoms of major depression are disabling and interfere with everyday activities such as studying, eating, and sleeping. People with this disorder may have only one episode of major depression in their lifetimes. But more often, depression comes back repeatedly.

- **Dysthymic disorder, also called dysthymia:** Dysthymia is mild, chronic depression. The symptoms of dysthymia last for a long time—two years or more. Dysthymia is less severe than major depression, but it can still interfere with everyday activities. People with dysthymia may also experience one or more episodes of major depression during their lifetimes.

Other types of depression include the following:

- **Psychotic depression:** Psychotic depression is a severe depression accompanied by some form of psychosis, such as hallucinations and delusions.

- **Seasonal affective disorder (SAD):** SAD is a depression that begins during the winter months and lifts during spring and summer.

What causes depression?

Depression does not have a single cause. Several factors can lead to depression. Some people carry genes that increase their risk of depression. But not all people with depression have these genes, and not all people with these genes have depression. Environment—your surroundings and life experiences—also affects your risk for depression. Any stressful situation may trigger depression. And high school students encounter a number of stressful situations!

How can I find out if I have depression?

The first step is to talk with your parents or a trusted adult who can help you make an appointment to speak with a doctor or mental health care provider.

Some school counselors may also be able to help you find appropriate care.

The doctor or mental health care provider can do an exam to help determine if you have depression or if you have another health or mental health problem. Some medical conditions or medications can produce symptoms similar to depression.

The doctor or mental health care provider will ask you about the following:

- Your symptoms
- Your history of depression
- Your family's history of depression
- Your medical history
- Alcohol or drug use
- Any thoughts of death or suicide

How is depression treated?

A number of very effective treatments for depression are available. The most common treatments are antidepressants and psychotherapy.

An NIMH-funded clinical trial of 439 teens with major depression found that a combination of medication and psychotherapy was the most effective treatment option. A doctor or mental health care provider can help you find the treatment that's right for you.

What are antidepressants?

Antidepressants work on brain chemicals called neurotransmitters, especially serotonin and norepinephrine. Other antidepressants work on the neurotransmitter dopamine. Scientists have found that these particular chemicals are involved in regulating mood, but they are unsure of the exact ways that they work.

If a doctor prescribes an antidepressant, how long will I have to take it?

You will need to take regular doses of antidepressants for four to six weeks before you feel the full effect of these medicines. Some people need to take antidepressants for a short time. If your depression is long lasting or comes back again and again, you may need to take antidepressants longer.

What is psychotherapy?

Psychotherapy involves talking with a mental health care professional to treat a mental illness. Types of psychotherapy often used to treat depression include the following:

- Cognitive-behavioral therapy (CBT) helps people change negative styles of thinking and behavior that may contribute to depression.
- Interpersonal therapy (IPT) helps people understand and work through troubled personal relationships that may cause or worsen depression.

Depending on the type and severity of your depression, a mental health professional may recommend short-term therapy, lasting 10 to 20 weeks, or longer-term therapy.

How can I help myself if I am depressed?

If you have depression, you may feel exhausted, helpless, and hopeless. But it is important to realize that these feelings are part of the depression and do not reflect your real circumstances. Treatment can help you feel better.

To help yourself feel better, try the following:

- Engage in mild physical activity or exercise.

- Participate in activities that you used to enjoy.

- Break up large projects into smaller tasks and do what you can.

- Spend time with or call your friends and family.

- Expect your mood to improve gradually with treatment.

- Remember that positive thinking will replace negative thoughts as your depression responds to treatment.

How can I help a friend who is depressed?

If you think a friend may have depression, you can help him or her get diagnosed and treated. Make sure he or she talks to an adult and gets evaluated by a doctor or mental health provider. If your friend seems unable or unwilling to seek help, offer to go with him or her and tell your friend that his or her health and safety is important to you.

Encourage your friend to stay in treatment or seek a different treatment if he or she does not begin to feel better after six to eight weeks.

You can also do the following:

- Offer emotional support, understanding, patience, and encouragement.

- Talk to your friend, not necessarily about depression, and listen carefully.

- Never discount the feelings your friend expresses, but point out realities and offer hope.

- Never ignore comments about suicide.

- Report comments about suicide to your friend's parents, therapist, or doctor.

- Invite your friend out for walks, outings, and other activities—keep trying if your friend declines, but don't push him or her to take on too much too soon.

- Remind your friend that with time and treatment, the depression will lift.

What if I or someone I know is in crisis?

If you are thinking about harming yourself or having thoughts of suicide, or if you know someone who is, seek help right away:

- Call your doctor or mental health care provider.

- Call 911 or go to a hospital emergency room to get immediate help, or ask a friend or family member to help you do these things.

- Call your campus suicide or crisis hotline.

- Call the National Suicide Prevention Lifeline's toll-free, 24-hour hotline at 800-273-TALK (800-273-8255) or TTY: 800-799-4TTY (800-799-4889) to talk to a trained counselor.

- If you are in crisis, make sure you are not left alone.

- If someone else is in crisis, make sure he or she is not left alone.

Chapter 16

Depression in College Students

Many people experience the first symptoms of depression during their college years. Unfortunately, many college students who have depression aren't getting the help they need. They may not know where to go for help, or they may believe that treatment won't help. Others don't get help because they think their symptoms are just part of the typical stress of college, or they worry about being judged if they seek mental health care.

In reality, these are the facts:

- Most colleges offer free or low-cost mental health services to students.

- Depression is a medical illness and treatments can be very effective.

- Early diagnosis and treatment of depression can relieve depression symptoms, prevent depression from returning, and help students succeed in college and after graduation.

What is depression?

Depression is a common but serious mental illness typically marked by sad or anxious feelings. Most college students occasionally feel sad or anxious, but these emotions usually pass quickly—within a couple

From "Depression and College Students," by the National Institute of Mental Health (NIMH, www.nimh.nih.gov), part of the National Institutes of Health, 2011.

of days. Untreated depression lasts for a long time, interferes with day-to-day activities, and is much more than just being "a little down" or "feeling blue."

How does depression affect college students?

In 2009, the American College Health Association-National College Health Assessment (ACHA-NCHA)—a nationwide survey of college students at two- and four-year institutions—found that nearly 30 percent of college students reported feeling "so depressed that it was difficult to function" at some time in the past year.

Depression can affect your academic performance in college. Studies suggest that college students who have depression are more likely to smoke. Research suggests that students with depression do not necessarily drink alcohol more heavily than other college students. But students with depression, especially women, are more likely to drink to get drunk and experience problems related to alcohol abuse, such as engaging in unsafe sex. It is not uncommon for students who have depression to self-medicate with street drugs.

Depression is also a major risk factor for suicide. Better diagnosis and treatment of depression can help reduce suicide rates among college students. In the Fall 2009 ACHA-NCHA survey, about 6 percent of college students reported seriously considering suicide, and about 1 percent reported attempting suicide in the previous year. Suicide is the third leading cause of death for teens and young adults ages 15 to 24. Students should also be aware that the warning signs can be different in men vs. women.

Are there different types of depression?

Yes. The most common depressive disorders are the following:

- **Major depressive disorder, also called major depression:** The symptoms of major depression are disabling and interfere with everyday activities such as studying, eating, and sleeping. People with this disorder may have only one episode of major depression in their lifetimes. But more often, depression comes back repeatedly.

- **Dysthymic disorder, also called dysthymia:** Dysthymia is mild, chronic depression. The symptoms of dysthymia last for a long time—two years or more. Dysthymia is less severe than major depression, but it can still interfere with everyday activities.

People with dysthymia may also experience one or more episodes of major depression during their lifetimes.

- **Minor depression:** Symptoms of minor depression are similar to major depression and dysthymia, but they are less severe and/ or are usually shorter term. Without treatment, however, people with minor depression are at high risk for developing major depressive disorder.

Other types of depression include the following:

- **Psychotic depression:** Psychotic depression is severe depression accompanied by some form of psychosis, such as hallucinations and delusions.

- **Seasonal affective disorder (SAD):** SAD is depression that begins during the winter months and lifts during spring and summer.

What are the signs and symptoms of depression?

The symptoms of depression vary. If you are depressed, you may feel the following:

- Sad
- Empty
- Guilty
- Helpless
- Restless

- Anxious
- Hopeless
- Worthless
- Irritable

You may also experience one or more of the following:

- Loss of interest in activities you used to enjoy

- Lack of energy

- Problems concentrating, remembering information, or making decisions

- Problems falling sleep, staying asleep, or sleeping too much

- Loss of appetite or eating too much

- Thoughts of suicide or suicide attempts

- Aches, pains, headaches, cramps, or digestive problems that do not go away

What causes depression?

Depression does not have a single cause. Several factors can lead to depression. Some people carry genes that increase their risk of depression. But not all people with depression have these genes, and not all people with these genes have depression. Environment—your surroundings and life experiences, such as stress—also affects your risk for depression. Stresses of college may include the following:

• Living away from family for the first time

• Missing family or friends

• Feeling alone or isolated

• Experiencing conflict in relationships

• Facing new and sometimes difficult school work

• Worrying about finances

How can I find out if I have depression?

The first step is to talk with a doctor or mental health care provider. He or she can perform an exam to help determine if you have depression or if you have another health or mental health problem. Some medical conditions or medications can produce symptoms similar to depression.

A doctor or mental health care provider will ask you about the following:

• Your symptoms

• Your history of depression

• Your family's history of depression

• Your medical history

• Alcohol or drug use

• Any thoughts of death or suicide

How is depression treated?

A number of very effective treatments for depression are available. The most common treatments are antidepressants and psychotherapy. Some people find that a combination of antidepressants and psychotherapy works best. A doctor or mental health care provider can help you find the treatment that's right for you.

What are antidepressants?

Antidepressants work on brain chemicals called neurotransmitters, especially serotonin and norepinephrine. Other antidepressants work on the neurotransmitter dopamine. Scientists have found that these particular chemicals are involved in regulating mood, but they are unsure of the exact ways that they work.

If a doctor prescribes an antidepressant, how long will I have to take it?

Always follow the directions of the doctor or health care provider when taking medication. You will need to take regular doses of antidepressants and the full effect of these medications may not take effect for several weeks or months. Some people need to take antidepressants for a short time. If your depression is long-lasting or comes back repeatedly, you may need to take antidepressants longer.

What is psychotherapy?

Psychotherapy involves talking with a mental health care professional to treat a mental illness. Types of psychotherapy often used to treat depression include the following:

- Cognitive-behavioral therapy (CBT) helps people change negative styles of thinking and behavior that may contribute to depression.
- Interpersonal therapy (IPT) helps people understand and work through troubled personal relationships that may cause or worsen depression.

Depending on the type and severity of your depression, a mental health professional may recommend short-term therapy, lasting 10 to 20 weeks, or longer-term therapy.

If I think I may have depression, where can I get help?

Most colleges provide mental health services through counseling centers, student health centers, or both. Check out your college website for information.

Counseling centers offer students free or very low-cost mental health services. Some counseling centers provide short-term or long-term counseling or psychotherapy, also called talk therapy. These centers may also refer you to mental health care providers in the community for additional services.

Student health centers provide basic health care services to students at little or no cost. A doctor or health care provider may be able to diagnose and treat depression or refer you to other mental health services.

If your college does not provide all of the mental health care you need, your insurance may cover additional mental health services. Many college students have insurance through their colleges, parents, or employers. If you are insured, contact your insurance company to find out about your mental health care coverage.

How can I help myself if I am depressed?

If you have depression, you may feel exhausted, helpless, and hopeless. But it is important to realize that these feelings are part of the illness. Treatment can help you feel better.

To help yourself feel better:

- Try to see a professional as soon as possible. Research shows that getting treatment sooner rather than later can relieve symptoms quicker and reduce the length of time treatment is needed.

- Break up large tasks into small ones, and do what you can as you can. Try not to do too many things at once.

- Spend time with other people and talk to a friend or relative about your feelings.

- Do not make important decisions until you feel better. Discuss decisions with others whom you trust and who know you well.

How can I help a friend who is depressed?

If you suspect a friend may have depression, you can help him or her get diagnosed and treated. You may need to help your friend find a doctor, mental health care provider, or mental health services on your college campus.

You can also do the following:

- Offer support, understanding, patience, and encouragement.

- Talk to your friend and listen carefully.

- Never ignore comments about suicide, and report them to your friend's therapist or doctor.

- Invite your friend out for walks, outings, and other activities. If they refuse keep trying, but don't push.

- Ensure that your friend gets to doctor's appointments and encourage him or her to report any concerns about medications to their health care professional.

- Remind your friend that with time and professional treatment, the depression will lift.

What if I or someone I know is in crisis?

If you are thinking about harming yourself or having thoughts of suicide, or if you know someone who is, seek help right away:

- Call your doctor or mental health care provider.

- Call 911 or go to a hospital emergency room to get immediate help, or ask a friend or family member to help you do these things.

- Call your campus suicide or crisis hotline.

- Call the National Suicide Prevention Lifeline's toll-free, 24-hour hotline at 800-273-TALK (800-273-8255) or TTY: 800-799-4TTY (800-799-4889) to talk to a trained counselor.

- Call your college counseling center or student health services.

- If you are in crisis, make sure you are not left alone.

- If someone else is in crisis, make sure he or she is not left alone.

Chapter 17

Depression in Older Adults

Everyone feels blue now and then. It's part of life. But, if you no longer enjoy activities that you usually like, you may have a more serious problem. Being depressed, without letup, can change the way you think and feel. Doctors call this clinical depression.

Being down in the dumps over a period of time is not a normal part of getting older. But, it is a common problem, and medical help may be needed. For most people, depression will get better with treatment. Talk therapy, medicine, or other treatment methods can ease the pain of depression. You do not need to suffer.

There are many reasons why depression in older people is often missed or untreated. As a person ages, the signs of depression are much more varied than at younger ages. It can appear as increased tiredness, or it can be seen as grumpiness or irritability. Confusion or attention problems caused by depression can sometimes look like Alzheimer disease or other brain disorders. Mood changes and signs of depression can be caused by medicines older people may take for arthritis, high blood pressure, or heart disease. The good news is that people who are depressed usually feel better with the right treatment.

What Causes Depression?

There is no one cause of depression. For some people, a single event can bring on the illness. Depression often strikes people who felt fine

From "AgePage: Depression," by the National Institute on Aging (NIA, www .nia.nih.gov), part of the National Institutes of Health, April 25, 2011.

but who suddenly find they are dealing with a death in the family or a serious illness. For some people, changes in the brain can affect mood and cause depression. Sometimes, those under a lot of stress, like caregivers, can feel depressed. Others become depressed for no clear reason.

People with serious illnesses, such as cancer, diabetes, heart disease, stroke, or Parkinson disease, may become depressed. They may worry about how their illness will change their lives. They might be tired and not able to deal with things that make them sad. Treatment for depression can help them manage their depressive symptoms and improve their quality of life.

Genetics, too, can play a role. Studies show that depression may run in families. Children of depressed parents may be at a higher risk for depression. And, depression tends to be a disorder that occurs more than once. Many older people who have been depressed in the past will be at an increased risk.

What to Look For

How do you know when you need help? After all, as you age, you may have to face problems that could cause anyone to feel depressed. Perhaps you are dealing with the death of a loved one or friend. Maybe you are having a tough time getting used to retirement, and you feel lonely. Possibly, you have a chronic illness. Or, you might feel like you have lost control over your life.

After a period of feeling sad, older people usually adjust and regain their emotional balance. But, if you are suffering from clinical depression and don't get help, your depression might last for weeks, months, or even years. Here is a list of the most common signs of depression. If you have several of these and they last for more than two weeks, see a doctor.

- An empty feeling, ongoing sadness, and anxiety

- Tiredness, lack of energy

- Loss of interest or pleasure in everyday activities, including sex

- Sleep problems, including trouble getting to sleep, very early morning waking, and sleeping too much

- Eating more or less than usual

- Crying too often or too much

- Aches and pains that don't go away when treated

- A hard time focusing, remembering, or making decisions
- Feeling guilty, helpless, worthless, or hopeless
- Being irritable
- Thoughts of death or suicide or a suicide attempt

If you are a family member, friend, or healthcare provider of an older person, watch for clues. Sometimes depression can hide behind a smiling face. A depressed person who lives alone may appear to feel better when someone stops by to say hello. The symptoms may seem to go away. But, when someone is very depressed, the symptoms usually come back.

Don't ignore the warning signs. If left untreated, serious depression can lead to suicide. Listen carefully if someone of any age complains about being depressed or says people don't care. That person may really be asking for help.

Getting Help

The first step is to accept that you or your family member needs help. You may not be comfortable with the subject of mental illness. Or, you might feel that asking for help is a sign of weakness. You might be like many older people, their relatives, or friends who believe that a depressed person can quickly "snap out of it" or that some people are too old to be helped. They are wrong.

A healthcare provider can help you. Once you decide to get medical advice, start with your family doctor. Your doctor should check to see if your depression could be caused by a health problem (such as hypothyroidism or vitamin B12 deficiency) or a medicine you are taking. After a complete exam, your doctor may suggest you talk to a mental health worker, for example, a social worker, mental health counselor, psychologist, or psychiatrist. Doctors specially trained to treat depression in older people are called geriatric psychiatrists.

Don't avoid getting help because you may be afraid of how much treatments might cost. Often, only short-term psychotherapy (talk therapy) is needed. Treatment for depression is usually covered by private insurance and Medicare. Also, some community mental health centers may offer treatment based on a person's ability to pay.

Be aware that some family doctors may not understand about aging and depression. If your doctor is unable or unwilling to help, you may want to talk to another healthcare provider.

155

Are you the relative or friend of a depressed older person who won't go to a doctor for treatment? Try explaining how treatment may help the person feel better. In some cases, when a depressed person can't or won't go to the doctor's office, the doctor or mental health specialist can start by making a phone call. A phone call can't take the place of the personal contact needed for a complete medical checkup, but it might inspire the person to go for treatment.

Treating Depression

Your doctor or mental health expert can often treat your depression successfully. Different therapies seem to work for different people. For instance, support groups can provide new coping skills or social support if you are dealing with a major life change. Several kinds of talk therapies are useful as well. One method might help you think in a more positive way. Always thinking about the sad things in your life or what you have lost might have led to your depression. Another method works to improve your relations with others so you will have more hope about your future. Getting better takes time, but with support from others and with treatment, you will get a little better each day.

Antidepressant drugs (medicine to treat depression) can also help. These medications can improve your mood, sleep, appetite, and concentration.

There are several types of antidepressants available. Some of these medicines can take up to 12 weeks before you feel like they are working. Your doctor may want you to continue medications for six months or more after your symptoms disappear. Some antidepressants can cause unwanted side effects, although newer medicines have fewer side effects. Any antidepressant should be used with great care to avoid this problem. Remember the following:

- The doctor needs to know about all prescribed and over-the-counter medications, vitamins, or herbal supplements you are taking.

- The doctor should also be aware of any other physical problems you have.

- Be sure to take antidepressants in the proper dose and on the right schedule.

If you are still very depressed after trying different treatments, electroconvulsive therapy (ECT) may be an option. Don't be misled by the way some movies and books have portrayed ECT (also called electroshock therapy). ECT may be recommended if medicines or other therapies do not work for you. ECT is given as a series of treatments over a few weeks.

Like other antidepressant therapies, follow-up treatment is often needed to help prevent a return of depression.

Help from Family and Friends

Family and friends can play an important role in treatment. You can help your relative or friend stay with the treatment plan. If needed, make appointments for the person or go along to the doctor, mental health expert, or support group.

Be patient and understanding. Ask your relative or friend to go on outings with you or to go back to an activity that he or she once enjoyed. Encourage the person to be active and busy but not to take on too much at one time.

Preventing Depression

What can be done to lower the risk of depression? How can people cope? There are a few steps you can take. Try to prepare for major changes in life, such as retirement or moving from your home of many years. One way to do this is to try and keep friendships over the years. Friends can help ease loneliness if you lose a spouse. You can also develop a hobby. Hobbies may help keep your mind and body active. Stay in touch with family. Let them help you when you feel sad. If you are faced with a lot to do, try to break it up into smaller jobs that are easy to finish.

Regular exercise may also help prevent depression or lift your mood if you are somewhat depressed. Older people who are depressed can gain mental as well as physical benefits from mild forms of exercise like walking outdoors or in shopping malls. Gardening, dancing, and swimming are other good forms of exercise. Pick something you like to do. Begin with 10–15 minutes a day, and increase the time as you are able. Being physically fit and eating a balanced diet may help avoid illnesses that can bring on disability or depression.

Remember, with treatment, most people will begin to feel better soon. Expect your mood to improve slowly. Feeling better takes time. But, it can happen.

Chapter 18

Mental Health Problems in Minority Populations

Chapter Contents

Section 18.1

Facts about Latino Mental Health

"Latino Community Mental Health Fact Sheet," © 2011
NAMI, the National Alliance on Mental Illness, www.nami.org.
Reprinted with permission.

Rates of Mental Illness

- Latinos are identified as a high-risk group for depression, anxiety, and substance abuse.[1]

- Women and Latinos are more likely to experience a major depressive episode.[2]

- Prevalence of depression is higher in Latino women (46%) than Latino men (19.6%).[3]

- The Commonwealth Fund Survey revealed that surveyed Latino and Asian American girls exhibited more depressive symptoms than the African American or white girls.[4]

- Among female high-school students in 1997, the rate of attempted suicide among Latino girls (14.9%) was one-and-a-half times that of African American (9.0%) and non-Hispanic white (10.3%) girls.[5]

- Close to one out of every three Latino female (30.3%) high-school students in 1997 had seriously considered committing suicide.[6]

- There are higher rates of mental illness among U.S. born and long-term residents than among recent Latino immigrants.

- Place of birth has a significant correlation with the subsequent risk for most psychiatric disorders.[7]

- A study found conclusively that long-term residence in the United States significantly increased rates in mental disorders, with particularly dramatic increases in the rates of substance abuse.[8]

- Research on suicidal ideation found that foreign-born Mexican Americans are at significantly lower risk of suicide and depression than those born in the United States.[9]

Barriers to Treatment

- Latinos are twice as likely to seek treatment for mental disorders in other settings, such as general health care or the clergy, than in mental health specialty settings.

- Among Latinos with mental disorders, fewer than one in 11 contact mental health care specialists, while fewer than one in five contact general health care providers.[10]

- The statistics become more alarming among Latino immigrants with mental disorders. Fewer than one in 20 Latino immigrants use services from mental health specialists, while less than one in 10 use services from general health care providers.[11]

- The existing studies about language skills of mental health professionals reveal that there are few Spanish-speaking and Latino providers.

- A national survey revealed that out of 596 licensed psychologists with active clinical practices who are members of the American Psychological Association, only 1% of the randomly selected sample identified themselves as Latino.[12]

- In 1999 CMHS [Center for Mental Health Services] reported the existence of 29 Latino mental health professionals for every 100,000 Latinos in the United States.

- The U.S. Bureau of the Census in 1993 reports that more than one in four Hispanics lives in a "linguistically isolated household" in the United States. This reality plus the lack of bilingual mental health providers makes access to care harder for Latinos.

- Living in poverty has the most measurable effect on the rates of mental illness. People in the lowest socioeconomic status are about two to three times more likely than those in the highest strata to have a mental disorder.[13]

- The lack of services for Latinos worsens when dealing with Latino children and youth.

- The Centers for Disease Control and Prevention (CDC) Youth Risk Survey found a 10.7% attempted suicide rate among Latino youth, compared with a 7.3% rate among African American youth and a 6.3% rate for White, non-Latino youth.

- Tragically, due to lack of cultural knowledge, Latino youth with mental illness are generally misdiagnosed as having anger problems or just conduct disorders.

- Latinos are over-represented in the criminal and juvenile justice system. Many of these Latinos have a misdiagnosed or not diagnosed mental illness.

- The Building Blocks for Youth report *Dónde Está La Justicia? A Call for Action on Behalf of Latino and Latina Youth in the U.S. Justice System* (2002) recently highlighted the alarmingly disproportionate rates of Latino youth in the juvenile justice system. The report found that in almost every state, Latinos and African Americans are over-represented in the justice system and receive harsher treatment than Caucasian youth charged for the same types of offenses.

- Different studies estimate that 50% to 70% of all youth in the juvenile justice system have mental health problems that usually go untreated or badly treated.

1. Quality Health Services for Hispanics: The Cultural Competency Component. National Alliance for Hispanic Health, 2001.

2. Mental Health: A Report of the Surgeon General. 1999.

3. Vega, W. and Amaro, H. Lifetime Prevalence of *DSM-III-R* Psychiatric Disorders among Rural and Urban Mexican Americans in California. *Archives of General Psychiatry*; 55, pp. 771–782, 1998.

4. Schoen C, Davis K, Collins KS, Greenberg L, Des Roches C, Abrams M. The Commonwealth Fund Survey of the Health of Adolescent Girls. New York, NY: Commonwealth Fund; 1997.

5. CDC. Youth Risk Behavior Surveillance—United States, 1997. *MMWR*; 1998, 47: 47.

6. Ibid.

7. Vega WA, Kolody B, Aguilar-Gaxiola S, et. al. Lifetime Prevalence of *DSM-III-R* Psychiatric Disorders Among Urban and Rural Mexican Americans in California. *Archives of General Psychiatry*. 1998; 55(9): 771–778.

8. Vega WA, Kolody B, Aguilar-Gaxiola S, et. al. Lifetime Prevalence of *DSM-III-R* Psychiatric Disorders Among Urban and Rural Mexican Americans in California. *Archives of General Psychiatry*. 1998; 55(9): 771–778.

9. Swanson JW, Linskey AO, Quintero-Salinas R, Pumariega AJ, Holzer CE. A Bi-National School Survey of Depressive

Symptom, Drug Use and Suicidal Ideation. *Journal of the American Academy of Child and Adolescent Psychiatry*. 1992; 31: 669–678.

10. Mental Health: Culture, Race, and Ethnicity. A Supplement to Mental Health: A Report of the Surgeon General. 2001.

11. Ibid.

12. Williams, S. and Kohout, J. L. *A Survey of Licensed Practitioners of Psychology: Activities, Roles, and Services.* American Psychological Association, Washington D.C., 1999.

13. Mental Health: A Report of the Surgeon General. 1999.

Section 18.2

Facts about African American Mental Health

"African American Community Mental Health," © 2011 NAMI, the National Alliance on Mental Illness, www.nami.org. Reprinted with permission.

- African Americans in the United States are less likely to receive accurate diagnoses than their Caucasian counterparts. Schizophrenia, for instance, has been shown to be overdiagnosed in the African-American population.

- Culture biases against mental health professionals and health care professionals in general prevent many African Americans from accessing care due to prior experiences with historical misdiagnoses, inadequate treatment, and a lack of cultural understanding; only 2 percent of psychiatrists, 2 percent of psychologists, and 4 percent of social workers in the United States are African American.

- African Americans tend to rely on family, religious, and social communities for emotional support rather than turning to health care professionals, even though this may at times be necessary. The health care providers they seek may not be aware of this important aspect of a person's life.

- Mental illness is frequently stigmatized and misunderstood in the African-American community. African Americans are much more likely to seek help though their primary care doctors as opposed to accessing specialty care.

- African Americans are often at a socioeconomic disadvantage in terms of accessing both medical and mental health care: in 2006, one-third of working adult African Americans were uninsured in the preceding year.

- Experiences of mental illness vary across cultures, and there is a need for improved cultural awareness and competence in the health care and mental health workforce.

- Across a recent 15-year span, suicide rates increased 233 percent among African Americans aged 10–14 compared to 120 percent among Caucasian Americans in the same age group across the same span of time.

- Somatization—the manifestation of physical illnesses related to mental health—occurs at a rate of 15 percent among African Americans and only 9 percent among Caucasian Americans.

- Some studies suggest that African Americans metabolize some medications more slowly than Caucasian Americans, yet they often receive higher doses of psychiatric medications, which may result in increased side effects and decreased medication compliance.

- Social circumstances often serve as an indicator for the likelihood of developing a mental illness. African Americans are disproportionately more likely to experience social circumstances that increase their chances of developing a mental illness.

- African Americans comprise 40 percent of the homeless population and only 12 percent of the U.S. population. People experiencing homelessness are at a greater risk of developing a mental illness.

- Nearly half of all prisoners in the United States are African American. Prison inmates are at a higher risk of developing a mental illness.

- Children in foster care and the child welfare system are more likely to develop mental illnesses. African-American children comprise 45 percent of the public foster care population.

- Exposure to violence increases the risk of developing a mental illness; over 25 percent of African-American children exposed to violence meet criteria for posttraumatic stress disorder.

- With the implementation of various programs and innovations, African Americans' patronization rates for mental health services may be improved.

- Programs in African-American communities sponsored by respected institutions, such as churches and local community groups, can increase awareness of mental health issues and resources and decrease the related stigma.

- Programs that improve enrollment rates in safety net health care providers can result in increased mental health care due to improved mental health coverage in the African-American community.

- Encouragement in the community to join mental health related professions can increase the number of African-American mental health care providers and increase social sensitivity among the provider community.

- Overall sensitivity to African-American cultural differences, such as differences in medication metabolization rates, unique views of mental illness, and propensity towards experiencing certain mental illnesses, can improve African Americans' treatment experiences and increase utilization of mental health care services.

Section 18.3

Facts about Asian American and Pacific Islander Mental Health

"Asian American and Pacific Islander (AA/PI) Community and Mental Health," © 2011 NAMI, the National Alliance on Mental Illness, www.nami.org. Reprinted with permission.

Did you know . . .

- There is very little research about mental health issues in these populations.

- Overall prevalence rates of diagnosable mental illnesses among AA/PIs are similar to those of the Caucasian population.

- Asian Americans and Pacific Islanders have the lowest rates of utilization of mental health services among ethnic populations.[1]

- AA/PIs show higher levels of depressive symptoms than whites. South Asian refugees reported the highest rates among Asian groups.[2]

- The Chinese American Psychiatric Epidemiologic Study (CAPES study) found a lifetime prevalence rate of about 7 percent (lifetime) and a 3 percent rate over 1 year.

- The National Comorbidity Study (NCS) reported even higher rates of major depression among Chinese Americans (17 percent for lifetime and 10 percent current).[3]

- The word depression does not exist in certain Asian languages (e.g., Chinese).

- The suicide rates for Filipino (3.5 percent), Chinese (8.3 percent), and Japanese (9.1 percent) Americans are substantially lower than the suicide rate of white Americans (12.8 percent).[4]

- Among elderly women of all ethnic or racial groups, Asians have the highest suicide rate.[5]

- According to mental health care providers: Asian American women ages 15–24 have a higher rate of suicide than Caucasians, African Americans, and Latinos in that age group.[6]

- The Commonwealth Fund Survey of the Health of Adolescent Girls reported that Asian American adolescent girls had the highest rates of depressive symptoms of all racial/ethnic and gender groups.[7]

- Southeast Asians suffer from particularly high rates of depression and post-traumatic stress disorder and exhibit more than twice the need for outpatient mental health services than the general Asian population.[8]

- Suicide rates are higher than the national average for some groups of Asian Americans.

- The suicide rate among Asian Americans and Pacific Islanders in California is similar to that of the total population.[9]

- Many Southeast Asian refugees are at risk for post-traumatic stress disorder (PTSD) associated with trauma experienced before and after immigration to the United States.

- One study found that 70 percent of Southeast Asian refugees receiving mental health care met diagnostic criteria for PTSD.

- In a study of Cambodian adolescents who survived Pol Pot's concentration camps, nearly half experienced PTSD and 41 percent suffered from depression 10 years after leaving Cambodia.[10]

- Approximately 70 AA/PI providers are available for every 100,000 AA/PIs in the United States, compared to 173 per 100,000 Caucasians.[11]

- AA/PIs appear to have the extremely low utilization of mental health services relative to other U.S. populations.

- In the CAPES study, only 17 percent of those experiencing problems sought care.[12]

- A national study concluded that Asian Americans were one quarter as likely as whites to seek mental health services and half as likely as Latinos and African Americans.[13]

Created by the NAMI Multicultural & International Outreach Center, June 2003.

References

1. Karen L. Koh, MPH and Margaret W. Leung, MPH. Asian Pacific Psychological Services, 431 30th Street, Suite 6A, Oakland, CA 94609.

2. Mental Health: Culture, Race, Ethnicity Supplement to Mental Health: Report of the Surgeon General.

3. Breaking the Silence. A Study of Depression Among Asian American Women. National Asian Women's Health Organization, 2001.

4. Mental Health: Culture, Race, Ethnicity Supplement to Mental Health: Report of the Surgeon General.

5. The Surgeon General's Call to Action to Prevent Suicide, 1999.

6. Monthly Vital Statistics Report. Center for Disease Control and Prevention/National Center for Health Statistics; Vol. 46, No. 1. August 17, 1997.

7. Louis Harris and Associates, Inc., 1997.

8. Karen L. Koh, MPH and Margaret W. Leung, MPH. Asian Pacific Psychological Services, 431 30th Street, Suite 6A, Oakland, CA 94609.

9. The Surgeon General's Call to Action to Prevent Suicide, 1999.

10. Mental Health: Culture, Race, Ethnicity Supplement to Mental Health: Report of the Surgeon General.

11. Mental Health: Culture, Race, Ethnicity Supplement to Mental Health: Report of the Surgeon General.

12. Mental Health: Culture, Race, Ethnicity Supplement to Mental Health: Report of the Surgeon General.

13. Snowden, LR. African American service use for mental health problems. *Journal of Community Psychology.*

Section 18.4

Facts about American Indian and Alaska Native Mental Health

"American Indian and Alaska Natives Communities Mental Health Facts," © 2011 NAMI, the National Alliance on Mental Illness, www.nami.org. Reprinted with permission.

Cultural differences exist in seeking mental health services and in reporting distress.

- An historical distrust of the outside population exists among many American Indian communities. Individuals tend to have negative opinions of non-Indian health service providers, and traditional healing is used by a majority of Native Americans.[1]

- Compared to the general population, AI/AN individuals tend to underutilize mental health services, have higher therapy drop-out rates, are less likely to respond to treatment.[1]

- A study of adult American Indians of a Northwest Coast Tribe demonstrated little differentiation between physical and emotional distress.[2]

- The words "depressed" and "anxious" are absent from some American Indian and Alaska Native languages. Different expression of illness, such as ghost sickness and heartbreak syndrome, do not correspond to *DSM* [*Diagnostic and Statistical Manual*] diagnoses.[2]

Living in a stressful environment has potentially negative mental health consequences.

- Approximately 26% of AI/AN live in poverty, as compared to 13% of the general population and 10% of white Americans.[3]

- In the Northern Plains study, 61% of the children had experienced a traumatic event.[2]

- The American Indian and Alaska Native population reports higher rates of frequent distress than the general population.[2]

High prevalence of substance abuse and alcohol dependence is tied to a high risk for concurrent mental health problems.

- Alcohol abuse is a problem for a substantial portion of the American Indian adult population, but widely varies among different tribes.[2]

- The Great Smoky Mountain study found that though prevalence of psychotic disorders is similar among American Indian and Caucasian American youth in the same geographic area, there are significantly higher rates of substance abuse in American Indian children.[2]

- A study of Alaska Natives in a community mental health center found substance abuse was the reason for 85% of men and 65% of women to seek mental health care.[2]

- In a study of Northern Plains youth, of those diagnosed with any depressive disorder 60% also had substance disorders.[2]

The prevalence of suicide is a strong indication of the necessity of mental health services in the AI/AN community.

- Alaska Native males have had one of the highest documented suicide rates in the world.

- Suicide rates are particularly high among Native American males ages 15–24, who account for 64% of all suicides by AI/AN individuals.[2]

- A study of Eskimo children in Nome, Alaska found previous suicide attempts to be one of the most common problems for those seeking mental health care.[2]

Mental health services are available for the AI/AN community, but are in need of improvement.

- The Indian Health Service funds 34 urban Indian health organizations, which operate at 41 sites located in cites throughout the United States offering a variety of care including mental health services and alcohol and drug abuse prevention. Approximately 605,000 American Indians and Alaska Natives are eligible to utilize this program.[4] However, only one in five American Indians reported access to this care in 2000.[2]

- Because Native tribes are not defined by state boundaries and many Native families have inadequately addressed dual-nationality issues, many tribal and intertribal family-run organizations face difficulty in obtaining critical funds through Federal grants.[5]

- Grassroots organizations such as InterTribal Voices of Children and Families create a network to connect Native families across tribes to influence the improvement of mental health services.[5]

References

1. *American Indian and Alaska Native Resource Manual.* NAMI, 2003.

2. Mental Health: Culture, Race, Ethnicity Supplement to Mental Health: Report of the Surgeon General. US Department of Health and Human Services, 2001.

3. Dolores Subia BigFoot, PhD, & Barbara L. Bonner, PhD, Trauma in Native Children. Indian Country Child Trauma Center, Oklahoma City, OK.

4. The Office of Minority Health, US Department of Health and Human Services.

5. Elaine Slaton, Offering Technical Assistance to Native Families: Clues From a Focus Group. Federation of Families for Children's Mental Health, 2000.

Chapter 19

Depression Related to Occupation

Chapter Contents

Section 19.1

Depression among Adults Employed Full-Time

Excerpted from "Depression among Adults Employed Full-Time, by Occupational Category," a National Survey on Drug Use and Health (NSDUH) report by the Substance Abuse and Mental Health Services Administration (SAMHSA, www.oas.samhsa.gov), part of the U.S. Department of Health and Human Services, October 11, 2007.

Depression can seriously impact a person's ability to perform routine activities at work. It negatively affects U.S. industry through lost productivity, employee absenteeism, and low morale. U.S. companies lose an estimated $30 to $44 billion dollars per year because of employee depression. Research shows that the rate of depression varies by occupation and industry.

The National Survey on Drug Use and Health (NSDUH) includes questions for adults aged 18 or older to assess lifetime and past year major depressive episode (MDE). In NSDUH, MDE is defined using the diagnostic criteria set forth in the 4th edition of the *Diagnostic and Statistical Manual of Mental Disorders (DSM-IV)*, which specifies a period of 2 weeks or longer during which there is either depressed mood or loss of interest or pleasure and at least four other symptoms that reflect a change in functioning, including problems with sleep, eating, energy, concentration, and self-image. NSDUH also asks respondents about their current employment situation and the type of occupation and industry in which they work. NSDUH defines full-time employed respondents as those who usually work 35 or more hours per week and who worked in the past week or had a job despite not working in the past week. This text uses data from the combined 2004 to 2006 surveys to present estimates of past-year MDE among full-time workers aged 18 to 64 by occupational category.

MDE, by Employment Status

Combined data from 2004 to 2006 indicate that the prevalence of past-year MDE among adults aged 18 to 64 was higher among the unemployed and those of "Other" employment status than among persons employed part time or full time. Among adults aged 18 to 64, an estimated 12.7 percent of those who were unemployed and 12.7 percent of those in the "Other" group experienced an MDE in the past year compared with 9.3 percent of those employed part time and 7.0 percent of those employed full time.

Reflecting the fact that over half of the adult population (64.3 percent) were employed full time, a majority of those who experienced an MDE in the past year also were employed full time. From 2004 to 2006, over half of all persons aged 18 to 64 who experienced a past-year MDE (52.4 percent) were employed full time.

MDE, by Occupational Category

Among the 21 major occupational categories, the highest rates of past year MDE among full-time workers aged 18 to 64 were found in the personal care and service occupations (10.8 percent) and the food preparation and serving related occupations (10.3 percent). The occupational categories with the lowest rates of past year MDE were engineering, architecture, and surveying (4.3 percent); life, physical, and social science (4.4 percent); and installation, maintenance, and repair (4.4 percent).

MDE, by Demographic Characteristics and Occupational Category

Among full-time workers aged 18 to 64, females were more likely than males to have a past year MDE (10.1 vs. 4.7 percent). The highest rates of past-year MDE among female full-time workers aged 18 to 64 were found in the food preparation and serving related occupations (14.8 percent) and community and social service occupations (13.3 percent). The highest rates of past year MDE among male full-time workers aged 18 to 64 were found in the arts, design, entertainment, sports, and media occupations (6.7 percent).

The lowest rates of past year MDE among both males and females were found in life, physical, and social science occupations (2.3 percent for males and 7.2 percent for females).

Full-time workers aged 18 to 25 were more likely to have a past-year MDE than full-time workers in all other age groups (8.9 percent for those aged 18 to 25; 7.6 percent for those aged 26 to 34; 7.2 for those aged 35 to 49; and 5.1 percent for those aged 50 to 64). Among full-time workers aged 18 to 25, the highest rates of past-year MDE were found in the health care practitioners and technical occupations (11.9 percent) and the lowest in the life, physical, and social science occupations (4.3 percent).

Section 19.2

Depression in Military Veterans

"Depression and Veterans Fact Sheet," © 2011 NAMI, the National Alliance on Mental Illness, www.nami.org. Reprinted with permission.

Depression is one of the most common and expensive mental disorders, costing the United States an estimated $66 billion per year. Veterans diagnosed with depression account for slightly more than 14 percent of the total. From 2000–2007, the medical records of more than 206,000 veterans entering the VA [Veterans Administration] health care system were assessed. Findings revealed that one in three patients was diagnosed with at least one mental health disorder—41 percent were diagnosed with either a mental health or a behavioral adjustment disorder. The diagnosis rate for posttraumatic stress disorder (PTSD) was 20 percent followed by 14 percent for depression, yet studies show that depression is under-diagnosed in this population.

What Is Depression?

Clinical depression is a serious medical illness that is much more than temporarily feeling sad or blue. It involves disturbances in mood, concentration, sleep, activity level, interests, appetite, and social behavior. Although depression is highly treatable, it is frequently a life-long condition in which periods of wellness alternate with recurrences of illness.

What Are Symptoms of Major Depression?

The onset of the first episode of major depression may not be obvious if it is gradual or mild. The symptoms of major depression characteristically represent a significant change from how a person functioned before the illness. The symptoms of depression include:

- persistently sad or irritable mood;
- pronounced changes in sleep, appetite, and energy;
- difficulty thinking, concentrating, and remembering;
- physical slowing or agitation;
- lack of interest in or pleasure from activities that were once enjoyed;
- feelings of guilt, worthlessness, hopelessness, and emptiness;
- recurrent thoughts of death or suicide; and
- persistent physical symptoms that do not respond to treatment such as headaches, digestive disorders, and chronic pain.

Like most groups, women have a higher rate of depression than men, and male veterans—regardless of their form of service—have nearly twice the rate of alcohol and drug use. In a study of approximately 100,000 returning veterans, 25 percent received a mental health diagnosis and more than 30 percent received a mental health diagnosis or had a behavioral adjustment problem. There was no correlation found between diagnosis and gender or ethnicity. However, older veterans had a higher rate of PTSD among the National Guard and reserve units while younger veterans had a higher rate among active-duty personnel.

Data shows that within the first year following a mental health diagnosis, two-thirds of patients receive very minimal or no psychiatric care. Without early intervention for specific subgroups of combat veterans, many veterans will go untreated and experience a several-month-long episode of depression—a period that will often repeat over a lifetime. This leaves them at risk for substance use, economic and relationship problems, and other consequences of untreated depression.

What Are the Causes for Major Depression?

There is no single cause of major depression. Psychological, biological, and environmental factors may all contribute to its development. Scientific research has firmly established that major depression is a biological, medical illness. There is also an increased risk for developing depression when there is a family history of the illness.

What Are the Risk Factors for Veterans?

A study found that the risk factors for suicide for U.S. veterans with depression differed in significant ways from those of the general population. Specifically, the risk for suicide generally increases with age, but in the veteran population, younger veterans are at the most risk. The study divided veterans into three age groups: 18–44, 45–64 and 65 or older. Among this population, younger veterans had moderately higher rates than middle-aged patients (about 95 percent versus 74 percent) and modestly higher rates than elderly patients (about 95 percent versus 90 percent). Other risk factors for suicide mirrored those found among the general population.

Veterans struggling with their diagnoses were more likely to commit suicide or battle with substance abuse. Depressed male veterans were three times as likely to commit suicide compared to females, and Caucasians were at a higher risk than African Americans or Latinos. Notably, people diagnosed with PTSD were less prone to suicide than those who were not diagnosed with PTSD. This is thought to be because compared to depression, PTSD had become a more acceptable set of symptoms and patients with the disorder more readily seek out psychiatric care.

Risk in Older Adult Veterans

Older adults comprise the fastest-growing segment of the U.S. population with the most significant growth among those over age 80. The percentage of older veterans is 38 percent of the total veteran population in 1999, and may number between 7.8 and 9 million until 2020. A considerable number of older veterans experience depression which is associated with substantial suffering, disability, suicide risk, and decreased health-related quality of life. Older adults receive treatment in primary care settings where depression is often inadequately treated or even diagnosed.

How Is Major Depression Treated?

Although major depression can be a devastating illness, it is highly treatable. Between 80–90 percent of persons diagnosed with major depression can be effectively treated and return to their usual daily activities and feelings. Many types of treatment are available, and the type chosen depends on the individual and the severity and patterns of his or her illness. There are three well-established types of treatment for depression: Medications, psychotherapy, and electroconvulsive therapy (ECT). For some people who have a seasonal component to their depression, light therapy may be useful. Transcranial magnetic stimulation (TMS) may be helpful for depression that has not responded to one medication trial. These treatments may be used alone or in combination. Additionally, peer education and support can promote recovery. Attention to lifestyle, including diet, exercise, and smoking cessation can result in better physical and mental health.

Medication

Research has shown that imbalances in neurotransmitters (chemicals in the brain) like serotonin, dopamine, and norepinephrine can be altered with antidepressants. It often takes 2 to 4 weeks for antidepressants to start having an effect, and 6 to 12 weeks for antidepressants to take full effect.

Individuals and their families must be cautious during the early stages of medication treatment because normal energy levels and the ability to take action often return before mood improves. At this time—when decisions are easier to make, but depression is still severe—the risk of suicide may temporarily increase. A greater risk of self-harm occurs in individuals taking antidepressants who are under 25. In 2004, the FDA [U.S. Food and Drug Administration] put a black box warning on antidepressants noting increased risk of suicidal thoughts and feelings in the first months of treatment.

Psychotherapy

There are several types of psychotherapy that have been shown to be effective for depression including cognitive-behavioral therapy (CBT) and interpersonal therapy (IPT). Research has shown that mild to moderate depression can often be treated successfully with either of these therapies used alone. However, severe depression appears more likely to respond to a combination of psychotherapy and medication.

Antidepressant treatment is just as effective in elderly patients as in younger adults. However, many elderly patients discontinue medication use prematurely, resulting in inconsistent recovery. Investigators have found that up to one-third of depressed older veterans did not consistently fill antidepressant prescriptions during treatment for reasons such as cognitive impairment and beliefs that are culturally influenced.

Group Support

Veterans often learn best from someone who has been there. The feeling of being unlike non-veterans—in terms of the experiences with combat and loss—can hamper individual treatment. Group sessions with veterans can offer support and understanding to each other that may lead to better outcomes.

As part of a comprehensive research agenda aimed at advancing the care of veterans with depression, Veterans Association (VA) researchers are developing, testing, and implementing new models of primary care to improve the outcomes among veterans affected by depression. Translating Initiatives for Depression into Effective Solutions (TIDES) is a model of care for veterans with depression that involves collaboration between primary care providers and mental health specialists with support from a depression-care manager.

The program has shown impressive results with eight out of 10 veterans effectively treated in three VA regions without the need for referrals to additional specialists. For more information about programs related to veterans and depression, visit the Veterans Health Administration at www.research.va.gov.

Chapter 20

Caregivers and Depression

Introduction

Could the sadness, loneliness, or anger you feel today be a warning sign of depression? It's possible. It is not unusual for caregivers to develop mild or more serious depression as a result of the constant demands they face in providing care.

Caregiving does not cause depression, nor will everyone who provides care experience the negative feelings that go with depression. But in an effort to provide the best possible care for a family member or friend, caregivers often sacrifice their own physical and emotional needs and the emotional and physical experiences involved with providing care can strain even the most capable person. The resulting feelings of anger, anxiety, sadness, isolation, exhaustion—and then guilt for having these feelings—can exact a heavy toll.

Everyone has negative feelings that come and go over time, but when these feelings become more intense and leave caregivers totally drained of energy, crying frequently, or easily angered by their loved one or other people, it may well be a warning sign of depression.

"Caregiving and Depression," © 2008 Family Caregiver Alliance. Reprinted with permission. To view the complete text of this article including a list of related organizations providing information and assistance, visit www.caregiver.org. The text that follows this document under the heading *"Health Reference Series* Medical Advisor's Notes and Updates" was provided to Omnigraphics, Inc. by David A. Cooke, MD, FACP, November 19, 2011. Dr. Cooke is not affiliated with the Family Caregiver Alliance.

Concerns about depression arise when the sadness and crying don't go away or when those negative feelings are unrelenting.

Unfortunately, feelings of depression are often seen as a sign of weakness rather than a sign that something is out of balance. Comments such as "snap out of it" or "it's all in your head" are not helpful, and reflect a belief that mental health concerns are not real. Ignoring or denying your feelings will not make them go away.

Early attention to symptoms of depression through exercise, a healthy diet, positive support of family and friends, or consultation with a trained health or mental health professional may help to prevent the development of a more serious depression over time.

Symptoms of Depression

People experience depression in different ways. Some may feel a general low-level sadness for months, while others suffer a more sudden and intense negative change in their outlook. The type and degree of symptoms vary by individual and can change over time. Consider these common symptoms of depression. Have you experienced any of the following for longer than two weeks?

- A change in eating habits resulting in unwanted weight gain or loss
- A change in sleep patterns—too much sleep or not enough
- Feeling tired all the time
- A loss of interest in people and/or activities that once brought you pleasure
- Becoming easily agitated or angered
- Feeling that nothing you do is good enough
- Thoughts of death or suicide, or attempting suicide
- Ongoing physical symptoms that do not respond to treatment, such as headaches, digestive disorders, and chronic pain

Special Caregiver Concerns

What do lack of sleep, dementia, and whether you are male or female have in common? Each can contribute in its own way to a caregiver's increased risk for depression.

Dementia and Care

Researchers have found that a person who provides care for someone with dementia is twice as likely to suffer from depression as a person providing care for someone without dementia. The more severe the case of dementia such as that caused by Alzheimer's disease, the more likely the caregiver is to experience depression. It is critical for caregivers, especially in these situations, to receive consistent and dependable support.

- Caring for a person with dementia can be all consuming. It is different from other types of caregiving. Not only do caregivers spend significantly more hours per week providing care, they report more employment problems, personal stress, mental and physical health problems, less time to do the things they enjoy, less time to spend with other family members, and more family conflict than nondementia caregivers. As stressful as the deterioration of a loved one's mental and physical abilities may be for the caregiver, dealing with dementia-related behavior is an even bigger contributor to developing symptoms of depression. Dementia-related symptoms such as wandering, agitation, hoarding, and embarrassing conduct makes every day challenging and makes it harder for a caregiver to get rest or assistance in providing care.

- Women experience depression at a higher rate than men. Women, primarily wives and daughters, provide the majority of caregiving. In the United States, approximately 12 million women experience clinical depression each year, at approximately twice the rate of men. A National Mental Health Association survey on the public's attitude and beliefs about clinical depression found that more than one-half of women surveyed still believe it is normal for a woman to be depressed during menopause. The study also found that many women do not seek treatment for depression because they are embarrassed or in denial about being depressed. In fact, 41% of women surveyed cited embarrassment or shame as barriers to treatment.

- Men who are caregivers deal with depression differently. Men are less likely to admit to depression and doctors are less likely to diagnose depression in men. Men will more often self-treat their depressive symptoms of anger, irritability, or powerlessness with alcohol or overwork. Although male caregivers tend to be more willing than female caregivers to hire outside help for assistance with home care duties, they tend to have fewer friends to confide in or positive activities outside the home. The assumption that depressive symptoms are a sign of weakness can make it especially difficult for men to seek help.

- Lack of sleep contributes to depression. While sleep needs vary, most people need 8 hours a day. Loss of sleep as a result of caring for a loved one can lead to serious depression. The important thing to remember is that even though you may not be able to get your loved one to rest throughout the night, you can arrange to get much needed sleep. Hiring a respite worker to be with your loved one while you take a nap or finding a care center or scheduling a stay over with another family member for a few nights are ways to keep your caregiving commitment while getting the sleep you need.

- Depression can persist after placement in a care facility. Making the decision to move a loved one to a care center is very stressful. While many caregivers are finally able to catch up on much needed rest, loneliness, guilt, and monitoring the care a loved one receives in this new location can add new stress. Many caregivers feel depressed at the time of placement and some continue to feel depressed for a long time after.

People assume that once caregiving is over, the stress from providing hands-on care will go away. Yet, researchers found that even three years after the death of a spouse with dementia, some former caregivers continued to experience depression and loneliness. In an effort to return their life to normal, former caregivers may need to seek out help for depression as well.

What to Do If You Think You Have Depression

Depression deserves to be treated with the same attention afforded any other illness, such as diabetes or high blood pressure. If you feel uncomfortable using the term depression, tell the professional that you are feeling blue or feeling down. The professional will get the message. The important thing is to seek help.

Those with chronic illnesses also may suffer from depression. If you suspect this is the case with your loved one, look for an opportunity to share your concern with him or her. If they are reluctant to talk about it with you, encourage a trusted friend to talk with them or consider leaving a message for their doctor regarding your concern prior to their next appointment.

How Is Depression Treated?

The first step to getting the best treatment for depression is to meet with a mental health professional such as a psychiatrist, psychologist, or social worker. At the same time, schedule a physical exam with your doctor. Certain medications, as well as some medical conditions such as viral infection, can cause the same symptoms as depression, and can be evaluated by your physician during an exam. The exam should include lab tests and an interview that tests for mental status to determine if speech, memory, or thought patterns have been affected.

Although it's not unusual for a physician to prescribe antidepressant medication, medication alone may not be the most effective treatment for depression. The guidance of a mental health professional throughout your treatment is strongly recommended. The therapist or counselor will listen to your concerns, screen you for symptoms of depression, and assist you in setting up an appropriate course of treatment.

One way to find a professional is to ask a friend for the name of someone they know and trust. You may also find someone by asking your minister or rabbi, your doctor, or, if you are employed, you may check your employer's health insurance provider list or EAP [employee assistance] program. In addition, national organizations can provide contact information for mental health professionals in your community.

It is important to trust and feel comfortable with the professional you see. It is not uncommon to request a free introductory phone or in-person meeting to help determine if the professional is the right match for your particular needs and style. It is appropriate to clarify what the cost will be, how much your insurance will pay, and how many scheduled sessions you should expect to have with the mental health therapist. Any treatment should be evaluated regularly to ensure that it continues to contribute toward your improved health and growth.

Questions to Expect in a Mental Health Exam for Depression

- Tell me why you think you may be experiencing depression.

  - When did you first notice these symptoms? How long have you experienced them?

  - How do they affect you? Are there things you don't or can't do anymore?

  - Have you ever experienced these feelings before?

  - If you have, did you receive treatment? What type?

- How often do you use alcohol or drugs (both prescription and nonprescription) to help during the week?

- Have you had any thoughts about death or considered suicide?
- Do you have any family members who have experienced depression?
- If so, did they receive treatment? What type?
- Have you experienced any serious loss, difficult relationships, financial problems, or other recent changes in your life?
- Is there anything else you'd like to add to help me understand your situation better?

Treatment Options

Upon review of the physical and mental evaluation, a course of treatment will be recommended. Primary treatment options are psychotherapy (also referred to as mental health therapy) and antidepressant medication. These treatments are used alone or in combination with one another. (Electroconvulsive therapy or shock therapy is used for severe cases of depression and is recommended only when other approaches have not been effective.) The most frequent treatment for depressive symptoms that have progressed beyond the mild stage is antidepressant medication, which provides relatively quick symptom relief, in conjunction with ongoing psychotherapy, which offers new strategies for a more satisfying life. Following are the most common treatments used today.

Psychotherapy

- **Cognitive and behavioral therapy:** The therapist will focus on identifying and changing persistent, self-defeating thinking and behaviors. The ultimate goal is to help caregivers recognize and enjoy positive events in their lives and learn practical skills to deal with the problems they are facing.

- **Interpersonal therapy:** The therapist helps the caregiver self-evaluate problems in their communication, or lack of communication, with other people. The caregiver will come to better understand his or her own communication style and learn how to improve relationships with others.

- **Psychodynamic therapy:** Although sometimes used to treat depression, this therapy is thought to be less effective than the other two therapies already mentioned. Its goal is to surface deeply held conflicted feelings to better experience and understand them.

Medication and Electroconvulsive (ECT) Therapy

- **Selective serotonin reuptake inhibitors (SSRIs) (Examples: Prozac, Zoloft, Paxil):** Medications that work by stabilizing levels of serotonin, a neurotransmitter. Low levels of serotonin have been linked to depression. Fewer side effects than tricyclic medications.

- **Tricyclics (Examples: Norpramin, Pamelor, Sinequan):** An earlier family of antidepressant drugs, tricyclics increase levels of neurotransmitters in the brain. May cause more side effects.

- **Monoamine oxidase inhibitors (MAOI) (Examples: Nardil, Parnate):** These therapies are not often used today. MAOIs are drugs that increase the level of neurotransmitters in the brain. They are most often used when other medication isn't effective or tolerated.

- **Electroconvulsive therapy (ECT):** A brief pulse of electricity is delivered through electrodes on the scalp over a period of several days to produce changes in the brain function. ECT is used only for serious (possibly life-threatening) depression and when medication doesn't work.[1]

If drug therapy is recommended, a certain amount of trial and error is necessary to find the right type and dosage of medication for each individual and it may take several weeks before effects are felt. Good communication between patient and doctor is important.

Older adults should be especially careful to watch for medication side effects caused from too high a dosage or interactions with other medications.

Complementary and Alternative Therapies

St. John's wort: One of the most studied alternative treatments for depressive symptoms is St. John's wort (Hypericum perforatum). It is an herb used extensively in the treatment of mild to moderate depression in Europe and is now undergoing studies in the United States. St. John's wort extract is sold over the counter in the United States as a nutritional supplement.

It is promoted as a natural way to improve mood, and as a treatment for mild to moderate depression. Researchers are studying it for possibly having fewer and less severe side effects than antidepressant drugs.

Yet, questions remain regarding whether St. John's wort really does what its promoters claim. For nonprescription drugs in the United

States there are no established criteria for determining the amount of active ingredient a company puts in their product or what dose is right for a given person. The Food and Drug Administration issued a warning stating that St. John's wort may affect the metabolic pathway used by many prescription drugs prescribed to treat a number of conditions, including heart disease, depression, and HIV [human immunodeficiency virus] infections. If you are taking St. John's wort or considering its use, talk with your health care provider to ensure it will not interfere with any other treatment you are receiving.[2]

Seasonal affective disorder: Caregivers who feel "the blues" when confined indoors or in response to winter's gray days may suffer from seasonal affective disorder (SAD), also referred to as winter depression. As seasons change, there is a shift in our biological internal clocks or circadian rhythms, partly in response to the changes in sunlight patterns. This can cause our biological clocks to be out of sync with our daily schedules. People with SAD have a difficult time adjusting to the shortage of sunlight in the winter months. SAD symptoms are most pronounced in January and February, when the days are shortest. SAD is often misdiagnosed as hypothyroidism, hypoglycemia, infectious mononucleosis, and other viral infections.

Phototherapy, using specially designed bright fluorescent lights, has been shown to reverse SAD's depressive symptoms. Experts believe that the light therapy works by altering the levels of certain brain chemicals, specifically melatonin. Antidepressant medication along with other treatments, including exercise, may be helpful as well.

If you experience mild depressive symptoms seasonally, experiment with increasing the light in your surroundings, using lamps or other sources. If the symptoms are strong enough to impair your day-to-day functioning, seek out a mental health professional with expertise in treating SAD.

Physical exercise: Exercise has been found to reduce the effects of depression. Walking three times a week for 30 to 45 minutes has been linked to reducing or alleviating symptoms of depression. It is unknown whether physical activity prevents the onset of depression or just helps modify the effects. Arranging time for exercise is sometimes difficult for caregivers. It is often seen as a value added activity— something to do when everything else is done. You might consider adding it to your to do list, asking a friend to give you a walk date each week as a gift, or requesting that your doctor write a prescription for walking or joining an exercise class. All the research shows that for a healthier life, it makes good sense to make time for exercise.

Paying for Treatment

Private health insurance and Medicare will typically pay for some mental health care. It's best to call the mental health professional directly to find out if they accept your insurance for payment. Health insurance providers will usually list mental health professionals in the same insurance material that lists health plan medical doctors. Medicare recipients will find the booklet titled, "Medicare and Your Mental Health Benefits" a helpful source of information. [See Chapter 41 for more information.]

The covered services of the insurance plan will specify mental health coverage for inpatient (hospital, treatment center) and outpatient (professional's office) care, how many visits are paid for, and at what rate of reimbursement. Employed caregivers may also have access to an Employee Assistance Program, where licensed professionals (usually psychologists and social workers) are available for confidential sessions to discuss personal or professional problems.

Caregivers without health insurance or who pay out of pocket for care will find that fees vary by professional, with psychiatrists charging at the higher end of the fee scale and psychologists and social workers offering their services at a more moderate rate. In some instances, a mental health center will apply a fee based on your ability to pay. In any case, find out what the fee is up front to avoid any misunderstandings later on.

Strategies to Help Yourself

Depressive disorders can make one feel exhausted, helpless, and hopeless. Such negative thoughts and feelings make some people feel like giving up. It is important to realize that these negative views are part of the depression and may not accurately reflect the situation. The National Institute of Mental Health offers the following recommendations for dealing with depression:

- Set realistic goals in light of the depression and assume a reasonable amount of responsibility.

- Break large tasks into small ones, set some priorities, and do what you can as you can.

- Try to be with other people and to confide in someone; it is usually better than being alone and secretive.

- Participate in activities that may make you feel better, such as mild exercise, going to a movie or ball game, or attending a religious, social, or community event.

- Expect your mood to improve gradually, not immediately. Feeling better takes time.

- It is advisable to postpone important decisions until the depression has lifted. Before deciding to make a significant transition—change jobs, get married, or divorced—discuss it with others who know you well and have a more objective view of your situation.

- People rarely snap out of a depression. But they can feel a little better day-by-day.

- Remember, positive thinking will replace the negative thinking that is part of the depression. The negative thinking will be reduced as your depression responds to treatment. Let your family and friends help you.

Direct assistance in providing care for your loved one, such as respite care relief, as well as positive feedback from others, positive self-talk, and recreational activities are linked to lower levels of depression. Look for classes and support groups available through caregiver support organizations to help you learn or practice effective problem-solving and coping strategies needed for caregiving. For your health and the health of those around you, take some time to care for yourself.

Health Reference Series Medical Advisor's Notes and Updates

1. Several additional types of antidepressants are now available, including serotonin-norepinephrine reuptake inhibitors (SNRIs) and unique agents such as bupropion and mirtazapine. These have complex effects on neurotransmitter levels involved in depression. A new treatment called transcranial magnetic stimulation has also become available in some centers for resistant depression. It uses magnetic fields to stimulate specific regions of the brain. It may be a good alternative to ECT, as it is gentler and has fewer side effects.

2. Several large studies have failed to demonstrate any benefit of St. John's wort in treating depression, as compared to sugar pills. Nevertheless, it remains popular with some alternative medicine practitioners. Life-threatening interactions have been reported when St. John's wort has been mixed with prescription antidepressants and many other drugs, so great caution needs to be exercised if you choose to take it.

Chapter 21

Mental Health Problems in Prison Inmates

At midyear 2005 more than half of all prison and jail inmates had a mental health problem, including 705,600 inmates in state prisons, 78,800 in federal prisons, and 479,900 in local jails. These estimates represented 56% of state prisoners, 45% of federal prisoners, and 64% of jail inmates. The findings in this text were based on data from personal interviews with state and federal prisoners in 2004 and local jail inmates in 2002.

Mental health problems were defined by two measures: A recent history or symptoms of a mental health problem. They must have occurred in the 12 months prior to the interview. A recent history of mental health problems included a clinical diagnosis or treatment by a mental health professional. Symptoms of a mental disorder were based on criteria specified in the *Diagnostic and Statistical Manual of Mental Disorders, Fourth Edition (DSM-IV)*.

More than two-fifths of state prisoners (43%) and more than half of jail inmates (54%) reported symptoms that met the criteria for mania. About 23% of state prisoners and 30% of jail inmates reported symptoms of major depression. An estimated 15% of state prisoners and 24% of jail inmates reported symptoms that met the criteria for a psychotic disorder.

Excerpted from "Mental Health Problems of Prison Inmates," by the U.S. Department of Justice, September 2006. Reviewed by David A. Cooke, MD, FACP, November 13, 2011.

A Quarter of State Prisoners Had a History of Mental Health Problems

Among all inmates, state prisoners were most likely to report a recent history of a mental health problem. About 24% of state prisoners had a recent history of a mental health problem, followed by 21% of jail inmates, and 14% of federal prisoners.

A recent history of mental health problems was measured by several questions in the inmate surveys. Offenders were asked about whether in the past 12 months they had been told by a mental health professional that they had a mental disorder or because of a mental health problem had stayed overnight in a hospital, used prescribed medication, or received professional mental health therapy. These items were classified as indicating a recent history of a mental health problem.

State prisoners (18%), federal prisoners (10%), and jail inmates (14%) most commonly reported that they had used prescribed medication for a mental problem in the year before arrest or since admission. They were least likely to report an overnight stay in a hospital for a mental health problem. Approximately, 5% of inmates in state prisons, 2% in federal prisons, and 5% in local jails reported an overnight stay in a hospital for a mental health problem.

Symptoms of Mental Disorder Highest among Jail Inmates

Jail inmates had the highest rate of symptoms of a mental health disorder (60%), followed by state (49%), and federal prisoners (40%). Symptoms of a mental health disorder were measured by a series of questions adopted from a structured clinical interview for diagnosing mental disorders based on the *DSM-IV*. The questions addressed behaviors or symptoms related to major depression, mania, or psychotic disorders that occurred in the 12 months before the interview.

To meet the criteria for major depression, inmates had to report a depressed mood or decreased interest or pleasure in activities, along with four additional symptoms of depression. In order to meet the criteria for mania, during the 12-month period inmates had to report three symptoms or a persistent angry mood. For a psychotic disorder, one symptom of delusions or hallucinations met the criteria.

The high rate of symptoms of mental health disorder among jail inmates may reflect the role of local jails in the criminal justice system. Jails are locally operated correctional facilities that receive offenders after an arrest and hold them for a short period of time, pending arraignment, trial, conviction, or sentencing. Among other functions, local jails hold mentally ill persons pending their movement to appropriate mental health facilities.

While jails hold inmates sentenced to short terms (usually less than 1 year), state and federal prisons hold offenders who typically are convicted and sentenced to serve more than 1 year. In general, because of the longer period of incarceration, prisons provide a greater opportunity for inmates to receive a clinical mental health assessment, diagnosis, and treatment by a mental health professional.

Mental Health Problems More Common among Female, White, and Young Inmates

Female inmates had much higher rates of mental health problems than male inmates. An estimated 73% of females in state prisons, compared to 55% of male inmates, had a mental health problem. In federal prisons, the rate was 61% of females compared to 44% of males; and in local jails, 75% of females compared to 63% of male inmates.

The same percentage of females in state prisons or local jails (23%) said that in the past 12 months they had been diagnosed with a mental disorder by a mental health professional. This was almost three times the rate of male inmates (around 8%) who had been told they had a mental health problem.

The prevalence of mental health problems varied by racial or ethnic group. Among state prisoners, 62% of white inmates, compared to 55% of blacks and 46% of Hispanics, were found to have a mental health problem. Among jail inmates, whites (71%) were also more likely than blacks (63%) or Hispanics (51%) to have a mental health problem.

The rate of mental health problems also varied by the age of inmates. Inmates age 24 or younger had the highest rate of mental health problems and those age 55 or older had the lowest rate. Among state prisoners, an estimated 63% of those age 24 or younger had a mental health problem, compared to 40% of those age 55 or older. An estimated 70% of local jail inmates age 24 or younger had a mental health problem, compared to 52% of those age 55 or older.

Homelessness, Foster Care More Common among Inmates Who Had Mental Health Problems

State prisoners (13%) and local jail inmates (17%) who had a mental health problem were twice as likely as inmates without a mental health problem (6% in State prisons; 9% in local jails) to have been homeless in the year before their incarceration.

About 18% of state prisoners who had a mental health problem, compared to 9% of state prisoners who did not have a mental problem, said that they had lived in a foster home, agency, or institution while growing up.

Among jail inmates, about 14% of those who had a mental health problem had lived in a foster home, agency, or institution while growing up, compared to 6% of jail inmates who did not have a mental health problem.

Low Rates of Employment and High Rates of Illegal Income among Inmates Who Had Mental Problems

An estimated 70% of State prisoners who had a mental health problem, compared to 76% of those without, said they were employed in the month before their arrest. Among federal prisoners, 68% of those who had a mental health problem were employed, compared to 76% of those who did not have a mental problem.

Among jail inmates, 69% of those who had a mental health problem reported that they were employed, while 76% of those without were employed in the month before their arrest.

Of state prisoners who had a mental health problem, 65% had received income from wages or salary in the month before their arrest. This percentage was larger for inmates without a mental health problem (71%). Over a quarter (28%) of state prisoners who had a mental health problem reported income from illegal sources, compared to around a fifth (21%) of state prisoners without a mental problem.

Past Physical or Sexual Abuse More Prevalent among Inmates Who Had Mental Health Problems

State prisoners who had a mental health problem (27%) were over two times more likely than those without (10%) to report being physically or sexually abused in the past.

Jail inmates who had a mental health problem were three times more likely than jail inmates without to have been physically or sexually abused in the past (24% compared to 8%).

Family Members of Inmates with Mental Problems Had High Rates of Substance Use and Incarceration

Inmates who had a mental health problem were more likely than inmates without to have family members who abused drugs or alcohol or both. Among state prisoners, 39% of those who had a mental health problem reported that a parent or guardian had abused alcohol, drugs, or both while they were growing up. In comparison, 25% of state prisoners without a mental problem reported parental abuse of alcohol, drugs, or both.

A third (33%) of federal prisoners who had a mental health problem, compared to a fifth (20%) of those without, reported that a parent or guardian had abused alcohol, drugs, or both while they were growing up.

An estimated 37% of jail inmates who had a mental health problem said a parent had abused alcohol, drugs, or both while they were growing up. This was almost twice the rate for jail inmates without a mental health problem (19%).

The majority of prison and jail inmates who had a mental health problem (52%) reported that they had a family member who had been incarcerated in the past. Among those without a mental health problem, about 41% of state inmates and 36% of jails inmates reported that a family member had served time.

Over a third of both state prisoners and local jail inmates who had a mental health problem (35%) had a brother who had served time in prison or jail. The rate for inmates without a mental health problem was 29% in state prisons and 26% in local jails.

Inmates Who Had Mental Health Problems Had High Rates of Substance Dependence or Abuse

Among inmates who had a mental health problem, local jail inmates had the highest rate of dependence or abuse of alcohol or drugs (76%), followed by state prisoners (74%), and federal prisoners (64%). Substance dependence or abuse was measured as defined in the *DSM-IV*.

Among inmates without a mental health problem, 56% in state prisons, 49% in federal prisons, and 53% in local jails were dependent on or abused alcohol or drugs. By specific type of substance, inmates who had a mental health problem had higher rates of dependence or abuse of drugs than alcohol. Among state prisoners who had a mental problem, 62% were dependent on or abused drugs and 51% alcohol. An estimated 63% of local jail inmates who had a mental problem were dependent on or abused drugs, while about 53% were dependent on or abused alcohol.

When dependence was estimated separately from abuse only, local jail inmates who had a mental health problem had the highest rate of drug dependence (46%). They were two and a half times more likely to be dependent on drugs than jail inmates without a mental problem (18%).

195

A larger percentage of state prisoners who had a mental health problem than those without were found to be dependent on drugs (44% compared to 26%). Among federal prisoners, 37% who had a mental health problem were found to be dependent on drugs, compared to 22% of those without.

State prisoners (30%) and local jail inmates (29%) who had a mental health problem had about the same rate of alcohol dependence. A quarter of federal prisoners (25%) who had a mental problem were dependent on alcohol.

Over a Third of Inmates Who Had Mental Health Problems Had Used Drugs at the Time of the Offense

Over a third (37%) of state prisoners who had a mental health problem said they had used drugs at the time of the offense, compared to over a quarter (26%) of state prisoners without a mental problem. Also, over a third (34%) of local jail inmates who had a mental health problem said they had used drugs at the time of the offense, compared to a fifth (20%) of jail inmates who did not have a mental problem.

Marijuana or hashish was the most common drug inmates said they had used in the month before the offense. Among inmates who had a mental health problem, more than two fifths of those in state prisons (46%), federal prisons (41%), or local jails (43%) reported they had used marijuana or hashish in the month before the offense.

Almost a quarter of inmates in state prisons or local jails who had a mental health problem (24%) reported they had used cocaine or crack in the month before the offense. A smaller percentage of inmates who had a mental health problem had used methamphetamines in the month before the offense—13% of state prisoners, 11% of federal prisoners, and 12% of jail inmates.

Binge Drinking Prevalent among Inmates Who Had Mental Problems

Inmates who had a mental health problem were more likely than inmates without a mental problem to report a binge drinking experience. Among state prisoners who had a mental health problem, 43% said they had participated in binge drinking in the past, compared to 29% of state prisoners without mental problems.

Similarly, jail inmates who had mental problems (48%) had a much higher rate of binge drinking than jail inmates without mental problems (30%).

Inmates who had a mental problem were more likely than inmates without to have been using alcohol at the time of the offense (state prisoners, 34% compared to 27%; federal prisoners, 22% compared to 15%; and jail inmates, 35% compared to 30%).

Violent Offenses Common among State Prisoners Who Had a Mental Health Problem

Among state prisoners who had a mental health problem, nearly half (49%) had a violent offense as their most serious offense, followed by property (20%) and drug offenses (19%). Among all types of offenses, robbery was the most common offense (14%), followed by drug trafficking (13%) and homicide (12%).

An estimated 46% of state prisoners without a mental health problem were held for a violent offense, including 13% for homicide and 11% for robbery. About 24% of state prisoners without a mental problem were held for drug offenses, particularly drug trafficking (17%).

Almost an equal percentage of jail inmates who had a mental health problem were held for violent (26%) and property (27%) offenses. About 12% were held for aggravated assault. Jail inmates who had a mental health problem were two times more likely than jail inmates without a mental problem to be held for burglary (8% compared to 4%).

Use of a Weapon Did Not Vary by Mental Health Status

Convicted violent offenders who had a mental health problem were as likely as those without to have used a weapon during the offense. An estimated 37% of both state prisoners who had a mental problem and those without said they had used a weapon during the offense.

By specific type of weapon, among convicted violent offenders in state prisons who had a mental health problem, slightly less than a quarter (24%) had used a firearm, while a tenth (10%) had used a knife or sharp object.

Violent Criminal Record More Prevalent among Inmates Who Had a Mental Health Problem

State prisoners who had a mental health problem (61%) were more likely than state prisoners without (56%) to have a current or past violent offense.

Among repeat offenders, an estimated 47% of state prisoners who had a mental health problem were violent recidivists, compared to 39% of state prisoners without a mental problem.

Nearly a third (32%) of local jail inmates who had a mental health problem were repeat violent offenders, while about a quarter (22%) of jail inmates without a mental problem were violent recidivists.

A larger proportion of inmates who had a mental health problem had served more prior sentences than inmates without a mental problem. An estimated 47% of state prisoners who had a mental health problem, compared to 39% of those without, had served three or more prior sentences to probation or incarceration. Among jail inmates, 42% of those with a mental health problem had served three or more prior sentences to probation or incarceration, compared to 33% of jail inmates without a mental problem.

State Prisoners Who Had Mental Health Problems Had Longer Sentences Than Prisoners Without

Overall, state prisoners who had a mental health problem reported a mean maximum sentence that was 5 months longer than state prisoners without a mental problem (146 months compared to 141 months). Among jail inmates, the mean sentence for those who had a mental problem was 5 months shorter than that for jail inmates without a mental problem (40 months compared to 45 months).

By most serious offense, excluding offenders sentenced to life or death, both violent state prisoners who had a mental health problem and those without had about the same mean sentence length. Violent state prisoners who had a mental health problem were sentenced to serve a mean maximum sentence length of 212 months and those without, 211 months.

Among prisoners sentenced to life or death, there was little variation in sentence length by mental health status. About 8% of state prisoners who had a mental health problem and 9% of those without were sentenced to life or death. Among federal prisoners, 3% of both those who had a mental health problem and those without were sentenced to life or death.

State Prisoners Who Had a Mental Health Problem Expected to Serve Four Months Longer Than Those Without

Overall, the mean time state prisoners who had a mental health problem expected to serve was 4 months longer than state prisoners without a mental problem (93 months compared to 89 months). Among convicted jail inmates who expected to serve their time in a local jail, there was little variation by mental health status in the amount of time expected to be served. About 55% of those who had a mental problem, and 54% of those without, expected to serve 6 months or less.

A Third of State Prisoners Who Had Mental Health Problems Had Received Treatment since Admission

State prisoners who had a mental health problem (34%) had the highest rate of mental health treatment since admission, followed by federal prisoners (24%) and local jail inmates (17%).

All federal prisons and most state prisons and jail jurisdictions, as a matter of policy, provide mental health services to inmates, including screening inmates at intake for mental health problems, providing therapy or counseling by trained mental health professionals, and distributing psychotropic medication.

More than a fifth of inmates (22%) in state prison who had a mental health problem had received mental health treatment during the year before their arrest, including 16% who had used prescribed medications, 11% who had professional therapy, and 6% who had stayed overnight in a hospital because of a mental or emotional problem. Among jail inmates who had a mental health problem, an estimated 23% had received treatment during the year before their arrest: 17% had used medication, 12% had received professional therapy, and 7% had stayed overnight in a hospital because of a mental or emotional problem.

Taking a prescribed medication for a mental health problem was the most common type of treatment inmates who had a mental health problem had received since admission to prison or jail. About 27% of state prisoners, 19% of federal prisoners, and 15% of jail inmates who had a mental problem had used prescribed medication for a mental problem since admission.

An overnight stay in a hospital was the least likely method of treatment inmates had received since admission. Among inmates who had a mental problem, about 5% of those in state prisons, 3% in federal prisons, and 2% in local jails had stayed overnight in a hospital for a mental problem.

Use of Medication for a Mental Health Problem by State Prisoners Rose between 1997 and 2004

The proportion of state prisoners who had used prescribed medication for a mental health problem since admission to prison rose to 15% in 2004, up from 12% in 1997. There was little change in the percentage of inmates who reported an overnight stay in a hospital since admission (around 3%), or in the percentage who had received professional mental health therapy (around 12%).

State prisoners who said they had ever used prescribed medication for a mental or emotional problem in the past rose to 24% in 2004, up from 19% in 1997. Overall, 31% of state prisoners said they had ever received mental health treatment in the past, up from 28% in 1997.

Among jail inmates, in 2002 around 30% said they had received treatment for a mental health problem in the past, up from 25% in 1996. The proportion who had received treatment since admission (11%) was unchanged.

Part Four

Causes and Risk Factors for Depression

Chapter 22

What Causes Depression?

Chapter Contents

Section 22.1

Overview of the Causes of Depression

It is important to understand that depression is not caused by one thing, but probably by a combination of factors interacting with one another. These factors can be grouped into two broad categories—biology and psychology. Many biological and psychological factors interact in depression, although precisely which specific factors interact may differ from person to person.

Biological Factors

The biological factors that might have some effect on depression include: Genes, hormones, and brain chemicals.

Genetic Factors

Depression often runs in families, which suggests that individuals may inherit genes that make them vulnerable to developing depression. However, one may inherit an increased vulnerability to the illness, but not necessarily the illness itself. Although many people may inherit the vulnerability, a great many of them may never suffer a depressive illness.

Hormones

Research has found that there are some hormonal changes that occur in depression. The brain goes through some changes before and during a depressive episode, and certain parts of the brain are affected. This might result in an over- or under-production of some hormones, which may account for some of the symptoms of depression. Medication treatment can be effective in treating these conditions.

Brain Chemicals (Neurotransmitters)

Nerve cells in the brain communicate to each other by specific chemical substances called neurotransmitters. It is believed that during depression, there is reduced activity of one or more of these neurotransmitter systems, and this disturbs certain areas of the brain that regulate functions such as sleep, appetite, sexual drive, and perhaps mood. The reduced level of neurotransmitters results in reduced communication between the nerve cells and accounts for the typical symptoms of depression. Many antidepressant drugs increase the neurotransmitters in the brain.

Psychological Factors

Thinking

Many thinking patterns are associated with depression. These thinking patterns include:

- overstressing the negative;
- taking the responsibility for bad events but not for good events;
- having inflexible rules about how one should behave;
- thinking that you know what others are thinking and that they are thinking badly of you.

Loss

Sometimes people experience events where loss occurs, and this can bring on depression. The experience of loss may include the loss of a loved one through bereavement or separation, loss of a job, loss of a friendship, loss of a promotion, loss of face, loss of support, etc.

Sense of Failure

Some people may stake their happiness on achieving particular goals, such as getting As on their exams, getting a particular job, earning a certain amount of profit from a business venture, or finding a life partner. If for some reason they are not able to achieve those goals, they might believe that they have failed somehow, and it is this sense of failure that can sometimes bring on, or increase, depression.

Stress

An accumulation of stressful life events may also bring on depression. Stressful events include situations such as unemployment, financial worries, serious difficulties with spouses, parents, or children, physical illness, and major changes in life circumstances.

Conclusion

While we cannot do much about the genes we have inherited, there are a number of things we can do to overcome depression, or to prevent us from becoming depressed. Your doctor may have suggested medications, especially in a severe depression. While taking medication can be of assistance in overcoming depression, psychological treatments are also available. Ask your doctor or mental health practitioner for more details.

Section 22.2

Probing the Depression-Rumination Cycle

The word "ruminate" derives from the Latin for chewing cud, a less than genteel process in which cattle grind up, swallow, then regurgitate and rechew their feed. Similarly, human ruminators mull an issue at length.

But while the approach might ease cows' digestion, it doesn't do the same for people's mental health: Ruminating about the darker side of life can fuel depression, said Yale University psychologist Susan Nolen-Hoeksema, PhD, in a Board of Scientific Affairs invited address at APA's 2005 Annual Convention.

What's more, rumination can impair thinking and problem-solving, and drive away critical social support, she said.

In work published in APA's *Journal of Personality and Social Psychology*, *JPSP* (Vol. 77, No. 4, pages 801–814), Nolen-Hoeksema and Christopher Davis, PhD, found that although ruminators report reaching for others' aid more than nonruminators, they receive less of it. In fact, many of them report more social friction—"things like people telling them to buck up and get on with their lives," said Nolen-Hoeksema.

People might respond to a ruminator compassionately at first, but their compassion can wear thin if the rumination persists.

"After a while they get frustrated, and even hostile, and start pulling away, which of course as a ruminator gives you a whole lot more to ruminate about: 'Why are they abandoning me, why are they being so critical of me?'" said Nolen-Hoeksema.

In her talk, she explored the roots of this cycle of rumination and depression, and what can be done to break it.

The Rumination-Depression Link

Numerous longitudinal studies point to rumination's negative effects: For example, research Nolen-Hoeksema conducted on Bay Area residents who experienced the 1989 San Francisco earthquake found that those who self-identified as ruminators afterward showed more symptoms of depression and post-traumatic stress disorder.

Another of her studies, conducted with Judith Parker, PhD, and Louise Parker, PhD, found rumination predicted major depression among 455 18- to 84-year-olds who had lost family members to terminal illnesses. Those who ruminated more often became depressed, and stayed depressed in follow-ups through 18 months later, according to the study, published in 1994 in *JPSP* (Vol. 67, No. 1, pages 92–104).

In addition, a community survey Nolen-Hoeksema conducted on 1,300 adults, ages 25 to 75, backed those results. It found that ruminators develop major depression four times as often as nonruminators: 20 percent versus 5 percent. (The results were significant even for ruminators who weren't depressed at baseline.)

Many ruminators stay in their depressive rut because their negative outlook hurts their problem-solving ability, said Nolen-Hoeksema. According to her research, they often struggle to find good solutions to hypothetical problems. For example, if a friend is avoiding them, they might say, "Well, I guess I'll just avoid them too."

In addition, ruminators express low confidence in their solutions and often fail to enact them—for example, failing to join a bereavement support group despite intending to, said Nolen-Hoeksema.

"Even when a person prone to rumination comes up with a potential solution to a significant problem, the rumination itself may induce a level of uncertainty and immobilization that makes it hard for them to move forward," she said.

Why People Ruminate

Such depressive rumination most often occurs in women as a reaction to sadness, according to research Nolen-Hoeksema conducted with Lisa Butler, PhD, of Stanford University. Men, by comparison, more often focus on their emotions when they're angry, rather than sad, she said.

The reason, Nolen-Hoeksema speculated, is largely cultural. "There are differences between what is OK for women versus men to focus on emotionally," she said.

Gender aside, ruminators share some common characteristics. They often:

- believe they're gaining insight through it;

- have a history of trauma;

- perceive that they face chronic, uncontrollable stressors;

- exhibit personality characteristics such as perfectionism, neuroticism, and excessive relational focus—"a tendency to so overvalue your relationships with others that you will sacrifice yourself to maintain them, no matter what the costs," Nolen-Hoeksema explained.

Bucking Rumination

It's hard to divert depressive ruminators from their negative thoughts, Nolen-Hoeksema's research indicates. However, distracting them by directing them to think about, for example, a plane flying overhead, the layout of their local mall, or a fan slowly rotating, does appear to decrease their rumination. Her studies with Sonja Lyubomirsky, PhD, of Stanford University—many of them published in *JPSP*—have found that distracted ruminators less often recall negative events, such as being dumped by a significant other, than nondistracted ruminators. Distraction also helps mitigate ruminators' tendency to focus on problems—and express self-blame and low confidence—when discussing their lives, the research suggests.

Practically speaking, people can use such distraction techniques as meditation and prayer to help break the rumination cycle, said Nolen-Hoeksema. Other cycle breakers she suggested include:

- taking small actions to begin solving problems;

- reappraising negative perceptions of events and high expectations of others;

- letting go of unhealthy or unattainable goals and developing multiple sources of self-esteem.

"For example, women who build their identity solely around family are rumination-prone" because they've got all of their self-esteem and social support in one basket, said Nolen-Hoeksema. "So helping them to develop multiple sources of gratification and social support can be helpful buffers against stressful events in any one of those domains."

Chapter 23

Stress, Resilience, and the Risk of Depression

Chapter Contents

Section 23.1

Stress and Your Health

Excerpted from "Frequently Asked Questions: Stress and Your Health,"
by the Office on Women's Health (www.womenshealth.gov), part of the
U.S. Department of Health and Human Services, March 17, 2010.

What is stress?

Stress is a feeling you get when faced with a challenge. In small
doses, stress can be good for you because it makes you more alert and
gives you a burst of energy. For instance, if you start to cross the street
and see a car about to run you over, that jolt you feel helps you to jump
out of the way before you get hit. But feeling stressed for a long time
can take a toll on your mental and physical health. Even though it may
seem hard to find ways to destress with all the things you have to do,
it's important to find those ways. Your health depends on it.

What are the most common causes of stress?

Stress happens when people feel like they don't have the tools to
manage all of the demands in their lives. Stress can be short-term or
long-term. Missing the bus or arguing with your spouse or partner
can cause short-term stress. Money problems or trouble at work can
cause long-term stress. Even happy events, like having a baby or getting married, can cause stress. Some of the most common stressful life
events include the following:

- Death of a spouse

- Death of a close family member

- Divorce

- Losing your job

- Major personal illness or injury

- Marital separation

- Marriage

- Pregnancy
- Retirement
- Spending time in jail

What are some common signs of stress?

Everyone responds to stress a little differently. Your symptoms may be different from someone else's. Here are some of the signs to look for:

- Not eating or eating too much
- Feeling like you have no control
- Needing to have too much control
- Forgetfulness
- Headaches
- Lack of energy
- Lack of focus
- Trouble getting things done
- Poor self-esteem
- Short temper
- Trouble sleeping
- Upset stomach
- Back pain
- General aches and pains

These symptoms may also be signs of depression or anxiety, which can be caused by long-term stress.

Do women react to stress differently than men?

One recent survey found that women were more likely to experience physical symptoms of stress than men. But we don't have enough proof to say that this applies to all women. We do know that women often cope with stress in different ways than men. Women "tend and befriend," taking care of those closest to them, but also drawing support from friends and family. Men are more likely to have the "fight or flight" response. They cope by escaping into a relaxing activity or other distraction.

Can stress affect my health?

The body responds to stress by releasing stress hormones. These hormones make blood pressure, heart rate, and blood sugar levels go up. Long-term stress can help cause a variety of health problems, including the following:

- Mental health disorders, like depression and anxiety
- Obesity
- Heart disease
- High blood pressure
- Abnormal heartbeats
- Menstrual problems
- Acne and other skin problems

Does stress cause ulcers?

No, stress doesn't cause ulcers, but it can make them worse. Most ulcers are caused by a germ called *H. pylori*. Researchers think people might get it through food or water. Most ulcers can be cured by taking a combination of antibiotics and other drugs.

What is posttraumatic stress disorder (PTSD)?

Posttraumatic stress disorder (PTSD) is a type of anxiety disorder that can occur after living through or seeing a dangerous event. It can also occur after a sudden traumatic event. This can include the following:

- Being a victim of or seeing violence
- Being a victim of sexual or physical abuse or assault
- The death or serious illness of a loved one
- Fighting in a war
- A severe car crash or a plane crash
- Hurricanes, tornadoes, and fires

You can start having PTSD symptoms right after the event. Or symptoms can develop months or even years later. Symptoms may include the following:

- Nightmares
- Flashbacks, or feeling like the event is happening again
- Staying away from places and things that remind you of what happened
- Being irritable, angry, or jumpy
- Feeling strong guilt, depression, or worry
- Trouble sleeping
- Feeling numb
- Having trouble remembering the event

Women are two to three times more likely to develop PTSD than men. Also, people with ongoing stress in their lives are more likely to develop PTSD after a dangerous event.

How can I help handle my stress?

Everyone has to deal with stress. There are steps you can take to help you handle stress in a positive way and keep it from making you sick. Try these tips to keep stress in check:

- **Become a problem solver.** Make a list of the things that cause you stress. From your list, figure out which problems you can solve now and which are beyond your control for the moment. From your list of problems that you can solve now, start with the little ones. Learn how to calmly look at a problem, think of possible solutions, and take action to solve the problem. Being able to solve small problems will give you confidence to tackle the big ones. And feeling confident that you can solve problems will go a long way to helping you feel less stressed.

- **Be flexible.** Sometimes, it's not worth the stress to argue. Give in once in a while or meet people halfway.

- **Get organized.** Think ahead about how you're going to spend your time. Write a to-do list. Figure out what's most important to do and do those things first.

- **Set limits.** When it comes to things like work and family, figure out what you can really do. There are only so many hours in the day. Set limits for yourself and others. Don't be afraid to say no to requests for your time and energy.

- **Take deep breaths.** If you're feeling stressed, taking a few deep breaths makes you breathe slower and helps your muscles relax.

- **Stretch.** Stretching can also help relax your muscles and make you feel less tense.

- **Massage tense muscles.** Having someone massage the muscles in the back of your neck and upper back can help you feel less tense.

- **Take time to do something you want to do.** We all have lots of things that we have to do. But often we don't take the time to do the things that we really want to do. It could be listening to music, reading a good book, or going to a movie. Think of this as an order from your doctor, so you won't feel guilty!

- **Get enough sleep.** Getting enough sleep helps you recover from the stresses of the day. Also, being well-rested helps you think better so that you are prepared to handle problems as they come up. Most adults need seven to nine hours of sleep a night to feel rested.

- **Eat right.** Try to fuel up with fruits, vegetables, beans, and whole grains.

- **Don't be fooled by the jolt you get from caffeine or high-sugar snack foods.** Your energy will wear off, and you could wind up feeling more tired than you did before.

- **Get moving.** Getting physical activity can not only help relax your tense muscles but improve your mood. Research shows that physical activity can help relieve symptoms of depression and anxiety.

- **Don't deal with stress in unhealthy ways.** This includes drinking too much alcohol, using drugs, smoking, or overeating.

- **Share your stress.** Talking about your problems with friends or family members can sometimes help you feel better. They might also help you see your problems in a new way and suggest solutions that you hadn't thought of.

- **Get help from a professional if you need it.** If you feel that you can no longer cope, talk to your doctor. She or he may suggest counseling to help you learn better ways to deal with stress. Your doctor may also prescribe medicines, such as antidepressants or sleep aids.

- **Help others.** Volunteering in your community can help you make new friends and feel better about yourself.

Section 23.2

Resilience Factors and the Risk of Developing Mental Health Problems

Excerpted from "Effects of Disasters: Risk and Resilience Factors," by the National Center for Posttraumatic Stress Disorder (NCPTSD, www.ptsd.va.gov), part of the Veterans Administration, March 16, 2011.

Every year, millions of people are affected by both human-caused and natural disasters. Disasters may be explosions, earthquakes, floods, hurricanes, tornados, or fires. In a disaster, you face the danger of death or physical injury. You may also lose your home, possessions, and community. Such stressors place you at risk for emotional and physical health problems.

Stress reactions after a disaster look very much like the common reactions seen after any type of trauma. Disasters can cause a full range of mental and physical reactions. You may also react to problems that occur after the event, as well as to triggers or reminders of the trauma.

Risk Factors

A number of factors makes it more likely that someone will have more severe or longer-lasting stress reactions after disasters.

Severity of Exposure

The amount of exposure to the disaster is highly related to risk of future mental problems. At highest risk are those that go through the disaster themselves. Next are those in close contact with victims. At lower risk of lasting impact are those who only had indirect exposure, such as news of the severe damage. Injury and life threat are the factors that lead most often to mental health problems. Studies have looked at severe natural disasters, such as the Armenian earthquake, mudslides in Mexico, and Hurricane Andrew in the United States. The findings show that at least half of these survivors suffer from distress or mental health problems that need clinical care.

217

Gender and Family

Almost always, women or girls suffer more negative effects than do men or boys. Disaster recovery is more stressful when children are present in the home. Women with spouses also experience more distress during recovery.

Having a family member in the home who is extremely distressed is related to more stress for everyone. Marital stress has been found to increase after disasters. Also, conflicts between family members or lack of support in the home make it harder to recover from disasters.

Age

Adults who are in the age range of 40–60 are likely to be more distressed after disasters. The thinking is that if you are in that age range, you have more demands from job and family. Research on how children react to natural disasters is limited. In general, children show more severe distress after disasters than do adults. Higher stress in the parents is related to worse recovery in children.

Other Factors Specific to the Survivor

Several factors related to a survivor's background and resources are important for recovery from disaster. Recovery is worse if you:

- were not functioning well before the disaster;
- have had no experience dealing with disasters;
- must deal with other stressors after the disaster;
- have poor self-esteem;
- think you are uncared for by others;
- think you have little control over what happens to you;
- lack the capacity to manage stress.

Other factors have also been found to predict worse outcomes:

- Bereavement (death of someone close)
- Injury to self or another family member
- Life threat
- Panic, horror, or feelings like that during the disaster
- Being separated from family (especially among youth)

- Great loss of property
- Displacement (being forced to leave home)

Developing Countries

These risk factors can be made worse if the disaster occurs in a developing country. Disasters in developing countries have more severe mental health impact than do disasters in developed countries. This is true even with less serious disasters. For example, natural disasters are generally thought to be less serious than human-caused. In developing countries, though, natural disasters have more severe effects than do human-caused disasters in developed countries.

Low or Negative Social Support

The support of others can be both a risk and a resilience factor. Social support can weaken after disasters. This may be due to stress and the need for members of the support network to get on with their own lives.

Sometimes the responses from others you rely on for support are negative. For example, someone may play down your problems, needs, or pain, or expect you to recover more quickly than is realistic. This is strongly linked to long-term distress in trauma survivors.

After a mass trauma, social conflicts, even those that have been resolved, may again be seen. Racial, religious, ethnic, social, and tribal divisions may recur as people try to gain access to much-needed resources. In families, conflicts may arise if family members went through different things in the disaster. This sets up different courses of recovery that often are not well understood among family members. Family members may also serve as distressing reminders to each other of the disaster.

Keep in mind that while millions of people have been directly affected by disasters, most of them do recover. Human nature is resilient, and most people have the ability to come back from a disaster. Plus, people sometimes report positive changes after disaster. They may rethink what is truly important and come to appreciate what they value most in life.

Resilience Factors

Human resilience dictates that a large number of survivors will naturally recover from disasters over time. They will move on without having severe, long-lasting mental health issues. Certain factors increase resilience after disasters.

Social Support

Social support is one of the keys to recovery after any trauma, including disaster. Social support increases well-being and limits distress after mass trauma. Being connected to others makes it easier to obtain knowledge needed for disaster recovery. Through social support, you can also find the following:

- Practical help solving problems
- A sense of being understood and accepted
- Sharing of trauma experiences
- Some comfort that what you went through and how you responded is not "abnormal"
- Shared tips about coping

Coping Confidence

Over and over, research has found that coping self-efficacy—"believing that you can do it"—is related to better mental health outcomes for disaster survivors. When you think that you can cope no matter what happens to you, you tend to do better after a disaster. It is not so much feeling like you can handle things in general. Rather, it is believing you can cope with the results of a disaster that has been found to help survivors to recover.

Hope

Better outcomes after disasters or mass trauma are likely if you have one or more of the following:

- Optimism (because you can hope for the future)
- Expecting the positive
- Confidence that you can predict your life and yourself
- Belief that it is very likely that things will work out as well as can reasonably be expected
- Belief that outside sources, such as the government, are acting on your behalf with your welfare at heart
- Belief in God
- Positive superstitious belief, such as "I'm always lucky"
- Practical resources, including housing, job, money

Section 23.3

DeltaFosB Mechanism Is Necessary for Resilience

Excerpted from "Resilience Factor Low in Depression, Protects Mice From Stress," by the National Institutes of Health (NIH, www.nih.gov), May 16, 2010.

Scientists have discovered a mechanism that helps to explain resilience to stress, vulnerability to depression, and how antidepressants work. The new findings, in the reward circuit of mouse and human brains, have spurred a high tech dragnet for compounds that boost the action of a key gene regulator there, called deltaFosB.

A molecular main power switch—called a transcription factor—inside neurons, deltaFosB turns multiple genes on and off, triggering the production of proteins that perform a cell's activities.

"We found that triggering deltaFosB in the reward circuit's hub is both necessary and sufficient for resilience; it protects mice from developing a depression-like syndrome following chronic social stress," explained Eric Nestler, MD, of the Mount Sinai School of Medicine, who led the research team, which was funded by the National Institute of Health's National Institute of Mental Health (NIMH).

"Antidepressants can reverse this social withdrawal syndrome by boosting deltaFosB. Moreover, deltaFosB is conspicuously depleted in brains of people who suffered from depression. Thus, induction of this protein is a positive adaptation that helps us cope with stress, so we're hoping to find ways to tweak it pharmacologically," added Nestler, who also directs the ongoing compound screening project.

Nestler and colleagues reported the findings that inspired the hunt online May 16, 2010 in the journal *Nature Neuroscience*.

"This search for small molecules that augment the actions of deltaFosB holds promise for development of a new class of resilience-boosting treatments for depression," said NIMH director Thomas R. Insel. "The project, funded under the American Recovery and Reinvestment Act of 2009, is a stunning example of how leads from rodent experiments can be quickly followed up and translated into potential clinical applications."

DeltaFosB is more active in the reward hub, called the nucleus accumbens, than in any other part of the brain. Chronic use of drugs of abuse—or even natural rewards like excess food, sex, or exercise—can gradually induce increasing levels of this transcription factor in the reward hub. Nestler and colleagues have shown that this increase in deltaFosB can eventually lead to lasting changes in cells that increase rewarding responses to such stimuli, hijacking an individual's reward circuitry—addiction.

The new study in mice and human postmortem brains confirms that the same reward circuitry is similarly corrupted (though to a lesser degree than with drugs of abuse) in depression via effects of stress on deltaFosB.

Depressed patients often lack motivation and the ability to experience reward or pleasure—and depression and addiction often go together. Indeed, mice susceptible to the depression-like syndrome show enhanced responses to drugs of abuse, the researchers have found.

But the similarity ends there. For, while an uptick in deltaFosB promotes addiction, the researchers have determined that it also protects against depression-inducing stress. It turns out that stress triggers the transcription factor in a different mix of nucleus accumbens cell types—working through different receptor types—than do drugs and natural rewards, likely accounting for the opposite effects.

The researchers explored the workings of deltaFosB in a mouse model of depression.

Much as depressed patients characteristically withdraw from social contact, mice exposed to aggression by a different dominant mouse daily for 10 days often become socially defeated; they vigorously avoid other mice, even weeks later. Key findings in the brain's reward hub include the following:

- The amount of deltaFosB induced by the stress determined susceptibility or resilience to developing the depression-like behaviors. It counteracted the strong tendency to learn an association, or generalize, the aversive experience to all mice.

- Induction of deltaFosB was required for the antidepressant fluoxetine (Prozac) to reverse the stress-induced depression-like syndrome.

- Prolonged isolation from environmental stimuli reduced levels of deltaFosB, increasing vulnerability to depression-like behaviors.

- Among numerous target genes regulated by deltaFosB, a gene that makes a protein called the AMPA [alpha-amino-3-hydroxy-5-methyl-4-isoxazolepropionic acid] receptor is critical for resilience—or protecting mice from the depression-like syndrome. The AMPA receptor is a protein on neurons that boosts the cell's activity when it binds to the chemical messenger glutamate.

- Increased activity of neurons triggered by heightened sensitivity of AMPA receptors to glutamate increased susceptibility to stress-induced depression-like behavior.

- Induction of deltaFosB calmed the neurons and protected against depression by suppressing AMPA receptors' sensitivity to glutamate.

- Postmortem brain tissue of depressed patients contained only about half as much deltaFosB as that of controls, suggesting that poor response to antidepressant treatment may be traceable, in part, to weak induction of the transcription factor.

Reduced deltaFosB in the reward hub likely helps to account for the impaired motivation and reward behavior seen in depression, said Nestler. Boosting it appears to enable an individual to pursue goal-directed behavior despite stress.

The high-tech screening for molecules that boost DeltaFosB, supported by the Recovery Act grant, could lead to development of medications that would help people cope with chronic stress. The molecules could also potentially be used as telltale tracers in brain imaging to chart depressed patients' treatment progress by reflecting changes in deltaFosB, said Nestler.

Source: DeltaFosB in brain reward circuits mediates resilience to stress and antidepressant responses. Vialou V, Robison AJ, LaPlant QC, Covington III HE, Dietz DM, Ohnishi YN, Mouson E, Rush III AJ, Watts EL, Wallace DL, Iniguez SD, Ohnishi YH, Steiner MA, Warren B, Krishnan V, Neve RL, Ghose S, Beron O, Tamminga CA, Nestler EJ. *NatNeurosci.* Epub 2010 May 16.

Chapter 24

Trauma as a Risk Factor for Depression

Chapter Contents

Section 24.1

Depression, Trauma, and Posttraumatic Stress Disorder (PTSD)

From "Depression, Trauma, and PTSD," by the National Center for Posttraumatic Stress Disorder (NCPTSD, www.ptsd.va.gov), part of the Veterans Administration, June 30, 2010.

Depression is a common problem that can occur following trauma. It involves feelings of sadness or low mood that last more than just a few days. Unlike a blue mood that comes and goes, depression is longer lasting. Depression can get in the way of daily life and make it hard to function. It can affect your eating and sleeping, how you think, and how you feel about yourself.

How common is depression following trauma?

In any given year, almost one in 10 adult Americans has some type of depression. Depression often occurs after trauma. For example, a survey of survivors from the Oklahoma City bombing showed that 23% had depression after the bombing. This was compared to 13% who had depression before the bombing. PTSD and depression are often seen together.

Results from a large national survey showed that depression is nearly three to five times more likely in those with PTSD than those without PTSD.

What are the symptoms of depression?

Depression is more than just feeling sad. Most people with depression feel down or sad more days than not for at least two weeks. Or they find they no longer enjoy or have interest in things anymore. If you have depression, you may notice that you're sleeping and eating a lot more or less than you used to. You may find it hard to stay focused. You may feel down on yourself or hopeless. With more severe depression, you may think about hurting or killing yourself.

How are depression and trauma related?

Depression can sometimes seem to come from out of the blue. It can also be caused by a stressful event such as a divorce or a trauma. Trouble coping with painful experiences or losses often leads to depression. For example, veterans returning from a war zone may have painful memories and feelings of guilt or regret about their war experiences. They may have been injured or lost friends. Disaster survivors may have lost a loved one, a home, or have been injured. Survivors of violence or abuse may feel like they can no longer trust other people. These kinds of experiences can lead to both depression and PTSD.

Many symptoms of depression overlap with the symptoms of PTSD. For example, with both depression and PTSD, you may have trouble sleeping or keeping your mind focused. You may not feel pleasure or interest in things you used to enjoy. You may not want to be with other people as much. Both PTSD and depression may involve greater irritability. It is quite possible to have both depression and PTSD at the same time.

How is depression treated?

There are many treatment options for depression. You should be assessed by a healthcare professional who can decide which type of treatment is best for you. In many cases, milder forms of depression are treated by counseling or therapy. More severe depression is treated with medicines or with both therapy and medicine.

Research has shown that certain types of therapy and medicine are effective for both depression and PTSD. Since the symptoms of PTSD and depression can overlap, treatment that helps with PTSD may also result in improvement of depression. Cognitive behavioral therapy (CBT) is a type of therapy that is proven effective for both problems. CBT can help patients change negative styles of thinking and acting that can lead to both depression and PTSD. A type of medicine that is effective for both depression and PTSD is a selective serotonin reuptake inhibitor (SSRI).

What can I do about feelings of depression?

Depression can make you feel worn out, worthless, helpless, hopeless, and sad. These feelings can make you feel as though you are never going to feel better. You may even think that you should just give up. Some symptoms of depression, such as being tired or not having the desire to do anything, can also get in the way of your seeking treatment.

It is very important for you to know that these negative thoughts and feelings are part of depression. If you think you might be depressed, you should seek help in spite of these feelings. You can expect them to change as treatment begins working. In the meantime, here is a list of things you can do that may improve your mood:

- Talk with your doctor or healthcare provider.

- Talk with family and friends.

- Spend more time with others and get support from them. Don't close yourself off.

- Take part in activities that might make you feel better. Do the things you used to enjoy before you began feeling depressed. Even if you don't feel like it, try doing some of these things. Chances are you will feel better after you do.

- Engage in mild exercise.

- Set realistic goals for yourself.

- Break up goals and tasks into smaller ones that you can manage.

Section 24.2

History of Childhood
Abuse or Neglect Increases Risk
of Major Depression

From "History of Childhood Abuse or Neglect Increases Risk of Major Depression," by the National Institute of Mental Health (NIMH, www .nimh.nih.gov), part of the National Institutes of Health, January 3, 2007.

People who were abused or neglected as children have increased risk of major depression, which often begins in childhood and has lingering effects as they mature, according to a study funded by NIMH. This was the first long-term study to examine the risk of depression in this population. The results were published in the January issue of the *Archives of General Psychiatry.*

Lead author Cathy Widom, PhD, formerly of New Jersey Medical School and currently at John Jay College in New York City, and colleagues compared 676 adults with a court-substantiated history of childhood physical and sexual abuse or neglect occurring before age 11 with 520 non-abused and non-neglected adults. The two groups were matched for age, race, sex, and approximate family social class during childhood. The average age of participants was 29 at the time of the study.

The researchers found that, overall, childhood physical abuse or multiple types of abuse increased the lifetime risk for depression. Neglect, which accounts for nearly two thirds of the reported and substantiated cases of child maltreatment in the United States, increased risk for current depression. Sexual abuse did not appear to increase risk of full-blown depression, but adults with a history of childhood sexual abuse reported more depression symptoms than people who did not experience such trauma. Previously abused or neglected study participants with depression were also more likely than matched control participants to meet the diagnostic criteria for at least one other mental disorder, such as post-traumatic stress disorder (PTSD), drug dependence, dysthymia (a less severe form of depression), or antisocial personality disorder. The researchers concluded that such results call for increased attention to the psychological health of abused and neglected children. Early diagnosis and treatment of mental disorders that may arise from maltreatment is important to prevent harmful, long-lasting effects on functioning.

References

Spatz Widom C, Dumont K, Czaja SJ. A prospective investigation of major depressive disorder and comorbidity in abused and neglected children grown up. *Arch Gen Psychiatry*. 2007 Jan;64(1):49–56.

U.S. Department of Health and Human Services, Administration for Children, Youth, and Families. *Child Maltreatment 2002: Reports from the States to the National Child Abuse and Neglect Data System*. Washington, DC: U.S. Government Printing Office; 2004.

Chapter 25

Unemployment, Poverty, and Depression

Chapter Contents

Section 25.1

People with Depression Less Likely to Be Employed

Excerpted from "Employment and Major Depressive Disorder," a National Survey on Drug Use and Health (NSDUH) report by the Substance Abuse and Mental Health Services Administration (SAMHSA, www.oas.samhsa.gov), part of the U.S. Department of Health and Human Services, August 6, 2009.

The inability to find and maintain meaningful employment is a major issue for individuals who experience mental disorders. Barriers to employment among those with mental disorders include lack of confidence, fear and anxiety, gaps in work history, social stigma, and workplace discrimination and inflexibility. The co-occurrence of mental disorders and unemployment can be a cycle in which a person's mental condition can make it difficult to get or maintain employment, and the strain of unemployment can worsen a person's mental condition. As a result, there is a need for additional services, such as supported employment programs, for those with mental disorders.

The National Survey on Drug Use and Health (NSDUH) includes questions about current employment (full time or part time), as well as about major depressive disorder (MDE). NSDUH defines "full-time employment" as usually working 35 or more hours per week and either working in the past week or having a job despite not working in the past week. "Part-time employment" is defined as usually working fewer than 35 hours per week and either working in the past week or having a job despite not working in the past week. "Any current employment" includes working either full or part time in the week prior to the interview. "MDE" refers to a period of 2 weeks or longer during which there is either depressed mood or loss of interest or pleasure, as well as other symptoms.

This text examines employment rates among adults aged 18 to 64 by MDE.

Trends in Employment Rates, by MDE

From 2004 to 2007, the rate of any current employment was lower in 2007 (63.2 percent) than in either 2004 (68.8 percent) or 2006 (66.9

percent) among adults aged 18 to 64 with MDE; this pattern was similar for full-time employment (i.e., a lower rate in 2007 compared with 2004 or 2006) (See Figure 25.1).

From 2004 to 2007, there were no statistically significant differences in the rates of part-time employment among those with MDE and among those without MDE.

In each year from 2004 to 2007, the rates of any current employment and full-time employment were lower for adults aged 18 to 64 with MDE compared with those without MDE. In each year, those with or without MDE had a similar rate of part-time employment.

Figure 25.1. *Current Employment Status among Adults Aged 18 to 64 with or without Major Depressive Episode (MDE)*: 2004 to 2007*

MDE, by Current Employment Status	2004	2005	2006	2007
Any Employment among Persons with MDE	68.8**	65.4	66.9**	63.2
Any Employment among Persons without MDE	79.1	78.9	78.5	78.7
Full-time Employment among Persons with MDE	54.3**	50.4	52.5**	48.0
Full-time Employment among Persons without MDE	65.7	65.4	65.2	65.0
Part-time Employment among Persons with MDE	14.5	15.1	14.4	15.2
Part-time Employment among Persons without MDE	13.4	13.5	13.3	13.6

* MDE is defined using the diagnostic criteria in the 4th edition of the *Diagnostic and Statistical Manual of Mental Disorders* (DSM-IV), which specifies a period of 2 weeks or longer during which there is either depressed mood or loss of interest or pleasure and at least four other symptoms that reflect a change in functioning, such as problems with sleep, eating, energy, concentration, and self-image. In assessing MDE, no exclusions were made for MDE caused by medical illness, bereavement, or substance use disorders. See the American Psychiatric Association. (1994). *Diagnostic and statistical manual of mental disorders* (4th ed.). Washington, DC: Author.

**Difference between estimate and estimate for 2007 is statistically significant at $p < .05$.

Source: 2004 to 2007 SAMHSA National Surveys on Drug Use and Health (NSDUHs).

Employment Status, by MDE and Demographic Characteristics

Combined data from 2004 to 2007 indicate that the rate of any current employment was lower among adults aged 18 to 64 with MDE than among those without MDE for both genders. However, there was less of a difference in the rate of any current employment by MDE for females than for males. Within each age group (18 to 25, 26 to 49, and 50 to 64), the rate of any current employment was lower for those with MDE than for those without MDE.

However, there was less of a difference in the current employment rate by MDE for those aged 18 to 25 than for those aged 26 to 49 and those aged 50 to 64.

The smaller impact of MDE on the employment of females compared with males and on those aged 18 to 25 compared with older age groups may be partially explained by the relatively high rate of part-time employment among those groups. The rate of part-time employment was higher for females than for males (18.2 vs. 8.8 percent) and was higher for those aged 18 to 25 than for those aged 26 to 49 or those aged 50 to 64 (25.4 vs. 10.6 and 11.8 percent, respectively).

Employment Status, by MDE and Geographic Characteristics

Combined data from 2004 to 2007 indicate that, within each region of the United States, the rate of any current employment was lower among adults aged 18 to 64 with MDE than among those without MDE. In both metropolitan and non-metropolitan counties, the rate of any current employment was lower among those with MDE than among those without MDE. However, there was less of a difference in the rate of current employment by MDE for those in metropolitan counties than for those in non-metropolitan counties.

Employment Status, by MDE and Receipt of Government Assistance

Combined data from 2004 to 2007 indicate that adults aged 18 to 64 with MDE had a lower rate of any current employment compared with their counterparts who did not have MDE, regardless of whether they had received government assistance in the past year. However, there was more of a difference in the rate of current employment by MDE for those who had received government assistance in the past year than for those who did not. Among those who received government assistance, the rate of any current employment was 40.6 percent for those with MDE.

Employment Status, by MDE and Substance Dependence or Abuse

Adults aged 18 to 64 with MDE had a lower rate of any current employment compared with those who did not have MDE, regardless of whether they had substance abuse or dependence in the past year. Additionally, the rate of any current employment was higher for those with substance dependence or abuse than for those without substance dependence or abuse, regardless of whether they had MDE.

Discussion

These data indicate that, from 2004 to 2007, adults aged 18 to 64 with MDE were less likely to be employed overall and less likely to be employed full time than those without MDE. This suggests that those who experience MDE may need additional services and support to find and maintain full-time employment and to transition from part-time to full-time work. These data also indicate that the difference in the overall employment rate between those who experienced MDE and those who did not was more marked for certain subgroups, including males, those aged 26 or older, those living in non-metropolitan areas, and those who received government assistance. The findings suggest that a concentration of employment services for persons from these subgroups who have experienced MDE may be an effective method of increasing the overall employment rate among those who have experienced this condition.

Section 25.2

Income Influences Postpartum Depression

A new study discovers more than half of low-income urban mothers meet the criteria for a diagnosis of depression at some point between 2 weeks and 14 months after giving birth. University of Rochester Medical Center researchers determined the prevalence of depression via a diagnostic interview performed when the low-income urban mothers were attending well-child care visits.

The study is the first of its kind to test the accuracy of three depression screening tools routinely used by physicians. The screening tools have high accuracy in identifying depression, the researchers concluded, but cutoff scores may need to be altered to identify depression more accurately among low-income urban mothers.

The study, found online in the journal *Pediatrics*, involved 198 mothers who were 18 years of age or older and whose children were no older than 14 months. The mothers attended well-child visits at the outpatient pediatric clinic at Golisano Children's Hospital at the Medical Center.

The researchers found that 56 percent of the mothers, after a diagnostic interview, met the criteria for a diagnosis of a major or minor depressive disorder.

"This is an unexpected, very high proportion to meet diagnostic criteria for depression," said Linda H. Chaudron, MD, associate professor of Psychology, Pediatrics, and of Obstetrics and Gynecology.

"This may be a group at high risk for depression. The message of this study is that pediatricians and other clinicians who work with low-income urban mothers have multiple screening tools that are easy to use and accurate. These tools can help clinicians identify mothers with depression so they can be referred for help."

Many women experience the so-called "baby blues." When the feelings persist or worsen it may be clinical depression. The symptoms include insomnia, persistent sadness, lack of interest in nearly all activity, anxiety, change in appetite, persistent feelings of guilt, and thoughts of harming oneself or the baby. Postpartum depression affects up to 14 percent of new mothers in the United States, with higher rates among poor and minority women.

The researchers evaluated three screening tools, the Edinburgh Postnatal Depression Scale, the Beck Depression Inventory II, and the Postpartum Depression Screening Scale, using the diagnostic interviews for validation.

The three screening tools have been evaluated in many populations, but one of the reasons the study was done was to test the tools with a group for whom there is not much data—low-income women, especially African-American women, Chaudron said. The researchers also evaluated the validity of the screening tools at various times during the postpartum year.

"The screening tools are valid when used anytime during the postpartum year," Chaudron said.

Use of traditional cutoff scores may not be as accurate as previously thought. Clinicians should be aware that scores two or three points below traditional cutoff scores may indicate a need for further evaluation, the researchers concluded.

The study was funded by a grant from the National Institute of Mental Health.

Chapter 26

Other Mental Health Disorders and the Relationship to Depression

Chapter Contents

Section 26.1

The Relationship between Depression and Anxiety

"Depression," by the Anxiety Disorders Association of America (ADAA, www.adaa.org). © 2011. Reprinted with permission.

Most people feel anxious or depressed at times. Losing a loved one, getting fired from a job, going through a divorce, and other difficult situations can lead a person to feel sad, lonely, scared, nervous, or anxious. These feelings are normal reactions to life's stressors.

But some people experience these feelings daily or nearly daily for no apparent reason, making it difficult to carry on with normal, everyday functioning. These people may have an anxiety disorder, depression, or both.

It is not uncommon for someone with an anxiety disorder to also suffer from depression or vice versa. Nearly one-half of those diagnosed with depression are also diagnosed with an anxiety disorder. The good news is that these disorders are both treatable, separately and together.

Read the following text to find out more about the co-occurrence of anxiety and depression[1,2] and how they can be treated.

Depression

Depression is a condition in which a person feels discouraged, sad, hopeless, unmotivated, or disinterested in life in general. When these feelings last for a short period of time, it may be a case of "the blues."

But when such feelings last for more than two weeks and when the feelings interfere with daily activities such as taking care of family, spending time with friends, or going to work or school, it's likely a major depressive episode.

Major depression is a treatable illness that affects the way a person thinks, feels, behaves, and functions. At any point in time, 3 to 5 percent of people suffer from major depression; the lifetime risk is about 17 percent.

Types of Depression

Three main types of depressive disorders—major depression, dysthymia, and bipolar disorder—can occur with any of the anxiety disorders.

Major depression involves at least five of these symptoms for a two-week period. Such an episode is disabling and will interfere with the ability to work, study, eat, and sleep. Major depressive episodes may occur once or twice in a lifetime, or they may re-occur frequently. They may also take place spontaneously, during or after the death of a loved one, a romantic breakup, a medical illness, or other life event.

Some people with major depression may feel that life is not worth living and some will attempt to end their lives.

Dysthymia is a less severe, long-term, and chronic form of depression. It involves the same symptoms as major depression, mainly low energy, poor appetite or overeating, and insomnia or oversleeping. It can manifest as stress, irritability, and mild anhedonia, which is the inability to derive pleasure from most activities.

People with dysthymia might be thought of as always seeing the glass as half empty.

Bipolar disorder, once called manic-depression, is characterized by a mood cycle that shifts from severe highs (mania) or mild highs (hypomania) to severe lows (depression).

During the manic phase, a person may experience abnormal or excessive elation, irritability, a decreased need for sleep, grandiose notions, increased talking, racing thoughts, increased sexual desire, markedly increased energy, poor judgment, and inappropriate social behavior.

During the depressive phase, a person experiences the same symptoms as would a sufferer of major depression. Mood swings from manic to depressive are often gradual, although occasionally they can occur abruptly.

Depression and Anxiety Disorders: Not the Same

Depression and anxiety disorders are different, but people with depression often experience symptoms similar to those of an anxiety disorder, such as nervousness, irritability, and problems sleeping and concentrating. But each disorder has its own causes and its own emotional and behavioral symptoms.

Many people who develop depression have a history of an anxiety disorder earlier in life. There is no evidence one disorder causes the other, but there is clear evidence that many people suffer from both disorders.

1. Barbee, J. G. (1998). Mixed symptoms and syndromes of anxiety and depression: Diagnostic, prognostic, and etiologic issues. *Annals of Clinical Psychiatry,* 10:15–29.

2. Regier, D. A., Rae, D. S., Narrow, W. E., Kaelber, C. T., & Schatzberg, A. F. (1998). Prevalence of anxiety disorders and their comorbidity with mood and addictive disorders. *British Journal of Psychiatry.* Supplement, 34: 24–28.

Section 26.2

Eating Disorders Frequently Coexist with Depression

Excerpted from "Eating Disorders," by the National Institute of Mental Health (NIMH, www.nimh.nih.gov), part of the National Institutes of Health, 2011.

What are eating disorders?

An eating disorder is an illness that causes serious disturbances to your everyday diet, such as eating extremely small amounts of food or severely overeating. A person with an eating disorder may have started out just eating smaller or larger amounts of food, but at some point, the urge to eat less or more spiraled out of control. Severe distress or concern about body weight or shape may also characterize an eating disorder.

Eating disorders frequently appear during the teen years or young adulthood but may also develop during childhood or later in life. Common eating disorders include anorexia nervosa, bulimia nervosa, and binge-eating disorder.

Eating disorders affect both men and women.

It is unknown how many adults and children suffer with other serious, significant eating disorders, including one category of eating disorders called eating disorders not otherwise specified (EDNOS). EDNOS includes eating disorders that do not meet the criteria for anorexia or bulimia nervosa.

Binge-eating disorder is a type of eating disorder called EDNOS. EDNOS is the most common diagnosis among people who seek treatment.

Eating disorders are real, treatable medical illnesses. They frequently coexist with other illnesses such as depression, substance abuse, or anxiety disorders.

Other symptoms can become life-threatening if a person does not receive treatment. People with anorexia nervosa are 18 times more likely to die early compared with people of similar age in the general population.

What are the different types of eating disorders?

Anorexia nervosa: Anorexia nervosa is characterized by the following:

- Extreme thinness (emaciation)

- A relentless pursuit of thinness and unwillingness to maintain a normal or healthy weight

- Intense fear of gaining weight

- Distorted body image, a self-esteem that is heavily influenced by perceptions of body weight and shape, or a denial of the seriousness of low body weight

- Lack of menstruation among girls and women

- Extremely restricted eating

Many people with anorexia nervosa see themselves as overweight, even when they are clearly underweight. Eating, food, and weight control become obsessions.

People with anorexia nervosa typically weigh themselves repeatedly, portion food carefully, and eat very small quantities of only certain foods. Some people with anorexia nervosa may also engage in binge eating followed by extreme dieting, excessive exercise, self-induced vomiting, and/or misuse of laxatives, diuretics, or enemas.

Some who have anorexia nervosa recover with treatment after only one episode. Others get well but have relapses. Still others have a more chronic, or long-lasting, form of anorexia nervosa, in which their health declines as they battle the illness.

Other symptoms may develop over time, including the following:

- Thinning of the bones (osteopenia or osteoporosis)

- Brittle hair and nails

- Dry and yellowish skin

- Growth of fine hair all over the body (lanugo)

- Mild anemia and muscle wasting and weakness

- Severe constipation

- Low blood pressure, slowed breathing, and pulse

- Damage to the structure and function of the heart

- Brain damage

- Multiorgan failure

- Drop in internal body temperature, causing a person to feel cold all the time

- Lethargy, sluggishness, or feeling tired all the time

- Infertility

Bulimia nervosa: Bulimia nervosa is characterized by recurrent and frequent episodes of eating unusually large amounts of food and feeling a lack of control over these episodes. This binge eating is followed by behavior that compensates for the overeating such as forced vomiting, excessive use of laxatives or diuretics, fasting, excessive exercise, or a combination of these behaviors.

Unlike anorexia nervosa, people with bulimia nervosa usually maintain what is considered a healthy or normal weight, while some are slightly overweight. But like people with anorexia nervosa, they often fear gaining weight, want desperately to lose weight, and are intensely unhappy with their body size and shape. Usually, bulimic behavior is done secretly because it is often accompanied by feelings of disgust or shame. The binge-eating and purging cycle happens anywhere from several times a week to many times a day.

Other symptoms include the following:

- Chronically inflamed and sore throat

- Swollen salivary glands in the neck and jaw area

- Worn tooth enamel and increasingly sensitive and decaying teeth as a result of exposure to stomach acid

- Acid reflux disorder and other gastrointestinal problems

- Intestinal distress and irritation from laxative abuse

- Severe dehydration from purging of fluids

- Electrolyte imbalance (too low or too high levels of sodium, calcium, potassium, and other minerals), which can lead to heart attack

Binge-eating disorder: With binge-eating disorder a person loses control over his or her eating. Unlike bulimia nervosa, periods of binge eating are not followed by purging, excessive exercise, or fasting. As a result, people with binge-eating disorder often are overweight or obese. People with binge-eating disorder who are obese are at higher risk for developing cardiovascular disease and high blood pressure. They also experience guilt, shame, and distress about their binge eating, which can lead to more binge eating.

How are eating disorders treated?

Adequate nutrition, reducing excessive exercise, and stopping purging behaviors are the foundations of treatment. Specific forms of psychotherapy, or talk therapy, and medication are effective for many eating disorders. However, in more chronic cases, specific treatments have not yet been identified. Treatment plans often are tailored to individual needs and may include one or more of the following:

- Individual, group, and/or family psychotherapy

- Medical care and monitoring

- Nutritional counseling

- Medications

Some patients may also need to be hospitalized to treat problems caused by malnutrition or to ensure they eat enough if they are very underweight.

How is anorexia nervosa treated?

Treating anorexia nervosa involves three components:

- Restoring the person to a healthy weight

- Treating the psychological issues related to the eating disorder

- Reducing or eliminating behaviors or thoughts that lead to insufficient eating and preventing relapse

Some research suggests that the use of medications, such as antidepressants, antipsychotics, or mood stabilizers, may be modestly effective in treating patients with anorexia nervosa. These medications may help resolve mood and anxiety symptoms that often occur along with anorexia nervosa. It is not clear whether antidepressants can prevent some weight-restored patients with anorexia nervosa from relapsing. Although research is still ongoing, no medication yet has shown to be effective in helping someone gain weight to reach a normal level.

Different forms of psychotherapy, including individual, group, and family based, can help address the psychological reasons for the illness. In a therapy called the Maudsley approach, parents of adolescents with anorexia nervosa assume responsibility for feeding their child. This approach appears to be very effective in helping people gain weight and improve eating habits and moods. Shown to be effective in case studies and clinical trials, the Maudsley approach is discussed in some guidelines and studies for treating eating disorders in younger, nonchronic patients.

Other research has found that a combined approach of medical attention and supportive psychotherapy designed specifically for anorexia nervosa patients is more effective than psychotherapy alone. The effectiveness of a treatment depends on the person involved and his or her situation. Unfortunately, no specific psychotherapy appears to be consistently effective for treating adults with anorexia nervosa. However, research into new treatment and prevention approaches is showing some promise. One study suggests that an online intervention program may prevent some at-risk women from developing an eating disorder. Also, specialized treatment of anorexia nervosa may help reduce the risk of death.

How is bulimia nervosa treated?

As with anorexia nervosa, treatment for bulimia nervosa often involves a combination of options and depends upon the needs of the individual. To reduce or eliminate binge eating and purging behaviors, a patient may undergo nutritional counseling and psychotherapy, especially cognitive behavioral therapy (CBT), or be prescribed medication. CBT helps a person focus on his or her current problems and how to solve them. The therapist helps the patient learn how to identify distorted or unhelpful thinking patterns, recognize, and change inaccurate beliefs, relate to others in more positive ways, and change behaviors accordingly.

CBT that is tailored to treat bulimia nervosa is effective in changing binge-eating and purging behaviors and eating attitudes. Therapy may be individual or group based.

Some antidepressants, such as fluoxetine (Prozac), which is the only medication approved by the U.S. Food and Drug Administration (FDA) for treating bulimia nervosa, may help patients who also have depression or anxiety. Fluoxetine also appears to help reduce binge-eating and purging behaviors, reduce the chance of relapse, and improve eating attitudes.

How is binge-eating disorder treated?

Treatment options for binge-eating disorder are similar to those used to treat bulimia nervosa. Psychotherapy, especially CBT that is tailored to the individual, has been shown to be effective. Again, this type of therapy can be offered in an individual or group environment.

Fluoxetine and other antidepressants may reduce binge-eating episodes and help lessen depression in some patients.

How are males affected?

Like females who have eating disorders, males also have a distorted sense of body image. For some, their symptoms are similar to those seen in females.

Others may have muscle dysmorphia, a type of disorder that is characterized by an extreme concern with becoming more muscular. Unlike girls with eating disorders, who mostly want to lose weight, some boys with muscle dysmorphia see themselves as smaller than they really are and want to gain weight or bulk up. Men and boys are more likely to use steroids or other dangerous drugs to increase muscle mass.

Although males with eating disorders exhibit the same signs and symptoms as females, they are less likely to be diagnosed with what is often considered a female disorder. More research is needed to understand the unique features of these disorders among males.

What is being done to better understand and treat eating disorders?

Researchers are finding that eating disorders are caused by a complex interaction of genetic, biological, behavioral, psychological, and social factors. But many questions still need answers. Researchers are using the latest in technology and science to better understand eating disorders.

One approach involves the study of human genes. Researchers are studying various combinations of genes to determine if any DNA variations are linked to the risk of developing eating disorders.

Neuroimaging studies are also providing a better understanding of eating disorders and possible treatments. One study showed different patterns of brain activity between women with bulimia nervosa and healthy women. Using functional magnetic resonance imaging (fMRI), researchers were able to see the differences in brain activity while the women performed a task that involved self-regulation (a task that requires overcoming an automatic or impulsive response).

Psychotherapy interventions are also being studied. One such study of adolescents found that more adolescents with bulimia nervosa recovered after receiving Maudsley model family-based treatment than those receiving supportive psychotherapy that did not specifically address the eating disorder.

Researchers are studying questions about behavior, genetics, and brain function to better understand risk factors, identify biological markers, and develop specific psychotherapies and medications that can target areas in the brain that control eating behavior. Neuroimaging and genetic studies may provide clues for how each person may respond to specific treatments for these medical illnesses.

Chapter 27

Depression, Substance Use, and Addiction

Chapter Contents

Section 27.1

Facts about Depression and Addiction

From "Facts about Addiction and Depression" by Hazelden
Foundation, Copyright 2007. Reprinted by permission of Hazelden
Foundation, Center City, MN.

Mental Health and Recovery

Individuals with untreated mental health issues may experience more difficulty in recovery. Sadness, despair, and depression are prevalent problems among alcoholics and addicts. It can be difficult to differentiate major depression from the emotional turbulence of addiction for any of the following reasons:

- Many drugs themselves are depressants, including alcohol, sedatives, and minor tranquilizers.

- Many symptoms of depression appear during withdrawal from drugs. For example, cocaine addicts typically experience a "crash" three to five days after their last use.

- Alcohol or drugs may provide a chemical cushion to ward off the emotional impact of everyday events. Without the drug, a person experiences feelings again and may think these feelings are not normal.

- The normal course of addiction may have brought about many tragedies (divorce, loss of custody of children) that cause intense, but normal, grief.

- Loss of relationship with the drug of choice can cause grief. Alcohol and other drugs often become a "best friend" that is always there to provide solace and relief.

Many symptoms of depression generally go away with abstinence from drugs and alcohol, and from utilizing the Twelve Steps to increase coping skills.

Prevalence of Depression

Most research suggests that the rate of major depression is two to four times higher among alcoholics and addicts than in the general population. About 30 to 40% of people seeking help for alcohol and drug problems suffer from major depression.

As in the general population, the rate of depression among female alcoholics and addicts is about twice as high as in males. When a person with alcohol or drug dependency has major depression, they require mental health treatment in addition to treatment for addiction.

Diagnosis of Depression

Careful diagnosis is critical. If you identify with these symptoms of depression, it is important that you have an assessment by a mental health professional that has expertise in alcohol and drug dependency.

Treatments Available

Typically depression for alcoholics and addicts is treated with psychotherapy and often antidepressants. Studies have demonstrated that antidepressant therapy is effective in reducing depression among alcoholics. The use of antidepressants is understood and supported by Alcoholics Anonymous. However, it is important that medication is just part of the treatment plan and does not replace the work of recovery. It is important to discuss medication options with a professional who has knowledge about substance abuse and dependency because some medications may be addictive.

Section 27.2

Depression and the Initiation of Cigarette, Alcohol, and Other Drug Use

Excerpted from "Depression and the Initiation of Cigarette, Alcohol, and Other Drug Use among Young Adults," by the Substance Abuse and Mental Health Services Administration (SAMHSA, www.oas.samhsa.gov), November 15, 2007.

Research has shown a strong association between mental disorders and substance use disorders. There is evidence that this linkage may be bidirectional: Depression may be associated with an escalation of substance use, and chronic substance abuse may be a factor in the development of depression.

The National Survey on Drug Use and Health (NSDUH) includes questions for adults aged 18 or older to assess lifetime and past year major depressive episode (MDE). For these estimates, MDE is defined using the diagnostic criteria set forth in the 4th edition of the *Diagnostic and Statistical Manual of Mental Disorders (DSM-IV)*, which specifies a period of 2 weeks or longer during which there is either depressed mood or loss of interest or pleasure and at least four other symptoms that reflect a change in functioning, such as problems with sleep, eating, energy, concentration, and self-image.

NSDUH also asks adults aged 18 or older to report on their use of cigarettes, alcohol, and illicit drugs in their lifetime and in the past year. Illicit drugs refer to marijuana/hashish, cocaine (including crack), inhalants, hallucinogens, heroin, or prescription-type drugs used nonmedically. Respondents who reported use of a given substance were asked how old they were when they first used it; responses to these questions were used to identify persons at risk for substance use initiation (i.e., persons who had never used the substance in their lifetime or used the substance for the first time within the 12 months preceding the survey) and to identify past year initiates (i.e., persons who used the substance for the first time in the 12 months prior to the survey).

This text examines past year MDE; past year initiation of cigarette, alcohol, and illicit drug use; and the association between MDE and the initiation of cigarette, alcohol, or other drug use in the past year among young adults aged 18 to 25. All findings presented in this report are based on combined 2005 and 2006 NSDUH data.

Past Year MDE

Combined data for 2005 and 2006 indicate that 9.4 percent of young adults aged 18 to 25 (3.0 million persons) experienced at least one MDE in the past year. Female young adults were nearly twice as likely as their male counterparts to have experienced a past year MDE (12.3 vs. 6.5 percent). Rates of past year MDE varied by racial/ethnic group, with the lowest rate among Asian young adults (6.1 percent) and the highest rate among those reporting two or more races (16.9 percent).

Initiation of Cigarette, Alcohol, and Illicit Drug Use in the Past Year

Combined data for 2005 and 2006 indicate that an estimated 943,000 adults aged 18 to 25 were past year initiates of cigarette use, which represents 8.0 percent of young adults who were at risk for initiating cigarette use. During that same period, 1.5 million young adults were past year initiates of alcohol use, representing 25.1 percent of young adults who were at risk for initiation of alcohol use. An estimated 870,000 young adults were past year initiates of illicit drug use, which represents 6.1 percent of young adults at risk for initiation of illicit drug use.

MDE and Substance Use Initiation in the Past Year

Among young adults aged 18 to 25 who had not previously used cigarettes, those who experienced a past year MDE were more likely to have initiated cigarette use in the past year than those who had not experienced a past year MDE (12.7 vs. 7.8 percent). Among young adults who had not previously used alcohol, those who experienced a past year MDE were more likely to have initiated alcohol use in the past year than those who had not experienced a past year MDE (33.7 vs. 24.8 percent). Similarly, among young adults aged 18 to 25 who had not previously used any illicit drug, those who experienced a past year MDE were twice as likely to have initiated use of any illicit drug in the past year as those who had not experienced a past year MDE (12.0 vs. 5.8 percent). This pattern was relatively consistent across specific drug types.

Section 27.3

Can Smoking Cause Depression?

Researchers have made bold claims about cigarette smoking leading to depression. It has long been known that smokers have higher rates of depression than nonsmokers, but researchers from the University of Otago in New Zealand investigated the link further, and say they have found a causal relationship.

The team took figures from over 1,000 men and women aged 18, 21, and 25 years. Smokers had more than twice the rate of depression. Using a computer modeling approach, their analysis supported a pathway in which nicotine addiction leads to increased risk of depression.

In the *British Journal of Psychiatry*, the researchers wrote, "The best-fitting causal model was one in which nicotine dependence led to increased risk of depression." They suggest two possible routes, one involving common risk factors, and the second a direct causal link.

According to the researchers, "this evidence is consistent with the conclusion that there is a cause and effect relationship between smoking and depression in which cigarette smoking increases the risk of symptoms of depression."

Professor David Fergusson, the study's lead researcher, said, "The reasons for this relationship are not clear. However, it's possible that nicotine causes changes to neurotransmitter activity in the brain, leading to an increased risk of depression." But he adds that the study "should be viewed as suggestive rather than definitive."

Writing in the same journal, Marcus Munafo, PhD, of Bristol University, United Kingdom, reports that cigarette smokers often talk about the antidepressant benefits of smoking. "But evidence suggests that cigarette smoking may itself increase negative affect [emotion], so the causal direction of this association remains unclear," he writes.

As Munafo points out, the role of nicotine in depression is complex, because smokers often feel emotionally uplifted following a cigarette. Bonnie Spring, PhD, at Hines Hospital, VA Medical Center, Illinois, looked at the link. Spring explains that depression-prone smokers are thought to self-administer nicotine to improve mood. But little evidence supports this view, so she examined nicotine's effect on depression.

Her team recruited 63 regular smokers with no history of diagnosed depression, 61 with past but not current depression, and 41 with both current and past depression. All were given either a "nicotinized" or a "denicotinized" cigarette following a positive mood trigger.

Those who had experienced depression showed an enhanced response to the positive mood trigger when smoking a nicotinized cigarette. The researchers wrote, "Self-administering nicotine appears to improve depression-prone smokers' emotional response to a pleasant stimulus." The reason for this effect is not clear.

This study was followed up in 2010 by scientists at the University of Pittsburgh. Kenneth A. Perkins, PhD, and colleagues looked at whether smoking can improve a negative mood.

Again using nicotinized and denicotinized cigarettes, they found that smokers do feel better after a cigarette, but only when they haven't smoked since the previous day. The improved mood after abstinence from smoking was a "robust" finding. However, cigarettes "only modestly" improved negative mood due to other sources of stress—in this case, a challenging computer task, preparing for a public speech, and watching negative mood slides.

The researchers say that relief from negative mood due to smoking depends on the situation rather than nicotine intake: "These results challenge the common assumption that smoking, and nicotine in particular, broadly alleviates negative affect."

One major factor must be the smoker's expectations. These were investigated by a team at the University of Montana. They write, "Expectancies about nicotine's ability to alleviate negative mood states may play a role in the relationship between smoking and depression."

They asked 315 undergraduate smokers to complete a survey, which supported the theory. Smokers believed that "higher levels of tobacco smoking will reduce negative emotions." This expectation "fully explained the link relationship between depressive symptoms and smoking," the researchers said.

Could the link between tobacco smoking and depression actually be due to other substance dependencies? A team from Switzerland thinks not. After surveying 1,849 men and women they found that alcohol and cocaine dependence were also significantly linked to depression. But when taking this into account, "the association between smoking and depression still remained statistically significant. This study adds support to the evidence that smoking is linked to depression," they concluded.

So it seems that the evidence is stacked against nicotine as a mood lifter, despite widely-held beliefs to the contrary.

References

Boden, J.M., Fergusson, D. M., and Horwood, L. J. Cigarette smoking and depression: Tests of causal linkages using a longitudinal birth cohort. *The British Journal of Psychiatry*, Vol. 196, June 2010, pp. 440–46.

Munafo, M. R. and Araya, R. Editorial: Cigarette smoking and depression: A question of causation. *The British Journal of Psychiatry*, Vol. 196, June 2010, pp. 425–26.

Spring, B. et al. Nicotine effects on affective response in depression-prone smokers. *Psychopharmacology*, Vol. 196, February 2008, pp. 461–71.

Schleicher, H. E. et al. The role of depression and negative affect regulation expectancies in tobacco smoking among college students. *The Journal of American College Health*, Vol. 57, March-April 2009, pp. 507–12.

Perkins, K. A. et al. Acute negative affect relief from smoking depends on the affect situation and measure but not on nicotine. *Biological Psychiatry*, Vol. 67, April 2010, pp. 707–14.

Wiesbeck, G. A. et al. Tobacco smoking and depression—results from the WHO/ISBRA study. *Neuropsychobiology*, Vol. 57, April 18, 2008, pp. 26–31.

Chapter 28

Other Depression Risk Factors

Chapter Contents

Section 28.1

Excessive Use of Internet Predicts Later Depression

Could excessive use of the internet mean teenagers are more likely to be depressed later in life?

According to new research, teens who spend an unreasonable amount of time on the internet could be at increased risk of depression.

"Young people who are initially free of mental health problems but use the internet pathologically could develop depression as a consequence," according to Dr. Lawrence T. Lam of the School of Medicine in Sydney and Zi-Wen Peng, MSc, of the Ministry of Education in Guangzhou, China.

Pathological use of the internet (uncontrolled or unreasonable use), commonly known as internet addiction, has become a widely discussed issue over the last several decades. Internet addiction is not an officially recognized diagnosis, but some have suggested it could affect up to one percent of the population.

Many research studies have shown that other psychological problems, such as depression, anxiety, social anxiety disorder, relationship problems, poor physical health, aggressive behavior, alcohol abuse, and ADHD [attention deficit hyperactivity disorder] occur at the same time as internet addiction.

Lam studied 1,041 teens aged 13 to 18 from high schools in Guangzhou, China, and measured internet use with the Pathological Use of the Internet Test (including questions such as "How often do you feel depressed, moody, or nervous when you are offline, which goes away once you are back online?"). Participants were also screened for depression and anxiety using the Zung Depression and Anxiety Scales, and after nine months, the teens were reassessed. Six point two percent of the teenagers (62 participants) were considered to have moderately pathological use of the internet at the beginning of the study, and 0.2 percent (2) were classified as high risk.

After nine months, when the teens were screened for anxiety and depression, 0.2 percent had symptoms of anxiety, and 8.4 percent had symptoms of depression.

The teens who had problematic use of the internet at baseline had two and a half times the rate of depression when assessed nine months later. No relationship was observed between pathological internet use and anxiety.

Those assessed as using the internet pathologically were also more likely to use it for entertainment purposes rather than for information.

Most prior studies on internet addiction have focused on association between current internet behaviors and mental health issues. That is, when both problems co-exist, it can be difficult to determine whether overuse of the internet leads to mental health problems, or if psychological problems cause internet addiction. These results are useful in suggesting that in some cases, misuse of the internet may precede mental health problems.

"Pathological use of the internet is predictive of depression at the nine-month followup," writes Lam. "This study has demonstrated a chronological sequence between pathological use of the internet and depression in healthy adolescents."

Dr. Lam's results can be found in the August online issue of the *Archives of Pediatric and Adolescent Medicine*.

Source: *Archives of Pediatric and Adolescent Medicine*

Section 28.2

Green Space Influences Depression and Anxiety

A new study documents that people living close to green space have lower rates of anxiety, depression, and poor physical health than those living in the concrete jungle.

The research, published in the [December 2009] *Journal of Epidemiology and Community Health* is based on the health records of people registered with 195 family doctors in 95 practices across the Netherlands. Between them, the practices serve a population of almost 350,000.

The percentages of green space within a 1- and 3-kilometer (roughly half a mile to 2-mile) radius of their home were calculated using the household's postcode. On average, green space accounted for 42 percent of the residential area within a 1-kilometer radius and almost 61 percent within a 3-kilometer radius of people's homes.

Green space within a kilometer radius of an individual's home had the most impact on rates of ill health.

The annual rates of 15 of 24 different disease clusters, categorized as cardiovascular disease, musculoskeletal disorders, mental ill health, respiratory disease, neurological disease, digestive disease, and miscellaneous complaints were significantly lower among those living close to more extensive areas of green space.

The impact was especially noticeable on rates of mental ill health. The annual prevalence of anxiety disorders among those living in a residential area containing 10 percent of green space within a 1-kilometer radius of their home was 26 per 1000, and for those living in an area containing 90 percent of green space it was 18 per 1000. Similarly, the figures for depression were, respectively, 32 and 24 per 1000 of the population.

The association was strongest for those who spent a lot of time in the vicinity—children and those with low levels of education and income—as well as those between the ages of 45 and 65. Exactly how the provision of green space affects health is not clear, but it may indicate better air quality as well as offering opportunities for relaxation, destressing, socializing, and exercise, suggest the authors.

"This study shows that the role of green space in the living environment for health should not be underestimated," they conclude, adding that many of the diseases and disorders on which green space seems to exert a positive influence are common and costly to treat.

Source: *The Journal of Epidemiology and Community Health*

Part Five

Depression and Chronic Illness

Chapter 29

Chronic Illness, Pain, and Depression

Chapter Contents

Section 29.1

Chronic Illness Related to Increased Symptoms of Depression

"Depression and Chronic Illness," © 2011 NAMI, the National Alliance
on Mental Illness, www.nami.org. Reprinted with permission.

Chronic (long-term) illness is related to increased symptoms of
depression. Examples of chronic illness include:

- heart disease;
- multiple sclerosis;
- cancer;
- chronic pain syndrome.

- Parkinson's disease;
- stroke;
- diabetes;

Depression should not be dismissed as a "normal" reaction to chronic
illness, but it is common. Depression is a problem for 15–25 percent of
cancer patients. One study found that one-third of patients with advanced
cancer and one-fifth with terminal cancer experience a depressive disorder. Sadly, less than half of those receive treatment for depression.

Facing a chronic illness naturally leads to feelings of uncertainty,
grief, sadness, anger, or fear. But when these feelings continue and
disrupt quality of life and day-to-day functioning, depression may be
the culprit. Both physical effects of illness and behavioral reactions
contribute to this risk.

Behavioral reactions during chronic illness associated with depression include:

- decreased adherence to treatment;
- being more likely to smoke and drink;
- lack of physical activity;
- poor eating habits.

Because of these behaviors, the effects of chronic illness and prospects of recovery may worsen.

When symptoms of depression are present alongside symptoms of chronic illness, it is necessary to treat both—not just the symptoms of chronic illness. The treatment is similar to the recommended treatment for other people with depression. Persons with depression should seek treatment as soon as depressive symptoms appear because early treatment is more likely to be effective.

Coping

- To cope with a chronic illness and depression, the first step is acceptance of the condition. Before depression and chronic illness can be treated, both must be accepted at least to a basic degree.

- Support groups can be a valuable way to fight depression. NAMI state and local affiliates offer several support and education programs for those with mental illness. (http://www.nami.org/Template.cfm?section=Find_Support) NAMI Connection recovery support groups are available in many communities across the country. A support group of others living with chronic conditions may also be helpful.

- Learn about your condition so that you can better manage it. Don't be afraid to ask for help. If you believe your medication is causing your depression, speak with your doctor about alternative treatments. If you are in chronic pain, speak with your doctor about alternative medications or strategies to address that concern.

- If possible, try to remain involved in the activities you've always enjoyed or learn new skills.

- Maintain a daily routine as best you can. Chronic illness is manageable and can be integrated into your life.

- Keep your support network active. Whether it is friends, family, church, golf, or another activity, connections to others are helpful to fight depression and isolation.

- Take proper care of yourself. Eating right, exercising, and quitting smoking and drinking can reduce the risk of depression and reduce negative effects of chronic illness.

For more information on coping with chronic illness: http://www.cc.nih.gov/ccc/patient_education/pepubs/copechron.pdf.

267

Section 29.2

Chronic Pain and Mental Health

From "Chronic Pain and PTSD: A Guide for Patients," by the National Center for Posttraumatic Stress Disorder (NCPTSD, www.ptsd.va.gov), part of the Veterans Administration, June 15, 2010.

What is chronic pain?

Chronic pain is when a person suffers from pain in a particular area of the body (for example, in the back or the neck) for at least three to six months. It may be as bad as, or even worse than, short-term pain, but it can feel like more of a problem because it lasts a longer time. Chronic pain lasts beyond the normal amount of time that an injury takes to heal.

Chronic pain can come from many things. Some people get chronic pain from normal wear and tear of the body or from aging. Others have chronic pain from various types of cancer, or other chronic medical illnesses. In some cases the chronic pain may be from an injury that happened during an accident or an assault. Some chronic pain has no explanation.

How common is chronic pain?

Approximately one in three Americans suffer from some kind of chronic pain in their lifetimes, and about one quarter of them are not able to do day-to-day activities because of their chronic pain. Between 80% and 90% of Americans experience chronic problems in the neck or lower back.

How do health care providers evaluate pain?

Care providers generally assess chronic pain during a physical exam, but how much pain someone is in is hard to determine. Every person is different and perceives and experiences pain in different ways. There is often very little consistency when different doctors try to measure a patient's pain. Sometimes the care provider may not believe the patient, or might minimize the amount of pain. All of these things can be frustrating for the person in pain. Additionally, this kind of experience often makes patients feel helplessness and hopeless, which in turn increases tension and pain and makes the person more upset. Conversation between the doctor and patient is important, including sharing information about treatment options. If no progress is made, get a second opinion.

What is the experience of chronic pain like physically?

There are many forms of chronic pain, including pain felt in the low back (most common); the neck; the mouth, face, and jaw; the pelvis; or the head (e.g., tension and migraine headaches). Of course, each type of condition results in different experiences of pain.

People with chronic pain are less able to function well in daily life than those who do not suffer from chronic pain. They may have trouble with things such as walking, standing, sitting, lifting light objects, doing paperwork, standing in line at a grocery store, going shopping, or working. Many patients with chronic pain cannot work because of their pain or physical limitations.

What is the experience of chronic pain like psychologically?

Research has shown that many patients who experience chronic pain (up to 100% of these patients) tend to also be diagnosed with depression. Because the pain and disability are always there and that may even become worse over time, many of them think suicide is the only way to end their pain and frustration. They think they have no control over their life. This frustration may also lead the person to use drugs or have unneeded surgery.

What is the connection between chronic pain and trauma?

Some people's chronic pain stems from a traumatic event, such as a physical or sexual assault, a motor vehicle accident, or some type of disaster. Under these circumstances the person may experience both chronic pain and PTSD [posttraumatic stress disorder]. The person in pain may not even realize the connection between their pain and a traumatic event. Approximately 15% to 35% of patients with chronic pain also have PTSD. Only 2% of people who do not have chronic pain have PTSD. One study found that 51% of patients with chronic low back pain had PTSD symptoms. For people with chronic pain, the pain may actually serve as a reminder of the traumatic event, which will tend to make the PTSD even worse. Survivors of physical, psychological, or sexual abuse tend to be more at risk for developing certain types of chronic pain later in their lives.

Chapter 30

Depression and Autoimmune Diseases

Chapter Contents

Section 30.1

Depression Often Coexists with Fibromyalgia

Excerpted from "Questions and Answers about Fibromyalgia," by the National Institute of Arthritis and Musculoskeletal and Skin Disorders (NIAMS, www.niams.nih.gov), part of the National Institutes of Health, July 2011.

Fibromyalgia syndrome is a common and chronic disorder characterized by widespread pain, diffuse tenderness, and a number of other symptoms. The word fibromyalgia comes from the Latin term for fibrous tissue (fibro) and the Greek ones for muscle (myo) and pain (algia).

Although fibromyalgia is often considered an arthritis-related condition, it is not truly a form of arthritis (a disease of the joints) because it does not cause inflammation or damage to the joints, muscles, or other tissues. Like arthritis, however, fibromyalgia can cause significant pain and fatigue, and it can interfere with a person's ability to carry on daily activities. Also like arthritis, fibromyalgia is considered a rheumatic condition, a medical condition that impairs the joints and/ or soft tissues and causes chronic pain.

In addition to pain and fatigue, people who have fibromyalgia may experience a variety of other symptoms including the following:

- Cognitive and memory problems (sometimes referred to as fibro fog)
- Sleep disturbances
- Morning stiffness
- Headaches
- Irritable bowel syndrome
- Painful menstrual periods
- Numbness or tingling of the extremities
- Restless legs syndrome
- Temperature sensitivity
- Sensitivity to loud noises or bright lights

Fibromyalgia is a syndrome rather than a disease. A syndrome is a collection of signs, symptoms, and medical problems that tend to occur together but are not related to a specific, identifiable cause. A disease, on the other hand, has a specific cause or causes and recognizable signs and symptoms.

A person may have two or more coexisting chronic pain conditions. Such conditions can include chronic fatigue syndrome, endometriosis, fibromyalgia, inflammatory bowel disease, interstitial cystitis, temporomandibular joint dysfunction, and vulvodynia. It is not known whether these disorders share a common cause.

How Is Fibromyalgia Treated?

Fibromyalgia can be difficult to treat. Not all doctors are familiar with fibromyalgia and its treatment, so it is important to find a doctor who is. Many family physicians, general internists, or rheumatologists (doctors who specialize in arthritis and other conditions that affect the joints or soft tissues) can treat fibromyalgia.

Fibromyalgia treatment often requires a team approach, with your doctor, a physical therapist, possibly other health professionals, and most importantly, yourself, all playing an active role. It can be hard to assemble this team, and you may struggle to find the right professionals to treat you. When you do, however, the combined expertise of these various professionals can help you improve your quality of life.

You may find several members of the treatment team you need at a clinic. There are pain clinics that specialize in pain and rheumatology clinics that specialize in arthritis and other rheumatic diseases, including fibromyalgia.

Only three medications, duloxetine (Cymbalta), milnacipran (Savella), and pregabalin (Lyrica) are approved by the U.S. Food and Drug Administration (FDA) for the treatment of fibromyalgia. Cymbalta was originally developed for and is still used to treat depression. Savella is similar to a drug used to treat depression, but is FDA approved only for fibromyalgia. Lyrica is a medication developed to treat neuropathic pain (chronic pain caused by damage to the nervous system).

Fibromyalgia and Antidepressants

Perhaps the most useful medications for fibromyalgia are several in the antidepressant class. These drugs work equally well in fibromyalgia patients with and without depression, because antidepressants elevate the levels of certain chemicals in the brain (including serotonin

273

and norepinephrine) that are associated not only with depression, but also with pain and fatigue. Increasing the levels of these chemicals can reduce pain in people who have fibromyalgia. Doctors prescribe several types of antidepressants for people with fibromyalgia.

Tricyclic antidepressants: When taken at bedtime in dosages lower than those used to treat depression, tricyclic antidepressants can help promote restorative sleep in people with fibromyalgia. They also can relax painful muscles and heighten the effects of the body's natural pain-killing substances called endorphins. Tricyclic antidepressants have been around for almost half a century. Some examples of tricyclic medications used to treat fibromyalgia include amitriptyline hydrochloride (Elavil, Endep), cyclobenzaprine (Cycloflex, Flexeril, Flexiban), doxepin (Adapin, Sinequan), and nortriptyline (Aventyl, Pamelor). Both amitriptyline and cyclobenzaprine have been proven useful for the treatment of fibromyalgia.

Selective serotonin reuptake inhibitors: If a tricyclic antidepressant fails to bring relief, doctors sometimes prescribe a newer type of antidepressant called a selective serotonin reuptake inhibitor (SSRI). As with tricyclics, doctors usually prescribe these for people with fibromyalgia in lower dosages than are used to treat depression. By promoting the release of serotonin, these drugs may reduce fatigue and some other symptoms associated with fibromyalgia. The group of SSRIs includes fluoxetine (Prozac), paroxetine (Paxil), and sertraline (Zoloft). Newer SSRIs such as citalopram (Celexa) or escitalopram (Lexapro) do not seem to work as well for pain as the older SSRIs. SSRIs may be prescribed along with a tricyclic antidepressant. Studies have shown that a combination therapy of the tricyclic amitriptyline and the SSRI fluoxetine resulted in greater improvements in the study participants' fibromyalgia symptoms than either drug alone.

Mixed reuptake inhibitors: Some newer antidepressants raise levels of both serotonin and norepinephrine and are therefore called mixed reuptake inhibitors. Examples of these medications include venlafaxine (Effexor) and duloxetine (Cymbalta). In general, these drugs work better for pain than SSRIs, probably because they also raise norepinephrine, which may play an even greater role in pain transmission than serotonin.

Section 30.2

Tests Prove Fibromyalgia Is Not Depression

Fibromyalgia can be distinguished from depression, according to a 2010 study by researchers at the University of Sherbrooke in Canada.

People with fibromyalgia not only have widespread pain, a large percentage also battle depression. This has led some investigators to argue that fibromyalgia might represent a form of depression, but pain system function tests prove otherwise.

The Canadian research team evaluated three groups of subjects: 40 healthy controls, 26 depressed patients, and 29 fibromyalgia patients. All participants were asked to determine when a heat probe changed from a warm sensation to pain.

The ability of the body to reduce the impact of pain was also measured. Prior studies by the corresponding author Serge Marchand, a professor in the department of surgery at the University of Sherbrooke in Canada, have shown that the body's natural ability to inhibit pain in fibromyalgia patients does not work. When the body is subjected to a lot of discomfort, the central nervous system should pour out pain relieving substances. This does not happen in people with fibromyalgia, but what about those with depression?

The temperature that healthy subjects rated the heat probe as painful was much higher than the ratings for fibromyalgia patients. The depressed subjects fell in between these two groups, so they do have some evidence of increased pain sensitivity.

Looking at the system that helps keep pain under control, the healthy and depressed groups both produced a similar response that led to pain relief. This same system did not work at all in the fibromyalgia patients.

According to Marchand, "this result shows that fibromyalgia can be distinguished from major depressive disorder." The system in the body that helps block out pain works efficiently in depressed patients,

275

but fails to function in people with fibromyalgia.

Fibromyalgia patients often struggle with symptoms of depression, and depressed patients report various pain complaints, such as headaches and back pain. Marchand suspects this overlap in symptoms may be related to the increased pain sensitivity in both groups. Despite this similarity, he emphasizes that the fibromyalgia patients were significantly more heat sensitive.

Source: Normand E, et al. "Pain Inhibition Is Deficient in Chronic Widespread Pain but Normal in Major Depressive Disorder" *Journal of Clinical Psychiatry* 2010; DOI: 10.4088/JCP.08m04969blu.

Section 30.3

Depression and Lupus

It is normal to experience feelings of unhappiness, frustration, anger, or sadness when you live with a chronic illness such as lupus. Life with lupus—with symptoms that come and go, disease flares and remissions, and the uncertainty of what each day will bring—can be difficult and challenging. And it is normal to grieve for the loss of the life you had before lupus. As you learn more about lupus, and how to adjust and adapt to necessary life changes, these sorts of negative feelings will lessen.

Sometimes, though, negative feelings can become overwhelming and long-lasting. How do you know if and when to seek professional help for these feelings? In this text, we will try to help you understand the difference between temporary mood swings and long-lasting feelings that signal a more serious illness, called clinical depression.

Clinical depression may not be recognized in people with lupus because its symptoms and the symptoms of active lupus can be so similar. For example, lack of energy, trouble sleeping, and diminished sexual interest can be attributed to the lupus itself. However, these are also symptoms of clinical depression.

Facts about Clinical Depression and Lupus

- Between 15 and 60 percent of people with a chronic illness will experience clinical depression.

- Clinical depression may be a result of the ways in which lupus physically affects your body.

- Some of the medicines to treat lupus—especially corticosteroids such as prednisone (and at higher doses of 20 mg or more)—play a role in causing clinical depression.

- Clinical depression may be a result of the continuous series of emotional and psychological stressors associated with living with a chronic illness.

- Clinical depression may be a result of neurologic problems or experiences unrelated to lupus.

- Clinical depression also produces anxiety, which may aggravate physical symptoms (headache, stomach pain, etc.).

- Two common feelings associated with clinical depression are hopelessness and helplessness. People who feel hopeless believe that their distressing symptoms may never improve. People who feel helpless believe they are beyond help—that no one cares enough to help them or could succeed in helping, even if they tried.

Symptoms

People are considered to be clinically depressed when they have a depressed or irritable mood, decreased energy, and other symptoms in the following list that last for more than a few weeks and are severe enough to disrupt daily life. Probably the best single marker for clinical depression is loss of interest in activities and responsibilities that used to be important. For example, if you find yourself saying, "I used to enjoy gardening, cooking, and going to church. I don't feel like doing any of those things anymore."

Clinical depression may be brought about by the lupus itself, by the various medications used to treat lupus, and/or by any of the factors and forces in a person's life that are not related to lupus. For reasons that are not entirely understood, this type of depression is often experienced by people with chronic disease. There is good news, however. If recognized and properly treated, you can recover from clinical depression.

Psychological and Physical Symptoms of Clinical Depression

- Feelings of helplessness or hopelessness
- Sadness
- Crying (often without reason)
- Insomnia or restless sleep, or sleeping too much
- Changes in appetite leading to weight loss or weight gain
- Feelings of uneasiness, anxiety, or irritability
- Feelings of guilt or regret
- Lowered self-esteem or feelings of worthlessness
- Inability to concentrate or difficulty thinking
- Diminished memory and recall
- Indecisiveness
- Lack of interest in things formerly enjoyed
- Lack of energy
- General slowing and clouding of mental functions
- Diminished sexual interest and/or performance
- Recurrent thoughts of death or suicide

Causes

A variety of factors can contribute to clinical depression in people with chronic illnesses. The most common cause is the emotional drain from the stress of coping with the complications of physical illness. Add to that economic, social, and workplace concerns. Various medications used to treat lupus—especially corticosteroids—may cause clinical depression. When certain organs or organ systems are affected by lupus (such as the brain, heart, or kidneys), clinical depression may occur. A flare of lupus also can trigger clinical depression, both because you feel ill, and because it may seem as though you are never going to be free of lupus.

What Can You Do?

Clinical depression generally improves with a combination of psychotherapy and medication.

- **Seek psychotherapy.** You should not feel embarrassed or hesitant about asking your doctor for a referral to a psychiatrist or psychologist. Psychotherapy, under the guidance of a trained professional, can help you learn to understand your feelings, your illness, and your relationships, and to cope more effectively with stress. Cognitive behavioral therapy—a special type of psychotherapy—can be very helpful when you are living with chronic illness. Support groups led by a therapist or trained counselor, such as those organized by the LFA network, also can be instrumental in helping you deal with symptoms of clinical depression. To find a group in your area, go to lupus.org/chapters or call toll-free 800-558-0121.

- **Take antidepressant medications.** Several classes of prescribed drugs can help ease the effects of clinical depression. Anti-anxiety medicines are also available to reduce worry and fearful feelings. These improvements can occur in a matter of weeks in some people once medication is started.

- **Find ways to reduce pain.** Chronic pain can be a factor in the development of clinical depression. Besides medication (which can also play a role in clinical depression), experts often recommend non-medication ways to conquer—or at least reduce—chronic pain, such as yoga, tai chi, Pilates, acupuncture, biofeedback, meditation, behavioral changes, play therapy, and chiropractic care. You may be considering over-the-counter treatments for your depression and/or pain. It is important to remember that all herbs and supplements should be discussed with your rheumatologist or primary care provider before you try them, as certain ingredients can cause reactions with your prescribed medications.

- **Improve your sleep habits.** Not getting enough sleep can cause many health problems, including symptoms of clinical depression. To improve your sleep, and, in turn, your mental well-being, try to:

  - Get seven to eight hours of sleep in a 24-hour period.

  - Do aerobic exercise every day, such as brisk walking—or whatever you can manage.

  - Avoid caffeine, nicotine, and alcohol several hours before bedtime.

  - Know which medications keep you from sleeping and take those early in the day.

  - Have a good mattress, comfortable bed linens, the right room temperature, and the right amount of darkness.

  - Include rest periods throughout your day when needed.

If you still aren't getting enough sleep, find a reputable sleep center and talk to your doctor about sleep medications.

Build a support system. Stay in touch with family members, former work buddies, or long-time friends. Make phone calls, join Facebook, or try videoconferencing.

Better Love Life

Some antidepressants may dampen the libido. But often, the bigger roadblock to a happy love life is depression itself. One study showed that 70 percent of people with depression reported a loss of sexual interest while not taking medicine. Treatment may help restore your self-confidence and strengthen your emotional connection with your partner.

Pain Relief

Treatment for your depression can make you feel better emotionally and may reduce pain. That's because depression can contribute to the discomfort of pain. Studies have found that people who have conditions like arthritis and migraines actually feel more pain—and are more disabled by it—if they're depressed. Seeking treatment may help provide relief.

Improved Health

If you are depressed, getting treatment may help prevent some serious diseases down the road. That's because depression can take a toll on your body. One study found that women who were depressed had double the risk of sudden cardiac death than women who weren't. Getting treatment may help lessen health risks.

Better Performance at Work

Depression can make it hard to hold a job. If you're depressed, you might lose focus at work and make more mistakes. If you think depression might be affecting you at work, getting help now could head off serious problems.

Sharper Thinking and Better Memory

Feeling forgetful? Does your thinking seem fuzzy? Experts have found that depression might cause structural changes to the areas of the brain involved in memory and decision-making.

The good news is that depression treatment may prevent or reverse these changes—clearing away the cobwebs and strengthening your recall.

Happier Home Life

Irritable and angry? Constantly snapping at your kids—and then feeling bad about it? Getting depression treatment can help boost your mood. And that can help reduce tension around the house and improve your relationship with your family.

Healthier Lifestyle

Why does depression cause some people to gain weight? In part, it's behavioral—you may withdraw and become less active, or turn to food for comfort. It's also physiological—low levels of certain brain chemicals can trigger a craving for carbs. Getting treatment may change that while giving you the energy to exercise and eat well.

Less Chaos, More Control

When depression zaps your energy, even the most basic tasks—like vacuuming or paying the bills—can become impossibly hard. The more chaotic things get, the less capable you feel. Depression treatment can restore the energy you need to take control of your life and get it organized.

Lower Risk of Future Depression

People who have been depressed have a higher risk of becoming depressed again. But ongoing therapy or medication may help prevent depression from coming back. Even if it does return, treatment now will prepare you. You'll know the early signs. You'll know some coping skills. And you'll know where to get help.

Stronger Ties with Friends and Family

Treating depression may improve your social life. Depression isolates people. It can sap your self-esteem, making you feel unlikeable. While therapy and medication can help restore some of that lost confidence, you still need to decide to reach out. Reconnecting to old friends when you're depressed—not to mention making new ones—is hard. But it's a crucial part of getting better.

Getting Help

Some people with depression try to wait it out, hoping it will get better on its own without treatment. That's a mistake. Studies have found that the longer depression lasts, the worse your symptoms may get and the harder it is to treat.

- See your doctor. Schedule an appointment with a therapist. The sooner you get help, the better your odds for a healthy future.

- Change your self-talk. Feelings of anger and self-pity can bring on unproductive thoughts; for example, "It's not fair. I haven't done anything wrong. Why me?" "I'm too weak even to fight off this illness." Replace negative, self-defeating inner language with truthful, productive thoughts, such as: "I feel lousy, but I have many blessings."

- You can also list the people and things in your life for which you are grateful: A loving spouse or significant other; your children, and the children of your extended family; caring relatives; good friends; a beloved pet; work or hobbies you enjoy and are able to do; a home you love; volunteer activities; fellowship at school, at a place of worship, or at a community center. Try to add to this list every day!

- Discover the values of volunteerism. Volunteerism can provide real emotional benefits. Helping with a charitable cause that is meaningful to you can create social, supportive connections. Helping others can have a positive impact on your sense of well-being.

- Strive to accept the new "you." Pace yourself, and don't feel badly about delegating some of your responsibilities. Ask for help, and accept help graciously. Finally, focus on what you have, not on what you don't have, and on what you can do, rather than what you can't do.

Conclusion

Just as clinical depression develops over time and not overnight, conquering clinical depression is a gradual process. However, most people with lupus find that, in time, their overall attitude and sense of well-being are greatly improved.

You will also find helpful suggestions for living well with lupus in the LFA Patient Education Series fact sheets, Living with Lupus and Coping with Lupus, and on the LFA website, lupus.org.

Chapter 31

Depression and Brain Injury

What is traumatic brain injury?

Traumatic brain injury (TBI) is the medical term for when your brain is injured by some force, such as:

- a direct hit to your head by an object;
- a fall to the ground or a hard surface;
- a car, motorcycle, or bike crash; or
- an explosion or a blast very close to your head.

Doctors can tell whether your injury is mild, moderate, or severe based on what happened at the time of your injury (if you were knocked out, if you had trouble seeing clearly, or lost some memory) and by other tests. Around 1.5 million people who are not in the military experience some form of TBI each year in the United States. It is likely that more people are affected, because many people with mild TBI do not go to the emergency room or report their injury.

Most TBI cases (75 percent) are mild.

Any injury to your brain—even if it is mild—can cause problems such as headaches, ringing in your ears, mood changes, or trouble remembering or thinking for long periods of time. You may have found that your sleeping habits are different or that you feel tired more often.

Excerpted from "Depression After Brain Injury: A Guide for Patients and Their Caregivers," by the Agency for Healthcare Research and Quality (AHRQ, www.effectivehealthcare.ahrq.gov), April 2011.

Even several months or years after your brain injury, you may notice other difficulties, including depression or anxiety.

What is depression?

Depression is more than feeling sad every now and then. It is normal for someone who has had a TBI to feel sad by the problems caused by this injury. But for some people, those feelings can extend beyond normal feelings of sadness. People with depression feel sad, lack energy or feel tired, or have difficulty enjoying routine events almost daily. Other symptoms include difficulty sleeping, loss of appetite, poor attention or concentration, feelings of guilt or worthlessness, or thoughts of suicide.

Depression is a serious but treatable problem that should not be ignored. Many people require some form of treatment by a doctor or other health care professional to relieve their depression.

How common is depression for people with TBI?

Research has found that patients with TBI are more likely to experience depression than those who have not had a brain injury.

For every 10 people who do not have a brain injury, approximately one person will have depression.

For every 10 people who do have a brain injury, approximately three people will have depression.

What increases my risk of depression?

The risk of depression after a TBI increases whether the injury is mild, moderate, or severe. Researchers cannot say if age, gender, the part of the brain that was injured, or the type of injury makes depression more likely.

How soon after my injury might I become depressed?

Researchers do not know when depression is most likely to occur after TBI. Some people experience depression right after their injury, whereas others develop depression a year or more later. It is important to tell your doctor about any symptoms of depression you may be having even if it has been a while since your head injury. Your doctor or health care professional will ask you a series of questions or have you fill out a questionnaire or form to see if you have depression.

How can I tell if I am depressed?

There are ways to tell if you are depressed:

- Feeling down, depressed, or sad most of the day
- Changes in your sleeping habits, such as sleeping poorly or sleeping more than usual
- Losing interest in usual activities such as favorite hobbies, time with family members, or activities with friends
- Increasing your use of alcohol, drugs, or tobacco
- Not eating as much or eating more, whether or not you are hungry
- Strong feelings of sadness, despair, or hopelessness
- Thoughts of suicide

You may not notice some of these symptoms, but people living and working around you may see them. You may want to ask the people close to you if they notice these signs in you.

What should I do if these symptoms start to occur?

Tell your doctor or health care professional as soon as you or others around you notice any symptoms.

When should I talk to my health care professional?

It is important that you contact your health care professional when you experience the following:

- Changes in sleeping or eating habits
- Frequent feelings of sadness, hopelessness, anxiety, or panic
- Disinterest in your favorite activities
- Thoughts about suicide

Here are some questions you may want to ask your health care professional if you are going to be treated for depression or anxiety following your brain injury:

- How often should we check to see if I am developing depression or an anxiety disorder?
- How long do you think I will need psychotherapy or medications to treat these problems?

Chapter 32

Depression and Cancer

Depression is a disabling illness that affects about 15% to 25% of cancer patients. It affects men and women with cancer equally. People who face a diagnosis of cancer will experience different levels of stress and emotional upset. Important issues in the life of any person with cancer may include the following:

- Fear of death
- Interruption of life plans
- Changes in body image and self-esteem
- Changes in social role and lifestyle
- Money and legal concerns

Everyone who is diagnosed with cancer will react to these issues in different ways and may not experience serious depression or anxiety.

Palliative care begins at diagnosis and continues throughout the patient's cancer care. Patients who are receiving palliative care for cancer during the last 6 months of life may have frequent feelings of depression and anxiety, leading to a much lower quality of life. During this time, patients in palliative care who suffer from depression report being more troubled about their physical symptoms, relationships, and beliefs about life. Depressed terminally ill patients have reported feelings of "being a burden" even when the actual amount of dependence on others is small.

PDQ® Cancer Information Summary. National Cancer Institute; Bethesda, MD. Depression (PDQ®): Patient Version. Updated August 2011. Available at: http://cancer.gov. Accessed November 7, 2011.

Just as patients need to be evaluated for depression throughout their treatment, so do family caregivers. Caregivers have been found to experience a good deal more anxiety and depression than people who are not caring for patients with cancer. Children are also affected when a parent with cancer develops depression. A study of women with breast cancer showed that children of depressed patients were the most likely to have emotional and behavioral problems themselves.

There are many misconceptions about cancer and how people cope with it, such as the following:

- All people with cancer are depressed.

- Depression in a person with cancer is normal.

- Treatment does not help the depression.

- Everyone with cancer faces suffering and a painful death.

Sadness and grief are normal reactions to the crises faced during cancer, and will be experienced at times by all people. Because sadness is common, it is important to distinguish between normal levels of sadness and depression. An important part of cancer care is the recognition of depression that needs to be treated. Some people may have more trouble adjusting to the diagnosis of cancer than others may. Major depression is not simply sadness or a blue mood. Major depression affects about 25% of patients and has common symptoms that can be diagnosed and treated. Symptoms of depression that are noticed when a patient is diagnosed with cancer may be a sign that the patient had a depression problem before the diagnosis of cancer.

All people will experience reactions of sadness and grief periodically throughout diagnosis, treatment, and survival of cancer. When people find out they have cancer, they often have feelings of disbelief, denial, or despair.

They may also experience difficulty sleeping, loss of appetite, anxiety, and a preoccupation with worries about the future. These symptoms and fears usually lessen as a person adjusts to the diagnosis. Signs that a person has adjusted to the diagnosis include an ability to maintain active involvement in daily life activities, and an ability to continue functioning as spouse, parent, employee, or other roles by incorporating treatment into his or her schedule. If the family of a patient diagnosed with cancer is able to express feelings openly and solve problems effectively, both the patient and family members have less depression. Good communication within the family reduces anxiety. A person who cannot adjust to the diagnosis after a long period of time, and who loses interest in usual activities, may be depressed. Mild symptoms of depression can be distressing and may be helped with counseling. Even patients without obvious symptoms of depression may benefit from counseling; however, when symptoms are intense and long-lasting, or when they keep coming back, more intensive treatment is important.

Diagnosis

The symptoms of major depression include the following:

- Having a depressed mood for most of the day and on most days
- Loss of pleasure and interest in most activities
- Changes in eating and sleeping habits
- Nervousness or sluggishness
- Tiredness
- Feelings of worthlessness or inappropriate guilt
- Poor concentration
- Constant thoughts of death or suicide

To make a diagnosis of depression, these symptoms should be present on most days for at least two weeks. The diagnosis of depression can be difficult to make in people with cancer due to the difficulty of separating the symptoms of depression from the side effects of medications or the symptoms of cancer. This is especially true in patients undergoing active cancer treatment or those with advanced disease. Symptoms of guilt, worthlessness, hopelessness, thoughts of suicide, and loss of pleasure are the most useful in diagnosing depression in people who have cancer.

Some people with cancer may have a higher risk for developing depression. The cause of depression is not known, but the risk factors for developing depression are known. Risk factors may be cancer-related and noncancer-related.

Cancer-Related Risk Factors

- Depression at the time of cancer diagnosis
- Poorly controlled pain
- An advanced stage of cancer
- Increased physical impairment or pain

- Pancreatic cancer

- Being unmarried and having head and neck cancer

- Treatment with some anticancer drugs

Noncancer-Related Risk Factors

- History of depression

- Lack of family support

- Other life events that cause stress

- Family history of depression or suicide

- Previous suicide attempts

- History of alcoholism or drug abuse

- Having many illnesses at the same time that produce symptoms of depression (such as stroke or heart attack)

The evaluation of depression in people with cancer should include a careful evaluation of the person's thoughts about the illness; medical history; personal or family history of depression or suicide; current mental status; physical status; side effects of treatment and the disease; other stresses in the person's life; and support available to the patient. Thinking of suicide, when it occurs, is frightening for the individual, for the health care worker, and for the family. Suicidal statements may range from an offhand comment resulting from frustration or disgust with a treatment course, such as "If I have to have one more bone marrow aspiration this year, I'll jump out the window," to a statement indicating deep despair and an emergency situation, such as, "I can't stand what this disease is doing to all of us, and I am going to kill myself."

Exploring the seriousness of these thoughts is important. If the thoughts of suicide seem to be serious, then the patient should be referred to a psychiatrist or psychologist, and the safety of the patient should be secured.

The most common type of depression in people with cancer is called reactive depression. This shows up as feeling moody and being unable to perform usual activities. The symptoms last longer and are more pronounced than a normal and expected reaction but do not meet the criteria for major depression. When these symptoms greatly interfere with a person's daily activities, such as work, school, shopping, or caring for a household, they should be treated in the same way that major depression is treated (such as crisis intervention, counseling, and medication, especially with drugs that can quickly relieve distressing symptoms). Basing the diagnosis on just these symptoms can be a problem in a person with advanced cancer since the illness may be causing decreased functioning. It is important to identify the difference between fatigue and depression since they can be assessed and treated separately. In more advanced illness, focusing on despair, guilty thoughts, and a total lack of enjoyment of life is helpful in diagnosing depression.

Medical factors may also cause symptoms of depression in patients with cancer. Medication usually helps this type of depression more effectively than counseling, especially if the medical factors cannot be changed (for example, dosages of the medications that are causing the depression cannot be changed or stopped). Some medical causes of depression in patients with cancer include uncontrolled pain; abnormal levels of calcium, sodium, or potassium in the blood; anemia; vitamin B12 or folate deficiency; fever; and abnormal levels of thyroid hormone or steroids in the blood.

Treatment

Major depression may be treated with a combination of counseling and medications (drugs), such as antidepressants. A primary care doctor may prescribe medications for depression and refer the patient to a psychiatrist or psychologist for the following reasons:

- A physician or oncologist is not comfortable treating the depression (for example, the patient has suicidal thoughts).

- The symptoms of depression do not improve after two to four weeks of treatment.

- The symptoms are getting worse.

- The side effects of the medication keep the patient from taking the dosage needed to control the depression.

- The symptoms are interfering with the patient's ability to continue medical treatment.

Antidepressants are usually effective in the treatment of depression and its symptoms. Unfortunately, antidepressants are not prescribed often for patients with cancer. About 25% of all patients are depressed, but only about 16% receive medication for the depression. The choice of antidepressant depends on the patient's symptoms, potential side effects of the antidepressant, and the person's individual medical problems and previous response to antidepressant drugs.

Patients with cancer may be treated with a number of drugs throughout their care. Some drugs do not mix safely with certain other drugs, foods, herbals, and nutritional supplements. Certain combinations may reduce or change how drugs work or cause life-threatening side effects. It is important that the patient's healthcare providers be told about all the drugs, herbals, and nutritional supplements the patient is taking, including drugs taken in patches on the skin. This can help prevent unwanted reactions.

Several psychiatric therapies have been found to be helpful in the treatment of depression related to cancer. Most therapy programs for depression are given in 4 to 30 hours and are offered in both individual and group settings. They may include sessions about cancer education or relaxation skills. These therapies are often used in combination and include crisis intervention, psychotherapy, and thought/behavior techniques. Patients explore methods of lowering distress, improving coping and problem-solving skills; enlisting support; reshaping negative and self-defeating thoughts; and developing a close personal bond with an understanding health care provider. Talking with a clergy member may also be helpful for some people.

Specific goals of these therapies include the following:

- These therapies assist people diagnosed with cancer and their families by answering questions about the illness and its treatment, explaining information, correcting misunderstandings, giving reassurance about the situation, and exploring with the patient how the diagnosis relates to previous experiences with cancer.

- These therapies assist with problem solving, improve the patient's coping skills, and help the patient and family to develop additional coping skills. Explore other areas of stress, such as family role and lifestyle changes, and encourage family members to support and share concern with each other.

- These therapies ensure that the patient and family understand that support will continue when the focus of treatment changes from trying to cure the cancer to relieving symptoms. The health care team will treat symptoms to help the patient control pain and remain comfortable, and will help the patient and his or her family members maintain dignity.

- Cancer support groups may also be helpful in treating depression in patients with cancer, especially adolescents. Support groups have been shown to improve mood, encourage the development of coping skills, improve quality of life, and improve immune response. Support groups can be found through the wellness community, the American Cancer Society, and many community resources, including the social work departments in medical centers and hospitals.

Recent studies of psychotherapy in patients with cancer, including training in problem solving, have shown that it helps decrease feelings of depression.

Chapter 33

Depression and Diabetes

Evidence suggests that an association between depression and diabetes exists, but it is not clear which comes first or why they are often linked. What is clear is that both depression and diabetes can be effectively managed and treated.

Anyone can develop depression, but people with diabetes may be at greater risk. Depression might result from the daily burden of having diabetes. Recent research has reported that depression is twice as common in people who have diabetes than it is in people who do not have this disease. In addition, the chances of becoming depressed increases as diabetes complications worsen.

Additional information from research on depression and diabetes suggests that depression alone may also increase the likelihood of a person developing type 2 diabetes. In fact, research shows that depressed adults have a 37% increased risk of developing type 2 diabetes.

Clinical depression is one of the most costly illnesses in the world. It is also a leading cause of disability in the United States and worldwide. Approximately 70% of people who have depression are employed; depression results in 400 million lost work days a year. It is estimated that the annual salary-equivalent cost of major depression due to work loss in the U.S. labor force is $44 billion per year.

Excerpted from "Diabetes at Work: What's Depression Got to Do with It?" by the National Diabetes Education Program (NDEP, www.diabetesatwork.org), a partnership of the National Institutes of Health and the Centers for Disease Control and Prevention, 2008.

Although depression can occur at any age, it tends to affect people in their prime working years, 25–44 years of age, and, if untreated, can last a lifetime.

Employers should know that there are several treatment options available to assist employees who are experiencing depression in the workplace. Research has shown that 80% of those who seek treatment show improvement. Depression does not have to be a debilitating disease.

Why Is Depression in Diabetes Serious?

Depression in diabetes is very concerning for several reasons:

- Individuals who are depressed may have more difficulty following the medical treatment that their health care team establishes. For example, depressed persons might not take their medication as prescribed or monitor their glucose levels as health care professionals recommend.

- Depression can result in poor physical and mental functioning, so a person is less likely to maintain regular physical activity.

- Individuals who are depressed might adopt unhealthy behaviors, such as a sedentary lifestyle and/or a poor diet.

- Social isolation is also common for people who are depressed, which decreases opportunities for social support that is often needed for self-management of diabetes.

Untreated depression in diabetes can result in the following:

- Hyperglycemia (high blood glucose)
- Poor metabolic control
- Decreased quality of life
- Increased health care usage and costs
- Increased risk of mortality

Untreated depression places people with diabetes at risk for complications that could be avoided. These complications include the following:

- Heart disease
- Blindness
- Amputations

- Erectile dysfunction

- Stroke

- Kidney disease

How Can an Employer Help an Employee Who Is Depressed?

If an employee is struggling with depression, the employer can be a valuable resource.

In reaching out to an employee who has disclosed that he or she is suffering from depression, employers should remember to handle this situation with confidentiality.

Employers should avoid trying to diagnose or treat a person with depression. Instead, the primary objective of the employer should be to assist the employee with receiving the appropriate, professional help needed, such as through an employee assistance program, which may be available at the work site.

In providing assistance to an employee with depression, employers should do the following:

- Be empathetic and understanding

- Avoid critical or shaming statements

- Emphasize that depression is treatable

- Provide information to employees about symptoms of depression and treatment options.

Employers can also raise awareness about depression by doing the following:

- Educating management and employees about depression and effective treatment options

- Informing employees of the availability of an employee assistance program

- Provide an easily accessible behavioral health system

- Including depression recognition screenings and stress management at health fairs

- Developing a return-to-work plan for employees who have been absent from work due to depression

Chapter 34

Depression and Heart Disease

Depression May Follow a Heart Attack

After a heart attack, most people experience a whirlwind of emotions. On the one hand, a patient may be grateful to still be alive, but he may also feel frightened and anxious about the future. Will he be able to go back to his former lifestyle? Will he have another heart attack? He may also feel angry and upset about the unfairness of it all.

- Feelings of sadness and anger are natural after a catastrophic illness like a heart attack. Survivors need to go through the grieving process, which involves a certain amount of unhappiness. But when those feelings linger and start affecting a patient's recovery, it's cause for concern. As many as one out of three heart attack survivors report feeling depressed.

- Depression can sap a person's will to recover and make him less likely to follow his doctor's recommendations.

- Heart patients with depression are less likely to eat a heart-healthy diet, give up smoking, or exercise regularly.

- Worse yet, depressed heart patients have a greater risk of suffering future heart attacks.

"How to Deal with Post Heart Attack Depression," © 2011 Caring, Inc. (www .Caring.com). All rights reserved. Reprinted with permission.

The good news is that depression can be treated. With the appropriate care, a patient will lead a happier life—and life will be easier for you, too. Here are some practical things you can do if you think a patient is depressed after a heart attack.

Knowing Whether It's Depression

Is it really depression or just a case of the blues? It's not always easy to tell the difference. And you may be thinking that the person in your care has good reason to feel down in the dumps. After all, he's just had a heart attack. But there's a difference between the normal grieving process and depression. The warning signs of depression include:

- frequent crying episodes;
- feelings of hopelessness or worthlessness;
- poor appetite or increased appetite;
- sleeping too much or not enough;
- increased agitation and restlessness;
- loss of interest in life;
- expressing thoughts of dying or suicide.

The patient should be evaluated for depression if he has had several of these symptoms for more than two weeks.

Encourage the Patient to Go for Testing

If you believe he's depressed, the first step is to talk to him about his feelings. This isn't always easy, especially if he isn't used to expressing emotions. Ask him if he's feeling sad or hopeless. Try to get an idea if it's really depression or just a temporary case of the blues.

The next step is to schedule an evaluation. His primary care physician may want to talk to him first, or she may refer him to a psychiatrist or counselor. In any case, the evaluating doctor will talk to him and assess his mood. She may also order screening tests to rule out other medical conditions that can mimic depression, such as a thyroid disorder or infection.

If he's resistant to the idea of testing because he's embarrassed or afraid, help him understand that a diagnosis of depression isn't the shameful secret it once was. It doesn't mean he's "crazy" or is going to be taken away to a nursing home. What's more, his test results are private, so no one but he and his doctor needs to know.

If he absolutely refuses to see a doctor, there's not a whole lot you can do. You can't force the issue unless he's psychotic or suicidal, or his depression has progressed to the point where he can no longer take care of himself. If none of those circumstances apply, your best bet is to enlist family members and friends to try to persuade him to seek help.

Supporting the Patient

If he's diagnosed with depression, the doctor may prescribe anti-depressant medications and/or psychotherapy. She may also recommend lifestyle changes. Even if a primary care doctor diagnosed his depression, a patient may still benefit from seeing a mental health professional. Not all primary care physicians are comfortable treating depression.

He may be anxious about taking antidepressants, either because of the stigma he associates with those medications or because he's afraid of potential side effects. Assure him that the doctor can work with him to find the medication that's most effective with the least severe side effects.

Other Ways You Can Help

Simply supporting someone as he struggles with depression can help him a great deal. Here are some other things you can do:

- Help him stay as physically active as possible. Talk to the doctor and rehabilitation team about what exercises are appropriate. Find activities you can do together, such as a morning walk around the neighborhood. Exposure to sunlight can help break the cycle of sleeping during the day that many depressed people fall into.

- Structure the day around activities that give him pleasure and a sense of purpose. For example, meet friends for lunch or enjoy a leisurely walk through the mall.

- Try to stay positive and upbeat, but don't foster unrealistic expectations. Instead of saying, "You'll be running a 10K next month," you might say, "The more we walk together, the easier it'll be."

- Join a support group—for either or both of you. Talking to other people who're struggling with similar issues can be enormously comforting and helpful. It's also a great way to connect with other heart attack survivors and caregivers.

In the end, it's really the patient's responsibility to get help for depression. If he won't talk to his doctor or comply with treatment, you can't make him—and you shouldn't blame yourself. Keep offering support and provide positive reinforcement when he takes those difficult steps toward recovery.

But there's only so much you can do. If feelings of guilt and sadness overwhelm you, you may need help coming to terms with the fact that the person you're caring for isn't going to get help. Ask his doctor for information about support groups and other resources to help you manage your own feelings.

Chapter 35

Depression and Human Immunodeficiency Virus

What Is Depression?

Depression is a mood disorder. It is more than sadness or grief.
Depression is sadness or grief that is more intense and lasts longer than it should. It has various causes:

- Events in your daily life

- Chemical changes in the brain

- A side effect of medications

- Several physical disorders

About 5% to 10% of the general population gets depressed. However, rates of depression in people with human immunodeficiency virus (HIV) are as high as 60%. Women with HIV are twice as likely as men to be depressed.

Being depressed is not a sign of weakness. It doesn't mean you're going crazy. You cannot "just get over it." Don't expect to be depressed because you are dealing with HIV. And don't think that you have to be depressed because you have HIV.

"Depression and HIV," Fact Sheet #558. © 2011 AIDS InfoNet. Reprinted with permission. InfoNet fact sheets are updated frequently. Please visit the website at http://www.aidsinfonet.org for the newest version.

Is Depression Important?

Depression can lead people to miss doses of their medication. It can increase high-risk behaviors that transmit HIV infection to others.

Depression might cause some latent viral infections to become active. Overall, depression can make HIV disease progress faster. It also interferes with your ability to enjoy life.

Depression often gets overlooked. Also, many HIV specialists have not been trained to recognize depression. Depression can also be mistaken for signs of advancing HIV.

What Are the Signs of Depression?

Symptoms of depression vary from person to person. Most health care providers suspect depression if patients report feeling blue or having very little interest in daily activities. If these feelings go on for two weeks or longer, and the patient also has some of the following symptoms, they are probably depressed:

- Fatigue or feeling slow and sluggish
- Problems concentrating
- Low sex drive
- Problems sleeping; waking very early or excessive sleeping
- Feeling guilty, worthless, or hopeless
- Decreased appetite or weight loss
- Overeating

What Causes Depression?

Some medications used to treat HIV can cause or worsen depression, especially efavirenz (Sustiva). Diseases such as anemia or diabetes can cause symptoms that look like depression. So can drug use, or low levels of testosterone, vitamin B6, or vitamin B12.

People who are infected with both HIV and hepatitis B or C are more likely to be depressed, especially if they are being treated with interferon.

Other risk factors include:

- being female;
- having a personal or family history of mental illness, alcohol and substance abuse;

- not having enough social support;
- not telling others you are HIV-positive;
- treatment failure (HIV or other).

Treatment for Depression

Depression can be treated with lifestyle changes, alternative therapies, and/or with medications. Many medications and therapies for depression can interfere with your HIV treatment. Your health care provider can help you select the therapy or combination of therapies most appropriate for you.

Do not try to self-medicate with alcohol or recreational drugs, as these can increase depression and create additional problems.

Lifestyle changes can improve depression for some people. These include:

- regular exercise;
- increased exposure to sunlight;
- stress management;
- counseling;
- improved sleep habits.

Alternative Therapies

Some people get good results from massage, acupuncture, or exercise. St. John's Wort is widely used to treat depression. However, it interferes with some HIV medications. Be sure to tell your health care provider if you are taking St. John's wort.

Valerian or melatonin may help improve your sleep. Supplements of vitamins B6 or B12 can help if you have a shortage.

Antidepressants

Some people with depression respond best to medication. Antidepressants can interact with ARVs [antiretrovirals]. They must be used under the supervision of a health care provider who is familiar with your HIV treatment. Protease inhibitors have many interactions with antidepressants.

The most common antidepressants used are selective serotonin reuptake inhibitors, called SSRIs. They can cause loss of sexual desire and function, lack of appetite, headache, insomnia, fatigue, upset stomach, diarrhea, and restlessness or anxiety.

The tricyclics have more side effects than the SSRIs. They can also cause sedation, constipation, and erratic heartbeat.

Some health care providers also use psychostimulants, the drugs used to treat attention deficit disorder.

A recent study showed that treatment with dehydroepiandrosterone (DHEA) can reduce depression in some HIV patients.

The Bottom Line

Depression is a very common condition for people with HIV. Untreated depression can cause you to miss medication doses and lower your quality of life.

Depression is a "whole body" issue that can interfere with your physical health, thinking, feeling, and behavior.

Chapter 36

Depression and Multiple Sclerosis

Introduction

According to the National Institute of Mental Health, nearly one in 10 American adults suffers from a depressive illness during any given one-year time period. Over the course of a lifetime, the prevalence of experiencing a depressive disorder may reach to nearly one in five for women, and one in eight for men—and some sources give even higher estimates.

Despite being a fairly common condition, depression is still a widely misunderstood and "stigmatized" disorder—causing some to feel a sense of disgrace or embarrassment. Providing accurate information to patients and their families is one of the best ways to help people recognize the symptoms of depression and to encourage treatment.

Depression often works its way quietly into people's lives. The very nature of depressive symptoms impedes someone's ability to realize that he or she is depressed. These same symptoms can even suppress one's desire to seek treatment. Symptoms often creep up slowly over time, and those suffering from depression may have trouble remembering what it's like to feel good.

Patients may describe depression as a black hole of despair, holding them down and shutting out any feelings of hope, excitement, or the possibility of future happiness. For many, joy disappears and everything is experienced as being bland or flat.

The prospect of continuing to feel this way day after day can be daunting. Many people who are depressed will find various ways to escape this reality. Some may self-medicate with drugs, alcohol, and/or food. Others may sleep the days away, avoiding contact with others and the outside world. Some may resort to suicide. Each year, approximately 500,000 Americans are treated for attempted suicide; each day, 85 die from these attempts.

Fortunately, depression is treatable. Once the illness is recognized and addressed, individuals with depression can rediscover the delights and pleasures of life.

Types of Depression and Diagnosis

Distinguishing between sadness and depression is important. Sadness is a normal emotion that everyone experiences at different points in his or her life. We feel sad when we experience a loss or tragedy—and this feeling is usually an appropriate reaction to the situation that has occurred. Feeling sad is a natural coping skill that is required for growth and maturity. Experiencing sadness helps us to move through painful events.

When sadness manifests itself physically we may feel tension in our chest, or our hearts may ache. We may also experience an overwhelming desire to cry; and some are strongly compelled to talk with others about their sorrow. After expressing and letting out our emotions, we normally begin to feel a sense of relief. Unlike depression, sadness typically passes within a few days and one begins to embrace life again, enjoying normal daily activities.

In contrast to sadness, depression can seemingly come from "out of the blue," and can last much longer. Someone may not even realize that he or she is depressed, and pinpointing any specific trigger for the depression can be difficult.

Different types of clinical depression have been identified. The first, which is commonly talked about, is major depressive disorder (also known as major depression). According to the *Diagnostic and Statistical Manual of Mental Disorders (DSM-IV)*, physicians will look for specific criteria when diagnosing a major depressive episode. These criteria dictate that five or more of the following symptoms must be present for at least a 2-week period (these symptoms are generally reported by either the patient or a family member who observes the patient):

1. A depressed mood for most of the day, nearly every day

2. Loss of interest or pleasure in all, or almost all, activities for most of the day

3. Significant change in weight or appetite

4. Insomnia or excessive sleepiness

5. Observable agitation or lethargy

6. Fatigue and loss of energy, nearly every day

7. Feelings of worthlessness, low self-esteem, or excessive guilt

8. Difficulty concentrating or indecisiveness

9. Recurrent thoughts of death or suicide

Additional symptoms may also be present, but these are not typically considered when making a diagnosis. Among others, these can include: A reduced interest in personal appearance and hygiene; complaints of aches and pains, with the worry of these symptoms being an indication of a serious health problem or disease; an increased sensitivity to noise; and bouts of crying or sobbing.

Another type of depression is known as dysthymic disorder, dysthymia, or chronic depression. Although this type of depression shares many symptoms with major depression, the symptoms tend to be less severe. These symptoms, however, are typically present for at least twp years rather than two weeks (as with major depressive episodes). This form of depression sneaks up on patients, slowly becoming a part of everyday life, and eventually can be perceived as a person's normal mood, often appearing unhappy. At least two of the following symptoms must be present to confirm a diagnosis of dysthymic disorder:

1. Poor appetite or overeating

2. Insomnia or excessive sleepiness

3. Low energy or fatigue

4. Poor concentration or indecisiveness; memory problems

5. Low self-esteem

6. Feelings of hopelessness

Bipolar disorder (previously known as manic-depressive illness) is a disorder which also falls under a separate category of depression. In this case, the patient will experience severe depressive episodes as well as periods of extreme euphoria. Additional categories of depression include postpartum depression and premenstrual dysphoria.

In general, the symptoms of depression can be divided into three categories: Physical, emotional, and mental. The physical symptoms include fatigue, poor appetite, insomnia, and agitation. The emotional symptoms include feelings of hopelessness, depressed mood, low self-esteem, guilt, and worthlessness. The mental symptoms include poor concentration, indecisiveness, and for some, thoughts of death or suicide. The severity of depression can vary from mild to moderate to severe. Regardless of how severe one's depression may be, it still affects us on all three levels: Physically, emotionally, and mentally.

In all types of depression, symptoms typically impair daily functioning such as our ability to work or take care of household responsibilities. Doing simple tasks such as bathing or cooking a meal can seem overwhelming.

You may recognize several depressive symptoms that are also symptoms of MS [multiple sclerosis]. Examples of shared symptoms include fatigue, insomnia or excessive sleepiness, and cognitive difficulties, as well as restlessness or slowing down. Because many of these symptoms mimic typical MS symptoms, they may not necessarily indicate depression for someone with MS. The similarities in symptoms do in fact make diagnosing depression challenging in MS patients. A trained professional who is familiar with both MS and depression is needed to make an accurate diagnosis of depression for an individual with MS.

One of the most commonly used tools for diagnosing and evaluating depression is the Beck Depression Inventory (BDI, BDI-II), which is a questionnaire aimed at measuring the severity of one's depression. The 21 multiple-choice questions allow adult patients to report on their depressive symptoms. Topics include: Physical symptoms such as fatigue, loss of libido, and loss of weight; emotional symptoms, such as hopelessness and irritability; as well as mental (or cognitive) symptoms, reflecting any negative thoughts about the world, oneself, or the future.

The BDI is named after its creator, Dr. Aaron T. Beck, and was first developed in 1961. The questionnaire was revised in 1971 (BDI-1A), and has since been revised again in 1996 (BDI-II). All versions of this inventory for depression translate the degree of severity into specific numbers from one to three for each symptom. The self-reported ratings are added together to determine a total score, which gives physicians an exact number for the evaluation of a patient's depression.

The Goldman Consensus Group (a panel of experts who reviewed the issue of depression in MS) recommends that individuals with

MS be routinely screened for depression using a tool such as the BDI. They also recommend individualized treatment plans (using therapy, medications, or an integrated approach), greater standardizations of treating depression in MS, as well as continuing clinical research.

Risk Factors for Depression

Individuals with MS have a greater risk of experiencing a depressive episode at some point in time. Fifty percent of individuals with MS will become depressed during their lifetime, compared to less than 20 percent of the American population. However, if you know you are at risk, you can be proactive: watching for signs and symptoms, and seeking help as soon as warning signs appear.

Women, who are twice as likely to have MS, are nearly twice as likely as men to experience depression. This is attributed to many factors. Hormonal fluctuations such as menopause, pregnancy, menstrual changes, miscarriage, and the postpartum period may trigger depressive episodes. Women who have multiple family responsibilities such as childrearing and caring for elderly parents are under tremendous stress, as are single moms. Mothers with disabilities face greater challenges and must wrestle with concern for their children, along with their own wellbeing. All of these challenges can make women vulnerable to depression as well as other illnesses.

One reason that fewer men are diagnosed with depression might be because they are less likely than women to seek appropriate treatment. As a result, they are more likely to self-medicate with drugs and alcohol, or develop a gambling addiction, rather than seek the help of a therapist and take prescribed antidepressants. Depressive symptoms for men may present as irritability or anger; for men who do seek therapy, these symptoms may be mistakenly treated as the primary issues, rather than the underlying depression.

Those who have a predisposition to depression prior to their MS diagnosis may be at an even higher risk for depression. Depressive disorders are one-and-a half to three times more common among those whose parents suffered from depression. Furthermore, other factors such as a chronic medical condition, lack of social supports, and substance dependence, may also contribute to the onset of depression. Understanding these risk factors, recognizing depressive symptoms, and seeking treatment, may play a significant role with improving one's quality of life, and possibly prevent potential thoughts of suicide.

Depression's Impact

Increased Risk of Suicide

Suicide is one of the leading causes of death among MS patients. The primary predictors of suicidal intent in those with MS include:

1. Severity of depression

2. Abuse of alcohol

3. Living alone

In addition, a family history of mental illness, higher perceived levels of social stress, and anxiety also contribute to suicidal intent. Although fewer men are diagnosed with depression, they are four times more likely to commit suicide than women.

In a study of individuals with MS who had suicidal intent, one-third had not received any psychological help and two thirds (all suicidal and with major depression) had not received any anti-depression medication. This research clearly points to the importance of seeking treatment for depression. When treatment is sought, the risk of suicide drops considerably.

Family Relationships Are Often Affected

Similar to the way in which MS affects the family, depression also has a strong impact on relationships. Family members will often say that they can handle the patient's physical MS symptoms, but they cannot deal with his or her depression. Others may feel helpless as they watch a loved one succumb to the grips of depression. Sometimes family members believe that they are somehow the cause of their loved one's unhappiness, but this is rarely the case, and this misperception puts an added strain on the relationship.

Since depression typically causes its victims to withdraw from others, family and friends can feel shunned or neglected. Similar to MS, the symptoms of depression are usually invisible, which can lead to misunderstandings. Unfortunately, when others cannot visibly see the cause of someone's pain, they may not be as sympathetic—as they may be unaware of how much the other person is suffering. Many people still believe that depression can be overcome by willpower or religious belief alone. They may have a "pull yourself up by your bootstraps" mentality, stemming from ignorance about the condition. These same people would never tell a cancer patient to just "try harder" or "snap out of it." Education is the best way to combat these misconceptions.

Children are not immune to a family member's depression. In fact, a recent Swiss study of children who have a parent with MS and depression found that these children are at a high risk of mental health problems themselves. These children were found to be two to three times as likely to experience anxiety or depression. Parents need to be aware of the impact that their own psychological state is having on their children, and to watch for symptoms in them as well. The symptoms of depression in children are more difficult to recognize. They may exhibit problems at school and with friends. They may be irritable and aggressive, or conversely, they may withdraw and isolate themselves from others. Children experiencing depression may not want to eat; they may also have trouble sleeping and have bad dreams, which may contribute to memory or learning problems that can also develop. When depression is present in one or more family members, seeing a family counselor as a group can help to bring about an emotionally healthy outlook.

Treatment Compliance and Health May Be Affected

Depression can compromise one's willpower to follow his or her MS treatment plan. Even simple activities, such as getting out of bed in the morning, may become difficult. Bigger tasks, such as getting to a doctor's appointment, may feel impossible. Following a treatment plan for MS includes taking medication on a regular basis. Taking the correct dosage at the scheduled times, especially with respect to injections, requires determination, discipline, and motivation. All of these traits are compromised when a patient is depressed. Other wellness strategies, such as following an exercise program, eating well, participating in support groups, and staying involved with positive people, may also fall by the wayside during depressive episodes.

Additionally, studies show that depression has been linked to many physical ailments. These can include (but are not limited to) such symptoms as: a lowered immune response, which could make someone more susceptible to colds and flu; an increased sensation of pain; mental and physical fatigue; weight gain or loss (according to changes in appetite and behavior); and an increased sensitivity to noise.

Loss of Libido

One of the chief complaints among individuals experiencing depression is a lack of interest in physical relationships. When someone is feeling tired, withdrawn, or unlovable, he or she is much less likely to be interested in physical intimacy. Naturally, this has a negative impact on relationships. Loved ones will often feel rejected and unwanted when their partner withdraws from them sexually.

Since 25 to 50 percent of men and 50 percent of women with MS report having some type of sexual dysfunction, depression only makes matters worse. However, these sexual issues can often be resolved when the underlying depression is treated.

Some worry that antidepressants may decrease their sexual desire, however, medications have been improved over the years and this has become less of an issue. Anyone taking a medication and experiencing reduced libido should discuss the situation with a medical professional. He or she may be able to adjust the prescription to minimize or eliminate this potential side effect.

Less Participation in Social Activities

Depression often causes people to turn inward, withdrawing from family and friends, and declining to take part in social activities. The thought of picking up the phone to call a friend or to hold a conversation can seem overwhelming for someone who is depressed. As a result, individuals with depression will often discontinue social activities and commitments. Friends may eventually become discouraged and stop calling to urge the depressed patient to join them.

Severely depressed people may feel that they have very little to give others, as they are often using all of their energy just to make it through the next few minutes. The net result is that support systems tend to crumble when they are needed the most. This is unfortunate, because connecting with others can often be of much benefit to the depressed patient.

Maintaining social contact is a necessity for both mental and physical health. According to the Centers for Disease Control and Prevention (CDC), a strong correlation exists between loving and supportive relationships, and the ability to cope with illness.

Losses in Employment

Although many mildly to moderately depressed patients are able to continue working, individuals who are severely depressed may have great difficulty going to the workplace, let alone being productive while there. In fact, the *Journal of the American Medical Association* estimates the annual cost of depression in the United States is $43 billion. Of that, $23 billion is lost through absenteeism or loss of productivity in the workplace. For the depressed individual with MS, the loss of employment and insurance benefits can have a devastating long-term impact.

Depression Is Under-Reported and Under-Treated

Despite all of the devastating implications of depression, this disease is still too often under-reported, and as a consequence, under-treated. Several factors contribute to this urgent situation.

One obstacle is the fact that depression, along with other psychological issues, is less tangible, especially given the relatively short times that a patient spends with his or her physician. Typically, both healthcare providers and patients may feel more comfortable discussing physical MS symptoms (which are easier to observe and evaluate), while ignoring the less obvious (and more sensitive) psychological issues.

This issue is further complicated by the demands placed on practitioners during a typical office visit. Most practitioners have good intentions, but they are challenged during office visits to complete a multitude of tasks. These include answering patients' questions, listening to their concerns, managing MS symptoms, tracking changes in the course of the disease, educating patients, evaluating treatment approaches, managing medications, and making referrals to other specialists. With all of the things a doctor must do, one can easily understand how a problem like depression may be overlooked.

In addition, individuals—including MS patients—may not recognize the symptoms of depression, particularly if they are experiencing irritation and anger, rather than the more common emotion of a depressed mood. Some patients may automatically assume that their feelings of depression are MS symptoms, and that they must simply live with the sadness and other negative emotions. Finally, some patients may not realize that treatments are available for depression, so they do not pursue the issue.

Addressing and Evaluating Your Depression

Because our bodies are ultimately our own responsibility, we often must advocate for ourselves when addressing depression. Writing down your concerns prior to a doctor's appointment, including a list of all the depressive symptoms you are experiencing, can be very helpful. Such a list may be given to the doctor or nurse during your visit.

Patients and family members need to understand that depression is not a weakness or a moral short-coming that people can simply get over. Depression is an illness, and just like MS, it deserves the time, attention, and treatment that any other illness would be given.

What Causes Depression in MS?

Why are MS patients at such a high risk for depression? The easy answer to this question is that living with MS in and of itself is depressing. Studies show, however, that those with other serious chronic medical conditions do not suffer from the same high rate of depression as do those with MS. By taking a closer look at what causes depression in MS, we can better target and treat its symptoms.

Disease Response

Experiencing a period of depression is not uncommon following the initial diagnosis of MS. Hearing the news that one has a chronic disease, which for now is incurable, has a tremendous impact on both the patient, as well as the family.

Psychologically "catching up" to this new information may take some time. One may initially assume that the prognosis will be the "worst case" scenario, at least until one has time to adjust to his or her unique symptoms and disease course. Prior to developing the skills needed to cope with the diagnosis, one may be susceptible to having depressive episodes, especially if he or she is already prone to depression. Many patients do not realize that most people do eventually adjust and adapt to the diagnosis of MS, but doing so just takes time.

Even after learning to cope with the initial diagnosis, patients will need to continually adjust to altered life circumstances. Some individuals may eventually experience losses which can occur as a result of disease progression. Examples include changes in physical abilities, employment, relationships, and plans for the future. During each of these losses, patients may be vulnerable to depression. Depression is an illness, and just like MS, it deserves the time, attention, and treatment that any other illness would be given.

Additionally, recent research shows that depression may be experienced during disease activity. Three predictors strongly correlate to the level of depression the patient experiences. These include:

1. Present state of illness (if the individual is currently experiencing an exacerbation)

2. Level of uncertainty about new symptoms and the future

3. Poor coping skills such as emotion-centered and escape avoidance reactions, rather than constructive problem solving

The uncertainty a patient experiences during an exacerbation strongly influences the level of depression that may result. During the course of MS, people can feel as if they have lost control not only of their bodies, but their thoughts and feelings as well. Healthcare providers may be able to reduce the level of depression that patients experience by offering reassurance, answering questions, and working to reduce uncertainty whenever possible.

Focusing on what the patient still has control over can also help to reduce the feelings of depression. Studies show that when individuals have the perception that they can influence their environment, they feel a greater sense of engagement, energy, and happiness.

Physiological Causes

Damage to the central nervous system caused by physiological changes may impact mood. In some cases, depression is thought to be caused by lesions in the right frontal and temporal lobes of the brain.

The authors of *Comprehensive Nursing Care in Multiple Sclerosis* (second edition, edited by J. Halper and N.J. Holland, Demos Medical Publishing, 2002) note, "Both clinical depression and less severe emotional distress are common in MS . . . [occurring at] a rate much higher than in the general population or in other conditions with similar disabilities, e.g., spinal cord injury. In fact, the very high frequency of depression in MS has led many to theorize that it may be due in part to damage to parts of the brain concerned with the regulation of emotions."

Chemical Changes

Chemical changes that occur within the body and the brain can affect mood. For instance, studies find that the expression of interferon-gamma (IFN-gamma) and other Th 1-type cytokines (pro-inflammatory protein molecules involved in cell-to-cell communications, shown to worsen MS) correlate with depression scores during an acute exacerbation. Another study showed that the level of depression, as well as IFN-gamma production, declined significantly in MS patients over a 16-week treatment period using cognitive behavioral therapy. These studies suggest that chemical changes caused by MS attacks may in fact cause depression. This would also help to explain why patients are more prone to depression during exacerbations.

Fatigue

Patients report that fatigue is the most disabling of all their MS symptoms. Between 75 and 90 percent of the MS population suffers from fatigue during the course of their illness. When we are exhausted, we are much more likely to feel depressed. We simply do not have the emotional energy to fight depression; we are too tired to do the things we might normally do to ward off depressive symptoms—such as socializing or exercising.

Similar to depression, fatigue impacts every aspect of life. As fatigue robs us of our ability to work, to help others, or to care for our children, we can fall victim to a painful spiral of fatigue causing depression and then depression compounding our fatigue.

You must also take responsibility for pacing yourself and pay attention to what causes your fatigue. Using a journal to rate your fatigue can be a useful exercise. The "Rating Your Fatigue" exercise found on page 145 of the book, *MS & Your Feelings: Handling the Ups and Downs of Multiple Sclerosis* (Hunter House Inc., 2006), can help give you a structured way to begin monitoring causes of your fatigue.

Medication Side Effects

Some of the medications prescribed to MS patients may be linked to depression. Steroids top the list. These are often prescribed during exacerbations when patients are already vulnerable to depressive symptoms. Steroids tend to induce a short-term euphoric steroid high when first given, followed by a plunge into depression once the medication is stopped.

Some neurologists recognize the emotional roller-coaster which steroids can cause and they are prescribing medications to lessen the emotional effects often associated with the treatment. These might include anti-anxiety and antidepressant drugs given prior to starting a steroid treatment.

Many relapsing-remitting MS patients are now taking interferons (Avonex, Betaseron, and Rebif) to help slow the progression of MS and reduce the number of attacks. Anecdotal reports suggest a possible association between this type of immunotherapy and increased depression. Recent follow-up studies, including data from SPECTRIMS [Secondary Progressive Efficacy Trial of Recombinant Interferon beta-1a in MS] and PRISMS [Prevention of Relapses and Disability by Interferon beta-1a Subcutaneously in Multiple Sclerosis] trials, failed to show a connection between these drugs and depression.

While this news is encouraging, the interferons have been shown to decrease the amount of serotonin formed in the brain. Decreased levels of this chemical in the brain may be linked to depression. Therefore, individuals who are taking an interferon and experience a change in their emotional state, are advised to talk with their doctor immediately.

Other medications given for MS symptom management may also cause depression. These include: Baclofen, prescribed for spasticity; benzodiazepines, taken for dizziness, vertigo, or spasticity; and other sedating drugs. When taking any of these medications, patients, family members, and the treating physician should closely monitor any changes in mood, watching for the signs of depression listed earlier.

Other Factors Increasing Susceptibility to Depression

In addition to the potential causes of depression already mentioned, other factors can make a person more vulnerable to depressive episodes. By being aware of these situations, you can be extra sensitive to your mood changes during these high risk times and seek treatment if you notice yourself slipping into a depressive episode before it becomes too severe.

Interruption of Routine

Some people find great comfort in sticking to a routine. They may believe that they have more influence over their MS symptoms when they are able to control their sleep, work, and exercise schedule, as well as having the freedom to choose when and what they eat. For these individuals, changing a routine can be a trigger for depression. Examples of changes that commonly affect routine include moving to another location, changing jobs, or traveling.

When someone clings to a routine and is forced to make a change, doing whatever is possible to maintain a normal schedule will help with the adjustment to the new circumstances. For example, if you typically exercise for 30 minutes each day, continue to do this even if circumstances are quite different, such as being on vacation or beginning a new job. Try not to change your activities when in a new situation.

Winter Weather

For many people, the winter season can trigger depression. This phenomenon is known as seasonal affective disorder, also referred to as SAD. If you recognize a tendency to get depressed in the winter, the following suggestions may be of help (with a doctor's approval):

1. Vacation in a sunny location.

2. Spend at least a half-hour outdoors.

3. Use some type of bright visible-spectrum light.

4. Talk with your doctor about your concerns and learn about additional strategies.

Changing Medications

Frequently when changing medications, one's mood is initially impacted. A few weeks may be needed to adjust to the new chemicals in your body. Informing your doctor of any mood changes when on a new medication is important to the success of a treatment as well as one's wellbeing.

Other Physical Conditions

One should not automatically assume that depression is caused by his or her MS. Individuals need to work with their doctor to rule out any other medical or physical issues that may be contributing to depression. Hormone or thyroid problems, changes in blood-sugar levels, and urinary tract or other infections, are among the types of medical conditions aside from MS that can cause depression.

Low Self-Esteem

Many people with chronic illness face challenges to their self-esteem. We may contend with issues such as poor body image, fewer social activities and friends, and the loss of a job or other responsibilities that made us feel worthy in the past. As our abilities change, we may begin to see ourselves as less valuable to both ourselves and others. Feelings of low self-esteem can lead to feelings of worthlessness and guilt—which can in turn lead to depression. One of the tasks that all people with MS must achieve in order to maintain mental health is the reinvention of a worthy self; despite physical disability.

The responsibility is on each of us to find ways that we can still contribute our talents and skills, regardless of the changes that have taken place within our bodies. Fortunately, we get to choose our self-image. This means that regardless of what our abilities are or how they change, we can consciously decide to adjust our expectations of ourselves and, in turn, adjust what we value about ourselves.

One positive way to combat low self-esteem as well as depression is to volunteer. Research shows that volunteers actually experience a helper's high. Frequently, volunteers report feeling physically, emotionally, and intellectually recharged after doing something for others. In fact, studies show that giving support to others can sometimes be more beneficial than receiving help.

Treatment Options for Depression

Seeking treatment for depression is just as important as getting help for one's MS. Depression rarely improves on its own and without treatment, it often gets worse.

Fortunately, depression is one of the most treatable of all MS symptoms, although specific treatment therapies are not the same for everyone. Individuals may need to try a few different approaches before finding a treatment plan that works best for them.

Taking a prescribed medication along with participating in psychological counseling appears to be the most effective treatment plan to alleviate depression. Treating depression with medication alone is generally not as effective as working in conjunction with a qualified professional therapist.

Many advances have been made with the drugs used to treat depression. The most frequently recommended medications for depression come from a class of drugs known as selective serotonin reuptake inhibitors (SSRIs). These antidepressant medications inhibit the reuptake of serotonin (a chemical produced within the body which is known to elevate mood), allowing it to remain in the body's system longer.

Some of the more commonly prescribed SSRIs include Celexa, Lexapro, Paxil, Prozac, and Zoloft. Unfortunately, some patients report experiencing side effects when taking these medications. Common side effects may include headache, nausea, sleeplessness, anxiety, drowsiness, and sexual dysfunction. These side effects may subside with time, or one's doctor may adjust the prescription or dosage. Newer antidepressants include serotonin and norepinephrine reuptake inhibitors (SNRIs), such as Cymbalta and Effexor, with side effects that are similar to the SSRIs.

Other drugs which are not SSRIs (belonging to other drug classes), such as Desyrel, Remeron, Serzone, and Wellbutrin, are options which may result in fewer side effects. Numerous other drugs are also FDA [U.S. Food and Drug Administration]-approved for the treatment of depression, many of which either augment another antidepressant, or are used to treat specific behaviors found in various types of depression—including anxiety, mood swings, manic episodes, insomnia, and excessive eating (among others). The key is to work closely with your treating physician and therapist to determine the correct drug and dosage that will work best for you.

When starting a prescribed treatment for depression, understanding that many of these drugs can take up to six weeks before reaching maximum effectiveness is important. If after six weeks you are not seeing any improvement in your symptoms, again consult with your doctor about adjusting your dose or switching to another medication.

Some patients find that monitoring their treatment progress by keeping a log of their symptoms is helpful. Since improvements may be gradual, this can be an effective way of documenting any changes you see in your mood. Suggestions include noting changes in appetite, energy, interest in activities, increases in socialization, increased sexual desire, as well as feelings of hope and optimism.

One note of caution, however, concerns the fact that patients often want to stop treatment once they start feeling better. Medications for depression usually need to be continued for at least four to nine months to prevent depression from quickly returning. For those with severe depression, medication may need to be continued indefinitely. Patients are advised not to alter the dose, stop taking medications, or combine a prescription with other medications, without first consulting their doctor. Of course, if a patient is experiencing an adverse reaction to the drug, a medical professional should be contacted immediately.

Some individuals may decide to try dietary supplements as a way to help improve their symptoms of depression. Examples of popular supplements which are promoted for depression include St. John's wort and ginkgo biloba. Anyone considering any type of supplement should first consult his or her physician, as these can cause serious side effects and/or interactions with other medications. Additionally, many supplements have not undergone the same rigorous studies as FDA-approved medications, which means that both safety and effectiveness may not be fully established.

Finding a Therapist

As mentioned earlier, the most successful treatment plan is to seek counseling in conjunction with a prescribed drug therapy. A variety of professionals are specifically trained to help those suffering from depression. Working with a psychiatrist, psychologist, social worker, psychiatric nurse, family therapist, or counselor can provide you and your loved ones with the guidance and support needed to help work through your depression.

These professionals can provide objective insight and concrete coping skills to help manage the symptoms of depression. A therapist may become one of the most important team players in assisting with the management of this debilitating disorder. Therefore, finding the right match for your specific needs is imperative. For those who have never worked with a mental health professional, one may feel a certain amount of anxiety over picking up the phone and beginning the process.

To follow are some points one should consider before starting the search for an appropriate therapist. Since a therapist may become a key player on one's treatment team, doing some research in advance may prove to be beneficial, before selecting the therapist that is right for you.

Your neurologist or physician should be able to give some referrals to mental health care providers. MS organizations, support group participants, and/or friends and family may also be able to offer recommendations. Understanding the differences between the types of professionals that offer counseling services is helpful as you begin the selection process.

The Interview Process

Ideally, patients should have the opportunity to interview potential therapists, just as they would when selecting other members of their medical team. As an empowered patient, you have the right to choose who treats you and to understand his or her treatment philosophy. If you don't click with the first person you speak with, meeting with more than one provider is reasonable when making this important decision. Some of the questions you might consider asking include:

1. Do you have experience working with MS patients?

2. What is your success rate in treating depression?

3. What is your psychological treatment approach?

4. What are your office hours?

5. Do you work closely with physicians?

6. How do you feel about using medications to treat depression?

7. Are your services covered by my insurance?

These questions will help give you the facts, but how you feel about the therapist at a gut level is the most important consideration. Does he or she listen to you? Do you feel that he or she cares about your concerns? Do you feel comfortable with the therapist? Does the therapist understand issues relating to chronic illness? The questions you ask, along with a certain amount of intuition, will help guide you toward the right match.

Once connected with the right therapist, a relationship can be established. This may ultimately help you to feel less alone as you gain a greater understanding of your emotions and how to feel better again.

Financial Considerations

Therapy can be expensive. Fees can range from $60 to more than $200 per hour, depending on where the patient lives and the professional credentials of the practitioner. If the patient has medical insurance, the insurer should be contacted directly to determine if any of the costs are covered for the specific therapist selected. Questions to ask the insurer include: What is the yearly deductible, how much will the company pay per visit, and how many visits are allowed each year.

If finances are an obstacle to treatment, other options may be available. Individuals may talk with their church, the city or county public health department, social service agencies, or an MS organization, to see if any of these agencies have programs which provide financial assistance and/or low-cost counseling. Some therapists offer a sliding-scale fee based on income. If the patient has Medicare or Medicaid, a mental health benefit may be available to pay for therapy. Exploring these avenues can sometimes uncover more affordable options.

Types of Therapeutic Approaches

A variety of therapeutic approaches may be used during the counseling process. These include: (1) talk therapy, which helps the patient gain insight and resolve problems through verbal exchange with a therapist; (2) behavioral therapy, which helps an individual find reinforcement through rewards based on his or her own actions; (3) interpersonal therapy, which concentrates on issues arising in relationships with others; (4) cognitive/behavioral therapy, which works to change negative ways of thinking and acting into more positive approaches; and (5) psychodynamic therapy, which helps to resolve internal conflicting feelings, often stemming from past experiences.

In addition to individual therapy, some clients benefit from family or couples therapy, while others find group therapy to be effective. Some less traditional, but increasingly popular therapy options also include phone therapy and therapy over the Internet. Although these options have limitations, the methods used can be very attractive for clients who are homebound or who live in remote areas, where finding qualified mental health professionals can be difficult.

Support groups and peer counseling are often particularly helpful for MS patients and a number of these programs are made available through MS organizations. These programs should not be substituted for professional therapy, but may be a nice adjunct. Talking to others who can relate first-hand to what it is like to live with MS and/or depression, helps to validate what you are experiencing.

Other Options When Traditional Therapies Fail

For a small number of individuals with significant depression who do not respond to the more traditional forms of therapy and medication, various procedures are sometimes performed. Examples include: Transcranial magnetic stimulation (presently being studied); vagus nerve stimulation (used since the late 1990s for epileptic patients and has since been approved for treatment-resistant depression); and electroconvulsive therapy (ECT), also known as electroshock treatment.

While this latter procedure (ECT) may sound extreme, patients may be reassured by the fact that this treatment method has been improved over the years. It is now considered to be safe and effective for many individuals. Patients receive anesthesia prior to treatment and each session lasts about 10 minutes. Individuals with MS must be cautious about this treatment course because ECT may have negative effects on the blood brain barrier. MS patients must carefully weigh the risks and benefits of this treatment technique with their physician.

Family Involvement

Often families feel helpless as they watch a loved one suffer from depression. Many will ask, "What can I do?" Family members may be pleased to learn that they can help in several ways. One of the first things to do is to encourage the patient to seek treatment. As a family member or close friend, you may want to specifically describe the changes that you have seen take place in the patient's life and explain the effect that this has on you. Doing research ahead of time, and having the names and numbers of therapists to call, can make that next step easier.

If the patient agrees to the idea, you may want to accompany your loved one to the doctor's office to discuss the changes you have seen and to obtain a referral for a therapist. This can help get the ball rolling. You may also offer to attend the first therapy appointment with the patient. Let him or her know that you will provide support in any way you can as he or she seeks treatment.

Patients may be encouraged to participate in activities, helping to draw them out of their depressed state. Family and friends may make plans for social activities, inviting their loved one to come along. Provide these individuals with opportunities to do the things that they previously enjoyed. Let them know that you love them, no matter how depressed they may feel.

If your family member is prescribed medication, help to make sure that he or she continues to take the drug(s). If you notice a change in personality after starting the medication, either positive or negative, talk with the patient and physician about those changes.

Finally, living with a depressed person can be extremely challenging, and quite frankly, depressing at times. Care partners (family or friends helping with the care of a patient) need to be sure to take care of themselves. As a care partner, you should try to keep balance in your life and to do the things that bring you pleasure. If experiencing depressive symptoms, a care partner should also seek professional help.

Immediate Positive Steps

While these tips have been highlighted throughout this text, to follow is a summary of these important positive steps:

1. Exercise. Exercise is proven to produce an increase in chemicals such as endorphins, which can make us feel less depressed—and can help to lessen fatigue as well.

2. Create a stress management program. Many strategies, such as meditation, yoga, and guided imagery, are available to manage stress, and can help with life's ups and downs.

3. Talk about your feelings. Confide in a trusted friend or family member.

4. Commit to one activity each week. Being accountable to a group can be a motivator to change your environment and get social support.

5. Journal your feelings. Take time to write down your emotions.

6. Develop a spiritual interest. Spend time in nature, prayer, meditation, religion, or some other form of spiritual practice.

7. Find your bliss. What is the one thing in your life that makes you want to get up in the morning?

8. Help others. Volunteering is a great way to improve self-esteem and combat feelings of worthlessness.

9. Reward yourself. Do something that makes you feel good (and causes no harm).

10. Adopt a pet. Pets provide unconditional love.

11. Create a gratitude list. Take the time to shift the focus from all that is going wrong, to all that is going right in your life.

12. Maintain a sense of humor. Laughing provides therapeutic value—even consciously smiling can help you to feel better.

Proven medications and therapy are now available to individuals who suffer from depression. Given the many resources that individuals with MS have to draw upon for support, we can see that this is a very hopeful time. By reading this text, you have taken an important first step toward healing your emotional pain. Having done so, you are greatly encouraged to take the next step . . . which is to seek treatment. Soon you will be on your way to a happier outlook in life.

Chapter 37

Depression and Neurological Disorders

Chapter Contents

Section 37.1

Depression and Alzheimer Disease

Introduction

Experts estimate that up to 40 percent of people with Alzheimer's
disease suffer from significant depression. Fortunately, there are many
effective non-drug and drug therapies available. Treatment of depression in Alzheimer's disease can improve a person's sense of well-being,
quality of life, and individual function.

Symptoms of Depression

Men and women with Alzheimer's experience depression with about
equal frequency. But identifying depression in someone with Alzheimer's can be difficult. There is no single test or questionnaire to detect
the condition, and diagnosis requires careful evaluation of a variety
of symptoms. Dementia itself can lead to certain symptoms commonly
associated with depression, including:

- apathy;
- loss of interest in activities and hobbies;
- social withdrawal;
- isolation.

The cognitive impairment experienced by people with Alzheimer's
often makes it difficult for them to articulate their sadness, hopelessness, guilt, and other feelings associated with depression.

Depression in Alzheimer's doesn't always look like depression in
people without the disorder. For example, depression in Alzheimer's is
sometimes less severe and may not last as long or recur as often.

Also, people with Alzheimer's and depression may be less likely to
talk openly about wanting to kill themselves, and they are less likely to

attempt suicide than depressed individuals without dementia. What's more, depressive symptoms in Alzheimer's may come and go, in contrast to memory and thinking problems that worsen steadily over time.

Diagnosing Depression in Alzheimer's Disease

The first step in diagnosis is a thorough professional evaluation. Side effects of medications or an unrecognized medical condition can sometimes produce symptoms of depression. Key elements of the evaluation will include:

- a review of the person's medical history;
- a physical and mental examination;
- interviews with family members who know the person well.

Because of the complexities involved in diagnosing depression in someone with Alzheimer's, it may be helpful to consult a geriatric psychiatrist who specializes in recognizing and treating depression in older adults.

To facilitate diagnosis and treatment of depression in people with Alzheimer's, the National Institute of Mental Health established a formal set of guidelines for diagnosing the condition. Although the criteria are similar to general diagnostic standards for major depression, they reduce emphasis on verbal expression and include irritability and social isolation.

For a person to be diagnosed with depression in Alzheimer's, he or she must have either depressed mood (sad, hopeless, discouraged, or tearful) or decreased pleasure in usual activities, along with two or more of the following symptoms over a two-week period:

- Social isolation or withdrawal
- Disruption in appetite that is not related to another medical condition
- Disruption in sleep
- Agitation or slowed behavior
- Irritability
- Fatigue or loss of energy
- Feelings of worthlessness or hopelessness, or inappropriate or excessive guilt
- Recurrent thoughts of death, suicide plans, or a suicide attempt

Treating Depression

The most common treatment for depression in Alzheimer's involves a combination of medicine, support, and gradual reconnection to activities and people the person finds pleasurable. Simply telling the person with Alzheimer's to "cheer up," "snap out of it," or "try harder" is seldom helpful. Depressed people with or without Alzheimer's are rarely able to make themselves better by sheer will, or without lots of support, reassurance, and professional help.

Non-Drug Approaches

- Schedule a predictable daily routine, taking advantage of the person's best time of day to undertake difficult tasks, such as bathing.

- Make a list of activities, people, or places that the person enjoys now and schedule these things more frequently.

- Help the person exercise regularly, particularly in the morning.

- Acknowledge the person's frustration or sadness, while continuing to express hope that he or she will feel better soon.

- Celebrate small successes and occasions.

- Find ways that the person can contribute to family life and be sure to recognize his or her contributions.

- Provide reassurance that the person is loved, respected, and appreciated as part of the family, and not just for what she or he can do now.

- Nurture the person with offers of favorite foods or soothing or inspirational activities.

- Reassure the person that he or she will not be abandoned.

- Consider supportive psychotherapy and/or a support group, especially an early-stage group for people with Alzheimer's who are aware of their diagnosis and prefer to take an active role in seeking help or helping others.

Medication to Treat Depression in Alzheimer's

Physicians may prescribe antidepressants for people with Alzheimer's who have depression. Examples include:

- bupropion (Wellbutrin®);

- citalopram (Celexa®);

- fluoxetine (Prozac®);

- mirtazapine (Remeron®);

- paroxetine (Paxil®);

- sertraline (Zoloft®);

- trazodone (Desyrel®);

- venlafaxine (Effexor®).

Antidepressants in a class called the tricyclics, which includes nortriptyline (Pamelor®) and desipramine (Norpramin®), are no longer used as first-choice treatments, but are sometimes used when individuals do not benefit from other medications.

Section 37.2

Depression and Parkinson Disease

"Combating Depression in Parkinson's Disease" by Matthew Menza, M.D. Parkinson's Disease Foundation News & Review, Spring 2009. © 2009 Parkinson's Disease Foundation (www.pdf.org). All rights reserved. Reprinted with permission.

Depression is one of the major, and most common, challenges for people living with Parkinson disease (PD). Everyone feels sad from time to time and it is normal to experience sadness and stress when faced with a difficult disease such as Parkinson disease. However, the sadness that is part of being human can become a significant problem if it crosses into the realm of clinical depression and is left untreated.

When this article was originally written, health professionals, researchers, and people living with or affected by PD were just beginning to recognize the extent of the prevalence of depression in Parkinson disease and its impact on daily life. Since that time, there has been a sharp and welcome increase in the awareness of depression as a common feature of the PD experience and of the importance of treating it.

Not only that, but new research has also advanced our understanding of how to treat PD-related depression and has increased the range of the treatment options we have available.

What is the difference between sadness and depression? While sadness is temporary, depression is persistent, and the people who experience it find that they cannot enjoy life as they used to. A person who is depressed may have little energy and may struggle to get out of bed in the morning. Other symptoms of depression can include poor appetite, sleep disturbances, fatigue, feelings of guilt, self-criticism and worthlessness, irritability, and anxiety. Some people may begin having persistent thoughts that they would be better off dead or may even begin planning on ending their life. The presence of these symptoms on most days for two weeks suggests a diagnosis of depression and should be discussed with a physician.

At least 40 percent of people with PD experience clinical depression at some time during the disease. It may occur early or late in the course of Parkinson disease, and may wax and wane in severity. It causes personal suffering and also appears to intensify problems with mobility and memory. A person with Parkinson disease, or his or her caregiver or physician, may at first dismiss the signs of depression because they assume that it is Parkinson disease that is causing the problem or because they assume it is normal to be depressed when faced with this illness. This can lead to feelings of helplessness and confusion, which may further exacerbate the problem.

What causes depression in PD? There is no clear answer but most specialists agree that it is probably a combination of living with the stress of a progressive chronic disease, along with changes in the neurochemistry of the brain that accompany Parkinson disease. The experience of depression early in the disease may be a natural reaction to an anticipated loss of ability and quality of life, but research suggests that it may also be directly due to PD-related chemical changes in the brain. Many of the areas of the brain that are affected in PD are also important in controlling mood. Specifically, Parkinson disease causes changes in areas of the brain that produce serotonin, norepinephrine, and dopamine — chemicals that are involved in regulating mood, energy, motivation, appetite, and sleep. In addition, the frontal lobe of the brain, which is important in controlling mood, is known to be underactive in Parkinson disease.

It is very important to address depression because of the effects it can have on other symptoms and on quality of life. If you are concerned that you or a loved one with Parkinson disease may be depressed, you should raise it with your doctor. If you have been diagnosed with clinical depression, there is no simple formula for treating it, but there are several principles that are true for nearly everyone.

First, it is extremely important that Parkinson disease itself be optimally treated. People with Parkinson disease who experience uncontrolled "on-off" periods and freezing episodes are more prone to depression, so it is important to talk with a doctor about the best approach to controlling these symptoms. The same is true of some other, nonmotor symptoms of PD—for example, poor sleep, constipation, and fatigue—that need to be treated to decrease the burden of living with the disease.

Second, it is important to make the effort to exercise regularly, to eat well, and to stay socially involved. Exercise is an effective tool in helping the symptoms of both depression and PD. The exercise does not need to be rigorous, but it does need to be regular. Eating a healthy diet is another lifestyle approach that can help your overall wellness. Staying involved in social and recreational activities is also very important. Everyone needs something to look forward to, whether it be working on a hobby or socializing with friends and family.

Third, people should consider taking advantage of psychological treatments such as stress management, relaxation, and cognitive behavioral therapy, as well as the kind of peer support that can be found in support groups. Receiving help from professionals and peers can help you learn to cope with stresses, improve social relationships, and find solutions to practical day-to-day impairments. For instance, your peers at a support group may have a lot of wisdom to share with you (and you with them) about the practical aspects of daily living with PD, such as handling finances or managing travel.

Lastly, people with Parkinson disease should be aware that many medications are available for depression in PD. Recent studies have suggested that one class of antidepressants, called dual reuptake inhibitors, which affect both serotonin and norepinephrine, do improve depressive symptoms in people with PD. These include medications such as Effexor®, Cymbalta®, and Pamelor®. Another class of antidepressants, called selective serotonin re-uptake inhibitors (SSRIs), work by making serotonin available for use by the brain. These are also sometimes useful. Among the most common SSRIs are Paxil® (paroxetine), Prozac® (fluoxetine), and Zoloft® (sertraline).

The pharmacological treatment of depression in Parkinson disease needs to be individualized and may involve a variety of strategies. If you or your loved one is currently taking an antidepressant that does not appear to be helping, talk to your doctor to see if a switch to a different agent may better benefit your symptoms.

There remain many unanswered questions about the causes and the treatments of depression in people with PD and the problem is receiving increasing attention from the scientific community. The National Institutes of Health, at the urging of clinicians and advocacy groups, have begun to fund studies on depression and some of these results are becoming available. (To learn more about clinical trials, visit www.PDtrials.org.)

One thing is certain: There is a clear consensus that awareness about depression in PD needs to be raised among people with PD, caregivers, and health professionals. More needs to be done to explore better ways to treat this illness in people living with Parkinson disease, and to better understand how the treatment of depression affects other aspects of life, including sleep, anxiety, memory, and concentration. In the meantime, if you or a loved one with PD experiences symptoms of depression, talk to your doctor and take advantage of the resources that are already available.

Ten Signs of Depression in Parkinson Disease

- Excessive worrying
- Persistent sadness
- Crying
- Loss of interest in usual activities and hobbies
- Increased fatigue and lack of energy
- Feelings of guilt
- Loss of motivation
- Complaints of aches and pains
- Feelings of being a burden to loved ones
- Ruminations about disability, death, and dying

People with these symptoms should discuss them with a physician.

Matthew Menza, MD, is a Professor of Psychiatry and Neurology at the Robert Wood Johnson Medical School.

Chapter 38

Depression and Stroke

Chapter Contents

Section 38.1

What to Do When Someone Experiences Depression after a Stroke

A Stroke Can Trigger Depression

For most people, the word "stroke" brings to mind a constellation of problems, including paralysis and difficulty with speech. But if someone has recently had a stroke, you're probably well aware that the effects go well beyond the physical. The emotional aftermath can be just as overwhelming and far more difficult to sort out.

Although depression can strike anyone, those who've suffered a catastrophic illness may be more susceptible than other people. And when you throw a brain injury into the mix, the risk of developing a mood disorder becomes even greater. As many as half of stroke survivors will become depressed, according to James Castle, a neurologist at Stanford University.

Depression isn't just miserable, it may also make a stoke survivor more susceptible to pain and fatigue and may even delay his recovery.

- In a study published in the journal *Stroke*, researchers reported that stroke survivors who were treated for depression demonstrated improved recovery in regular daily activities compared with those whose depression went untreated.

- People who are depressed also tend to be less compliant with rehabilitation and more resistant to making lifestyle changes to prevent a second stroke.

Fortunately, depression can be treated. With the appropriate care, a patient will lead a happier life—and life will be easier for you, too. Here are some practical things you can do if you think the person you're caring for is depressed after a stroke.

It's not always easy to recognize depression. In the case of someone who's had a stroke, the situation can be even more complicated. If a patient has trouble talking or understanding language, it might be especially difficult to recognize depression. Increased emotional lability—sudden and extreme mood swings, common after a stroke—may also hide symptoms of depression.

You may also think he has good reason to feel depressed. After all, he's just had a stroke and can't do the things he used to be able to do. But there's a difference between the normal grieving process and depression. The warning signs of depression include:

- frequent crying episodes;

- feelings of hopelessness or worthlessness;

- poor appetite or increased appetite;

- sleeping too much or not enough;

- increased agitation and restlessness;

- loss of interest in life;

- expressing thoughts of dying or suicide.

A stroke survivor should be evaluated for depression if he has had several of these symptoms for more than two weeks.

If you believe a patient is depressed, the first step is to talk to him about his feelings. This isn't always easy, especially if he isn't used to expressing emotions. Ask him if he's feeling sad or hopeless. Try to get an idea if it's really depression or just a temporary case of the blues.

The next step is to schedule an evaluation. His primary care physician may want to talk to him first, or she may refer him to a psychiatrist or counselor. In any case, the evaluating doctor will talk to him and assess his mood. She may also order screening tests to rule out other medical conditions that can mimic depression, such as a thyroid disorder or infection.

If he resists the idea of testing because he's embarrassed or afraid, help him understand that a diagnosis of depression isn't the shameful secret it once may have been. It doesn't mean he's "crazy" or is going to be taken away to a nursing home. And his test results are private, so no one but he and his doctor needs to know.

If he absolutely refuses to see a doctor, there's not a whole lot you can do. "There's no way to force the issue unless there are severe circumstances," says Castle. If he has become psychotic or suicidal, or if his depression has progressed to the point where he can no longer care for himself, Castle recommends that you notify his doctor or emergency medical services immediately. Otherwise, your best bet is to enlist family members and friends to try to persuade him to seek help.

If a patient is diagnosed with depression, the doctor may prescribe antidepressant medications and/or recommend psychotherapy. "Most doctors take a multidirected approach toward battling depression," says Castle. "Medicines can be highly effective, but often there's a role for psychotherapy and lifestyle changes."

Even if a primary care doctor diagnosed depression, a patient may still benefit from seeing a mental health professional, says Castle. "Some primary care physicians feel comfortable treating this disorder, but many would prefer the assistance of a psychiatrist or psychologist." Castle says this can be difficult for people who associate a stigma with mental health treatment. "It's important for the family to support the patient over that barrier."

The person in your care may also be nervous about taking antidepressants, but Castle points out that they present very little risk: "If anything, there's some evidence to suggest that these medicines might actually decrease the chance of having another stroke." Some of the common side effects, such as loss of libido or excessive sweating, can be annoying, but they're nothing compared to the misery of depression. And the doctor can work with the patient to find the most effective medication with the fewest side effects.

Simply supporting the patient as he struggles with depression can help him a great deal. Here are some other things you can do:

- Help him stay as physically active as possible. Talk to the doctor and rehabilitation team about what exercises are appropriate. Find activities you can do together, such as a morning walk around the neighborhood.

- Depressed people often want to sleep during the day. "As much as possible, don't allow a patient to slip into a depressed routine," says Castle. "Break the cycle by encouraging him to be awake during the day with exposure to sunlight." A simple walk outdoors or some time in the garden can really help.

- Structure the day around activities that give him pleasure and a sense of purpose. For example, meet friends for lunch or enjoy a leisurely walk through the mall.

- Try to stay positive and upbeat, but don't foster unrealistic expectations. Instead of saying, "You'll be hiking again in no time," you might say, "If we keep walking together every day, you'll notice that it gets a lot easier."

- Join a support group—for either or both of you. Talking to other people who're struggling with similar issues can be enormously comforting and helpful. It's also a great way to connect with other stroke survivors and caregivers. Remember that it's not all up to you.

In the end, it's really up to the stroke survivor to get help for depression. If he won't talk to his doctor or comply with treatment, you can't make him—and you shouldn't blame yourself. Keep offering support and provide positive reinforcement when he takes those difficult steps toward recovery.

But there's only so much you can do. If feelings of guilt and sadness overwhelm you, you may need help coming to terms with the fact that he isn't going to get help. Ask his doctor for information about support groups and other resources to help you manage your own feelings.

Source: E. Chemerinski et al. "Improved recovery in activities of daily living associated with remission of post stroke depression." *Stroke* 32, 2001.

Section 38.2

Behavioral Intervention Can Reduce Depression in Stroke Survivors

From "A Brief Behavioral Intervention Can Reduce Depression in Stroke Survivors," by the National Institutes of Health (NIH, www.nih.gov), August 6, 2009.

A nurse-led behavioral intervention can reduce the incidence of depression in stroke survivors, according to the results of a study published in the September 2009 issue of the journal *Stroke*. The intervention, called Living Well with Stroke (LWWS), provided individualized counseling sessions aimed at increasing pleasant social interactions and physical activity as a way to elevate mood, and was designed to be used alone or in conjunction with antidepressant medications. This study was funded by the National Institute of Nursing Research (NINR), a component of the National Institutes of Health (NIH).

A stroke occurs when the blood supply to a part of the brain becomes blocked or interrupted, leading to brain damage in the affected area. Stroke survivors can experience a range of aftereffects, including impaired mobility or paralysis, pain, speech and language problems, and altered cognition. As many as one-third of stroke survivors also develop post-stroke depression (PSD), which may include intense feelings of loss, anger, sadness, and/or hopelessness.

Compared to stroke survivors without depression, those with PSD tend to have a poorer response to rehabilitation, a longer delay in returning to work, more social withdrawal, and increased use of health care services. They are also at higher risk for subsequent strokes, cardiac events, and death. While antidepressant medications have shown varying degrees of short-term efficacy for PSD patients, few studies have examined non-pharmacologic interventions or long-term outcomes.

In a clinical trial involving over 100 stroke survivors who exhibited symptoms of PSD, Dr. Mitchell's research team compared LWWS against usual post-stroke care. The study participants ranged in age from 25 to 88 years, and 59 percent were male. In addition, over 70 percent had experienced at least one episode of depression prior to their stroke, and 60 percent were taking an antidepressant medication at entry into the study. All participants received standard post-stroke information and continued to see their primary care provider for ongoing medical care.

Those assigned to the LWWS program received nine counseling sessions over two months with a specially trained stroke rehabilitation nurse. In these sessions, the nurse taught the participants problem-solving skills and helped them develop realistic treatment goals. In addition, several sessions were devoted to improving mood by helping the participants identify and increase their participation in pleasant social events and physical activities, such as being with family, listening to music, reading, solving a puzzle, or learning something new.

"In designing LWWS, we reasoned that changing the behaviors commonly associated with depression through an individualized counseling program would lead to a more effective and longer-lasting elevation of mood than is often seen with medications alone," said Dr. Pamela Mitchell, the principal investigator of the study.

"Individuals who have suffered a stroke often must make adaptations in their lives and learn to cope with new limitations, both physical and cognitive. Depression during the recovery period can interfere with their ability to fully engage in their treatment regimen or return to family and work," noted Dr. Patricia A. Grady, the NINR Director.

Depression scores in the LWWS group were significantly lower after treatment and at a one-year follow-up compared to the control group.

In addition, more participants in the LWWS group achieved remission—with scores no longer meeting the criteria for depression—compared to the control group both immediately after treatment (47 percent vs. 19 percent), and at a one-year follow-up (48 percent vs. 27 percent). At 2 years, depression scores continued to decrease and remission rates continued to increase for both groups, although the gap narrowed so that the differences were no longer statistically significant.

For both the intervention and control groups, patients in remission at 1 year had significantly higher scores in perceived ability, recovery, and social participation than those who were not.

"The success of LWWS shows the importance of including behavioral strategies in the care of stroke survivors. We believe our study is the first to report a clinically significant reduction in depression in these patients over a long term," said Dr. Mitchell. "We also showed that achieving remission from depression by any means is an important treatment goal that could promote recovery and sociability."

"This study has the potential to add another tool for health care professionals to use in helping individuals cope following a stroke," added Dr. Grady. "Also of note, the LWWS program included instruction to help family members and other informal caregivers identify resources and support services as a way to reduce their caregiving burden, an important aspect of comprehensive post-stroke care."

Reference: Mitchell PH, Veith RC, Becker KJ, Buzaitis A, Cain KC, Fruin M, Tirschwell DL, and Teri L. *Stroke.* September 2009 (online ahead of print).

Part Six

Diagnosis and Treatment of Depression

Chapter 39

Depression Screening Self-Assessment

[*Editor's Note:* Only a health professional can diagnose and treat depression, but your responses to the following questions may indicate you need an evaluation for mental health disorders.]

Check the one response to each item that best describes you for the past seven days. During the past seven days . . .

Falling Asleep

- I never take longer than 30 minutes.
- I take at least 30 minutes to fall asleep, less than half the time.
- I take at least 30 minutes to fall asleep, more than half the time.
- I take more than 60 minutes to fall asleep, more than half the time.

Sleep during the Night

- I do not wake up at night.
- I have a restless, light sleep with a few brief awakenings each night.

Source: The Quick Inventory of Depressive Symptomatology 16-Item Self-Report (QIDS–SR16), University of Pittsburgh, http://www.ids-qids.org. Original Citation: Rush, A.J., Giles, D.E., Schlesser, M.A., Fulton, C.L., Weissenburger, J.E. and Burns, C.T. The Inventory of Depressive Symptomatology (IDS): Preliminary findings. *Psychiatry Research,* 18:65–87, 1986. Reviewed by David A. Cooke, MD, FACP, November 23, 2011.

- I wake up at least once a night, but I go back to sleep easily.
- I awaken more than once a night and stay awake for 20 minutes or more, more than half the time.

Waking up Too Early

- Most of the time, I awaken no more than 30 minutes before I need to get up.
- More than half the time, I awaken more than 30 minutes before I need to get up.
- I almost always awaken at least one hour or so before I need to, but I go back to sleep eventually.
- I awaken at least one hour before I need to, and can't go back to sleep.

Sleeping Too Much

- I sleep no longer than seven to eight hours/night, without napping during the day.
- I sleep no longer than 10 hours in a 24-hour period including naps.
- I sleep no longer than 12 hours in a 24-hour period including naps.
- I sleep longer than 12 hours in a 24-hour period including naps.

Feeling Sad

- I do not feel sad.
- I feel sad less than half the time.
- I feel sad more than half the time.
- I feel sad nearly all the time.

Appetite

- There is no change in my usual appetite.
- I've lost my appetite.
- I'm eating too much.

Decreased Appetite

- I eat somewhat less often or lesser amounts of food than usual.
- I eat much less than usual and only with a personal effort.
- I rarely eat within a 24-hour period, and only with extreme personal effort or when others persuade me to eat.

Increased Appetite

- I feel a need to eat more frequently than usual.
- I regularly eat more often and/or greater amounts of food than usual.
- I feel driven to overeat at mealtime and between meals.

Weight

- I have not had a change in my weight.
- I've lost weight.
- I've gained weight.

Decreased Weight (Within the Last Two Weeks)

- I feel as if I have had a slight weight loss.
- I have lost two pounds or more.
- I have lost five pounds or more.

Increased Weight (Within the Last Two Weeks)

- I feel as if I have had a slight weight gain.
- I have gained two pounds or more.
- I have gained five pounds or more.

Concentration/Decision Making

- There is no change in my usual capacity to concentrate or make decisions.
- I occasionally feel indecisive or find that my attention wanders.
- Most of the time, I struggle to focus my attention or to make decisions.

- I cannot concentrate well enough to read or cannot make even minor decisions.

View of Myself

- I see myself as equally worthwhile and deserving as other people.
- I am more self-blaming than usual.
- I largely believe that I cause problems for others.
- I think almost constantly about major and minor defects in myself.

Thoughts of Death or Suicide

- I do not think of suicide or death.
- I feel that life is empty or wonder if it's worth living.
- I think of suicide or death several times a week for several minutes.
- I think of suicide or death several times a day in some detail, or have actually tried to take my life.

General Interest

- There is no change from usual in how interested I am in other people or activities.
- I notice that I am less interested in people or activities.
- I find I have interest in only one or two of my formerly pursued activities.
- I have virtually no interest in formerly pursued activities.

Energy Level

- There is no change in my usual level of energy.
- I get tired more easily than usual.
- I have to make a big effort to start or finish my usual daily activities (for example, shopping, homework, cooking or going to work).
- I really cannot carry out most of my usual daily activities because I just don't have the energy.

Feeling Slowed Down

- I think, speak, and move at my usual rate of speed.

- I find that my thinking is slowed down or my voice sounds dull or flat.

- It takes me several seconds to respond to most questions and I'm sure my thinking is slowed.

- I am often unable to respond to questions without extreme effort.

Feeling Restless

- I do not feel restless.

- I'm often fidgety, wringing my hands, or need to shift how I am sitting.

- I have impulses to move about and am quite restless.

- At times, I am unable to stay seated and need to pace around.

To score your Depression Screening Quiz, go to www.smokefree.gov/depression_quiz.aspx.

Chapter 40

Diagnosing Depression

Chapter Contents

Section 40.1

Talking to Your Doctor about Depression

Excerpted from "Talk with Your Doctor about Depression," by
Healthfinder.gov, part of the National Health Information Center,
updated September 29, 2011.

If you think you might be depressed, talk with a doctor about how you are feeling. Depression is a serious illness.

The good news is that depression can be treated. Getting help is the best thing you can do for yourself and your loved ones. You can feel better.

Depression can be treated with talking therapy, medicine (called antidepressants), or both. Your doctor may refer you to a counselor or therapist.

Get a medical checkup. Ask to see a doctor or nurse who can test you for depression.

Screening for depression is covered under the new Affordable Care Act (ACA). Depending on your insurance plan, you may be able to get screened at no cost to you. Talk to your insurance company, and ask about the ACA. Even if you don't have insurance, there are free and low-cost mental health services.

Here are some places you can go to for help:

- Doctor's office or health clinic

- Family service or social service agency

- Church or clergy person

- Psychologist

- Counselor or social worker

- Psychotherapist

If someone you care about is depressed, get help. Get help right away if you or someone you know is thinking about suicide. Call 800-273-8255 or 911.

Section 40.2

Diagnostic Evaluation of Depression: What Your Doctor Should Do

Excerpted from "Men and Depression," by the National
Institute of Mental Health (NIMH, www.nimh.nih.gov), part of the
National Institutes of Health, January 23, 2009.

The first step to getting appropriate treatment for depression is a physical examination by a physician. Certain medications as well as some medical conditions such as a viral infection, thyroid disorder, or low testosterone level can cause the same symptoms as depression, and the physician should rule out these possibilities through examination, interview, and lab tests. If no such cause of the depressive symptoms is found, the physician should do a psychological evaluation or refer the patient to a mental health professional.

A good diagnostic evaluation will include a complete history of symptoms: i.e., when they started, how long they have lasted, their severity, and whether the patient had them before and, if so, if the symptoms were treated and what treatment was given. The doctor should ask about alcohol and drug use, and if the patient has thoughts about death or suicide. Further, a history should include questions about whether other family members have had a depressive illness and, if treated, what treatments they may have received and if they were effective. Last, a diagnostic evaluation should include a mental status examination to determine if speech, thought patterns, or memory has been affected, as sometimes happens with depressive disorders.

Treatment choice will depend on the patient's diagnosis, severity of symptoms, and preference. There are a variety of treatments, including medications and short term psychotherapies (i.e., "talk" therapies), that have proven effective for depressive disorders. In general, severe depressive illnesses, particularly those that are recurrent, will require a combination of treatments for the best outcome.

Medications

There are several types of medications used to treat depression. These include newer antidepressant medications—chiefly the selective serotonin reuptake inhibitors (SSRIs)—and older ones, the tricyclics and the monoamine oxidase inhibitors (MAOIs). The SSRIs (and other newer medications that affect neurotransmitters such as dopamine or norepinephrine) generally have fewer side effects than tricyclics. Sometimes the doctor will try a variety of antidepressants before finding the most effective medication or combination of medications for the patient. Sometimes the dosage must be increased to be effective. Although some improvements may be seen in the first couple of weeks, antidepressant medications must be taken regularly for three to four weeks (in some cases, as many as eight weeks) before the full therapeutic effect occurs.

Patients often are tempted to stop medication too soon. They may feel better and think they no longer need the medication, or they may think it isn't helping at all. It is important to keep taking medication until it has a chance to work, though side effects may appear before antidepressant activity does. Once the person is feeling better, it is important to continue the medication for at least four to nine months to prevent a relapse into depression. Some medications must be stopped gradually to give the body time to adjust, and many can produce withdrawal symptoms if discontinued abruptly. Therefore, you should never discontinue your medication without first talking to your doctor. For individuals with bipolar disorder and those with chronic or recurrent major depression, medication may have to be maintained indefinitely.

Despite the relative safety and popularity of SSRIs and other antidepressants, some studies have suggested that they may have unintentional effects on some people, especially adolescents and young adults. In 2004, the Food and Drug Administration (FDA) conducted a thorough review of published and unpublished controlled clinical trials of antidepressants that involved nearly 4,400 children and adolescents. The review revealed that 4% of those taking antidepressants thought about or attempted suicide (although no suicides occurred), compared to 2% of those receiving placebos.

This information prompted the FDA, in 2005, to adopt a "black box" warning label on all antidepressant medications to alert the public about the potential increased risk of suicidal thinking or attempts in children and adolescents taking antidepressants. In 2007, the FDA proposed that makers of all antidepressant medications extend the warning to include young adults up through age 24. A "black box" warning is the most serious type of warning on prescription drug labeling.

The warning emphasizes that patients of all ages taking antidepressants should be closely monitored, especially during the initial weeks of treatment. Possible side effects to look for are worsening depression, suicidal thinking or behavior, or any unusual changes in behavior such as sleeplessness, agitation, or withdrawal from normal social situations. The warning adds that families and caregivers should also be told of the need for close monitoring and report any changes to the physician. The latest information from the FDA can be found on their website at www.fda.gov.

Results of a comprehensive review of pediatric trials conducted between 1988 and 2006 suggested that the benefits of antidepressant medications likely outweigh their risks to children and adolescents with major depression and anxiety disorders. The study was funded in part by the National Institute of Mental Health. Also, the FDA issued a warning that combining an SSRI or SNRI antidepressant with one of the commonly-used triptan medications for migraine headache could cause a life-threatening serotonin syndrome, marked by agitation, hallucinations, elevated body temperature, and rapid changes in blood pressure. Although most dramatic in the case of the MAOIs, newer antidepressants may also be associated with potentially dangerous interactions with other medications.

Medications for depressive disorders are not habit forming. Nevertheless, as is the case with any type of medication prescribed for more than a few days, doctors must carefully monitor these treatments to determine if the patient is getting the most effective dosage. The doctor should check regularly the dosage of each medicine and its effectiveness.

For the small number of people for whom MAO inhibitors are the best treatment, it is necessary to avoid certain foods that contain high levels of tyramine, including many cheeses, wines, and pickles, as well as medications such as decongestants. The interaction of tyramine with MAOIs can bring on a hypertensive crisis (a sharp increase in blood pressure) that can lead to a stroke. The doctor should furnish a complete list of prohibited foods, and the patient should carry it at all times. Other forms of antidepressants require no food restrictions. Efforts are underway to develop a "skin patch" system for one of the newer MAOIs, selegiline. If successful, this may be a more convenient and safer medication option than the older MAOI tablets.

Medications of any kind—prescribed, over the counter, or borrowed—should never be mixed without consulting a doctor. Health professionals who may prescribe a medication, such as a dentist or other medical specialist, should be told of all the medications the patient is taking. Some medications, although safe when taken alone, can cause severe and dangerous side effects if taken in combination with others.

Alcohol—including wine, beer, and hard liquor—or street drugs may reduce the effectiveness of antidepressants and should be avoided. However, doctors may permit people who have not had a problem with alcohol abuse or dependence to use a modest amount of alcohol while taking one of the newer antidepressants.

Antianxiety drugs or sedatives are not antidepressants. They are sometimes prescribed along with antidepressants, but they are not effective when taken alone for a depressive disorder. Stimulants, such as amphetamines, are also not effective antidepressants, but they are used occasionally, under close supervision, in medically ill depressed patients.

Lithium has for many years been the treatment of choice for bipolar disorder, as it can be effective in smoothing out the mood swings common to this illness. Doctors must carefully monitor its use as the range between an effective dose and a toxic one is small. If a person has preexisting thyroid, kidney, or heart disorders or epilepsy, lithium may not be recommended. Fortunately, other medications have been found to be of benefit in controlling mood swings. Among these are two mood stabilizing anticonvulsants, valproate (Depakote®) and carbamazepine (Tegretol®). Both of these medications have gained wide acceptance in clinical practice, and the Food and Drug Administration has approved valproate for first line treatment of acute mania. Other anticonvulsants that are being used now include lamotrigine (Lamictal®), and topiramate (Topamax®); however, their role in the treatment of bipolar disorder is not yet proven and remains under study.

Most people who have bipolar disorder take more than one medication. In addition to lithium and/or an anticonvulsant, doctors often prescribe a medication for accompanying agitation, anxiety, depression, or insomnia. Finding the best possible combination of these medications is of utmost importance to the patient and requires close monitoring by the physician.

Questions about any medication prescribed, or problems that may be related to it, should be discussed with your doctor.

Side Effects

Before starting a new medication, ask the doctor to tell you about any side effects you may experience. Antidepressants may cause mild and, usually, temporary side effects (sometimes referred to as adverse effects) in some people. Typically, these are annoying, but not serious. However, any unusual reactions or side effects, or those that interfere with functioning, should be reported to the doctor immediately.

The most common side effects of the newer antidepressants (SSRIs and others) are the following:

- **Headache:** Headache will usually go away.

- **Nausea:** Nausea is also temporary, but even when it occurs, it is short lived after each dose.

- **Insomnia and nervousness** (trouble falling asleep or waking often during the night): These side effects may occur during the first few weeks but are usually resolved over time or with a reduction in dosage.

- **Agitation** (feeling jittery): Notify your doctor if this happens for the first time after the drug is taken and is persistent.

- **Sexual problems:** Consult your doctor if the problem is persistent or worrisome. Although depression itself can lower libido and impair sexual performance, SSRIs and some other antidepressants can provoke sexual dysfunction. These side effects can affect more than half of adults taking SSRIs. In men, common problems include reduced sexual drive, erectile dysfunction, and delayed ejaculation. For some men, dosage reductions or acquired tolerance to the medication reduce sexual dysfunction symptoms. Although changing from one SSRI to another has generally not been shown to be beneficial, one study showed that citalopram (Celexa®) did not seem to cause sexual impairment in patients who had experienced such events with another SSRI.

Some clinicians treating men with antidepressant associated sexual dysfunction report improvement with the addition of bupropion (Wellbutrin®) or sildenafil (Viagra®) to ongoing treatment. Be sure to discuss the various options with your doctor and inquire about other interventions that can help.

Tricyclic antidepressants have different types of side effects:

- **Dry mouth:** Drinking sips of water, chewing sugarless gum, and cleaning teeth daily is helpful.

- **Constipation:** Adding bran cereals, prunes, fruit, and vegetables to your diet should help.

- **Bladder problems:** Emptying the bladder may be troublesome, and the urine stream may not be as strong as usual; notify your doctor if there is marked difficulty or pain. This side effect may be particularly problematic in older men with enlarged prostate conditions.

- **Sexual problems:** Sexual functioning may change; men may experience some loss of interest in sex and difficulty in maintaining an erection or achieving orgasm. If they are worrisome, discuss these side effects your doctor.

- **Blurred vision:** This effect will pass soon and will not usually necessitate a new glasses prescription.

- **Dizziness:** Rising from the bed or chair slowly is helpful.

- **Drowsiness as a daytime problem:** This side effect usually passes soon. If you feel drowsy or sedated you should not drive or operate heavy equipment. The more sedating antidepressants are generally taken at bedtime to help sleep and minimize daytime drowsiness.

Psychotherapies

Several forms of psychotherapy, including some short term (10- to 20-week) therapies, can help people with depressive disorders. Two of the short-term psychotherapies that research has shown to be effective for depression are cognitive behavioral therapy (CBT) and interpersonal therapy (IPT). Cognitive behavioral therapists help patients change the negative thinking and behavior patterns that contribute to, or result from, depression. Through verbal exchange with the therapist, as well as "homework" assignments between therapy sessions, CBT helps patients understand their depression and resolve problems related to it. Interpersonal therapists help patients work through disturbed personal relationships that may be contributing to or worsening their depression.

Psychotherapy is offered by a variety of licensed mental health providers, including psychiatrists, psychologists, social workers, and mental health counselors.

For many depressed patients, especially those with moderate to severe depression, a combination of antidepressant medication and psychotherapy is the preferred approach to treatment. Some psychiatrists offer both types of intervention. Alternatively, two mental health professionals may collaborate in the treatment of a person with depression; for example, a psychiatrist or other physician, such as a family doctor, may prescribe medication while a nonmedical therapist provides ongoing psychotherapy.

Electroconvulsive Therapy

Electroconvulsive therapy (ECT) is another treatment option that may be particularly useful for individuals whose depression is severe or life threatening or who cannot take antidepressant medication. ECT often is effective in cases where antidepressant medications do not provide sufficient relief of symptoms. The exact mechanisms by which ECT exerts its therapeutic effect are not yet known.

In recent years, ECT has much improved. Before treatment, which is done under brief anesthesia, patients are given a muscle relaxant. Electrodes are placed at precise locations on the head to deliver electrical impulses. The stimulation causes a brief (about 30-second) generalized seizure within the brain, which is necessary for therapeutic efficacy. The person receiving ECT does not consciously experience the electrical stimulus.

A typical course of ECT entails six to 12 treatments, administered at a rate of three times per week, on either an inpatient or outpatient basis. To sustain the response to ECT, continuation treatment, often in the form of antidepressant and/or mood stabilizer medication, must be instituted. Some individuals may require maintenance ECT (M ECT), which is delivered on an outpatient basis at a rate usually of one treatment weekly, tapered off to bi-weekly to monthly for up to one year.

The most common side effects of ECT are confusion and memory loss for events surrounding the period of ECT treatment. The confusion and disorientation experienced upon awakening after ECT typically clear within an hour. More persistent memory problems are variable and can be minimized with the use of modern treatment techniques, such as application of both stimulus electrodes to the right side of the head (unilateral ECT). A recent study showed no adverse cognitive effects of M ECT after one year.

Herbal Therapy

In the past several years, there has been an increase in public interest in the use of herbs for the treatment of both depression and anxiety. The extract from St. John's wort (*Hypericum perforatum*), a wild growing plant with yellow flowers, has been used extensively in Europe as a treatment for mild to moderate depression, and it now ranks among the top selling botanical products in the United States. Because of the increase in Americans' use of St. John's wort and the need to answer important remaining questions about the herb's efficacy for long-term treatment of depression, the National Institutes of

Health (NIH) conducted a clinical trial to determine whether a well standardized extract of St. John's wort is effective in the treatment of adults suffering from major depression of moderate severity. The trial found that St. John's wort was no more effective for treating major depression of moderate severity than an inert pill (placebo). Another study is under way, looking at St. John's wort for the treatment of minor depression.

Research from NIH has shown that St. John's wort interacts with some drugs including certain drugs used to control HIV [human immunodeficiency virus] infection. The Food and Drug Administration issued a Public Health Advisory on February 10, 2000, which stated that the herb appears to affect an important metabolic pathway that many prescription drugs use to treat conditions such as heart disease, depression, seizures, certain cancers, and rejection of organ transplants. The same pathway is also responsible for the effectiveness of oral contraceptives to prevent pregnancy. Using the herb may limit the effectiveness of these medications.

People taking HIV medications should be especially careful since St. John's wort may reduce the HIV medication levels in the bloodstream and could allow the AIDS [acquired immunodeficiency syndrome] virus to rebound, perhaps in a drug resistant form. Health care providers should alert their patients about these potential drug interactions, and patients should always consult their health care provider before taking any herbal supplement.

Chapter 41

Paying for Mental Health Care

Chapter Contents

Section 41.1

Finding Low-Cost Mental Health Care and Help Paying for Prescriptions

"Finding Low-Cost Mental Health Care," September 2010, reprinted with permission from www.kidshealth.org. Copyright © 2010 The Nemours Foundation. This information was provided by KidsHealth, one of the largest resources online for medically reviewed health information written for parents, kids, and teens. For more articles like this one, visit www.KidsHealth.org, or www.TeensHealth.org.

What should you do if you're under a lot of stress or dealing with a mental health issue and you don't have the money for treatment?

You're not alone if you're concerned about paying for mental health care. Lots of people need help and worry that they can't afford it. Even if you have insurance, it can be challenging. Some insurance companies don't cover mental health services very much, if at all, and they often have expensive copays and deductibles.

Still, it is possible to find affordable—sometimes even free—mental health care or support.

Free or Low-Cost Counseling

When it comes to finding a counselor, start at school. School counselors and school psychologists can provide a good listening ear—for free. They can help you size up the situation you're dealing with and, if needed, refer you to more support in your county or community.

If your school counselor can't help, you'll need to do a little more research to figure out how to get help. Some of the free or low-cost mental health care possibilities to explore include:

- **Local mental health centers and clinics:** These groups are funded by federal and state governments so they charge less than you might pay a private therapist. Search online for "mental health services" and the name of the county or city where you live. Or, go to the website for the National Association of Free Clinics [http://www.freeclinics.us]. The U.S. Department of Health and Human Services' Health Resources and Services Administration [http://www.hrsa.gov] also provides a list of federally funded clinics by state. One thing to keep in mind: Not every mental health clinic will fit your needs. Some might not work with people your age. For example, a clinic might specialize in veterans or kids with developmental disabilities. It's still worth a call, though. Even if a clinic can't help you, the people who work there might recommend someone who can.

- **Hospitals:** Call your local hospitals and ask what kinds of mental health services they offer—and at what price. Teaching hospitals, where doctors are trained, often provide low- or no-cost services.

- **Colleges and universities:** If a college in your area offers graduate degrees in psychology or social work, the students might run free or low-cost clinics as part of their training.

- **On-campus health services:** If you're in college or about to start, find out what kind of counseling and therapy your school offers and at what cost. Ask if they offer financial assistance for students.

- **Employee Assistance Programs (EAPs):** These free programs provide professional therapists to evaluate people for mental health conditions and offer short-term counseling. Not everyone has access to this benefit: EAPs are run through workplaces, so you (or your parents) need to work for an employer that offers this type of program.

- **Private therapists:** Ask trusted friends and adults who they'd recommend, then call to see if they offer a "sliding fee scale" (this means they charge based on how much you can afford to pay). Some psychologists even offer certain services for free, if necessary. You can find a therapist in your area by going to the website for your state's psychological association or to the site for the American Psychological Association (APA). To qualify for low-cost services, you may need to prove financial need. If you still live at home, that could mean getting parents or guardians involved in filling out paperwork. But your therapist will keep everything confidential.

If you're in college, you may be covered under a parent's health insurance policy. (Depending on the rules in your state, you may even be covered if you are not in college.) It's worth a call to your parent's insurance company to find out.

Financial Help

Programs like Medicaid or the State Children's Health Insurance Program (SCHIP) offer free or reduced-fee medical insurance to teens who are not covered. To find out if you qualify for mental health assistance through these programs, call your doctor's office or hospital and ask to speak to a financial counselor. Your school counselor also might be able to help you figure out what kind of public medical assistance you could qualify for and guide you through the process of applying.

People under age 18 who live at home will need a parent or guardian to sign off on the paperwork for these programs. After that, though, your care will be confidential. A therapist won't tell parents what you've talked about—unless he or she thinks you may harm yourself or another person.

Getting Help in a Crisis

If you're feeling suicidal, very hopeless or depressed, or like you might harm yourself or others in any way, call a suicide or crisis hotline. These offer free help right away.

- **Suicide hotlines:** Toll-free confidential lines like 800-SUICIDE or 800-999-9999 are staffed 24 hours a day, seven days a week by trained professionals who can help you without ever knowing your name or seeing your face. They can often give you a referral to a mental health professional you can follow up with in your area.

- **Crisis hotlines:** These help survivors of rape, violence, and other traumas, Some may also provide short-term counseling. To find one, do an online search for your state and "crisis hotline."

Other cost-effective ways to help you work through crisis situations are:

- **Emergency rooms (ERs):** Emergency rooms are required to evaluate and care for people who have emotional emergencies as well as physical ones. If you think you might hurt yourself or someone else, you can also call 911.

- **Local crisis centers:** Some states have walk-in crisis centers for people coping with mental health problems, abuse, or sexual assault. They're a bit like ERs for people who are having an emotional crisis.

Each county and state does things differently. A few might not have crisis centers. Others may have mobile units that come to you in an emergency. Some crisis centers operate in hospitals, others are run by non-profits or county mental health services. To see if there's a crisis center near you, search online for your city, county, or state and terms like "crisis center," "crisis counseling center," "psychiatric emergency services," or "crisis intervention."

If you need help finding any kind of services, contact your state's mental health association or psychological association to find out where you can get therapy and treatment near you.

Prescriptions

Paying for prescriptions can really drain your wallet. Here are some ways to be smart about the money you spend on medicines:

- Find out if you can take generic or non-brand medicines. Ask your doctor or pharmacist if there are over-the-counter versions of the same kinds of prescription medications.

- Find out about prescription assistance programs (also called "patient assistance programs"). The Partnership for Prescription Association gives free or low-cost prescriptions to people who qualify based on income. Visit their website to learn more.

- Compare prices at local pharmacies. Call each to ask what they're charging for your prescriptions.

- Contact the pharmaceutical company that makes the medication. All the big pharmaceutical companies have prescription assistance numbers you can call for help.

- Beware of free prescription samples (or coupons and rebates). They sound appealing, but they are often for expensive, name-brand medications. That's fine while the samples last. But since doctors don't like to change a medication if it's working, you could get stuck paying full price after the samples run out. Before accepting a free sample, talk to your doctor about whether you can afford that medication in the long term. If it's something you'll only need for as long as the samples last, take advantage of the freebie!

If you're already taking medication, there are two things to know:

- Never stop taking a prescribed medication or reduce your dosage because you can't afford to fill the prescription. Some medications can cause side effects if they're adjusted or stopped without a doctor's advice.

- Never use someone else's medicine. Even if the person has the same health condition you do, medications work differently for different people.

- If you can't afford to refill a prescription, call the prescribing doctor. Say you're having a hard time affording your meds and need some advice.

- It's not unusual these days for people to ask for this kind of help, and doctor's offices often know how to get it or put you in touch with someone who can.

Parents and Other Adults

Navigating your way through the health care system can be confusing (even for adults). That's why it's a good idea to have a parent, relative, doctor, school counselor, or social worker help you connect with a mental health professional.

But what if you want to get counseling without a parent (or guardian) knowing? In many states, teens can be given mental health treatment without parental consent. When you call a clinic, hospital, or therapist, ask about your state's rules on parental consent for mental health services. And, when you see a counselor, find out about the rules when it comes to filling a prescription. Even if you can get confidential care, your parents may need to give the OK to fill prescriptions.

Whatever happens, don't let money hold you back from getting help. Affordable mental health care options are out there—it may just take some time and effort to find them. But don't give up. Stress and mental health problems don't usually get better on their own.

Section 41.2

Medicare and Your Mental Health Care Benefits

Excerpted from "Medicare and Your Mental Health Benefits," by the Center for Medicare and Medicaid Services (CMS, www.medicare.gov), December 2009.

Mental health conditions like depression or anxiety can come at any age and can happen to anyone. If you think you may have problems that affect your mental health, you can get help. Talk to your doctor or health care provider if you have any of the following symptoms:

- Sad, empty, or hopeless feelings

- A lack of energy

- Trouble concentrating

- Difficulty sleeping

- Little interest in things you used to enjoy

- Thoughts of ending your life

Mental health care includes services and programs to help diagnose and treat mental health conditions. These services and programs may be provided in outpatient and inpatient settings. Medicare helps cover outpatient and inpatient mental health care, as well as prescription drugs. This text gives you information about mental health benefits in Original Medicare.

If you get your Medicare benefits through a Medicare health plan, check your plan's membership materials and call the plan for details about your Medicare-covered mental health benefits. These plans provide all your Part A and Part B coverage.

If you need immediate help for yourself or someone in a crisis, call the National Suicide Prevention Lifeline at 800-273-TALK or 800-SUICIDE (800-273-8255). TTY users should call 800-799-4TTY (800-799-4889). Call the Lifeline for any reason such as the following:

- To speak with someone who cares

- If you feel you might be in danger of hurting yourself

- To speak to a crisis worker if you're concerned about someone

- To find referrals to mental health services in your area

How Original Medicare Covers Mental Health Services

Medicare Part A (Hospital Insurance) helps cover mental health care if you are a hospital inpatient. Medicare Part A covers your room, meals, nursing care, and other related services and supplies.

Medicare Part B (Medical Insurance) helps cover mental health services that you would generally get outside a hospital, including visits with a psychiatrist or other doctor, visits with a clinical psychologist or clinical social worker, and lab tests ordered by your doctor. Medicare Part B may also pay for partial hospitalization services, if you need intensive coordinated outpatient care.

Medicare Part D (Medicare prescription drug coverage) helps cover prescription drugs you may need to treat a mental health condition.

Outpatient Mental Health Care and Professional Services

What Original Medicare Covers

If you are in Original Medicare and have Medicare Part B (Medical Insurance), Medicare helps cover visits with these types of health professionals:

- A psychiatrist or other doctor

- Clinical psychologist

- Clinical social worker

- Clinical nurse specialist

- Nurse practitioner

- Physician's assistant

It's important to know that Medicare only covers these visits when they are provided by a health care provider who accepts Medicare payment. To pay even less, you should also ask your health care providers if they accept assignment before you schedule an appointment.

Medicare Part B helps cover outpatient mental health services. This includes services that are usually provided outside a hospital (like in a clinic, or doctor's or therapist's office), and those provided in a hospital's outpatient department. Medicare helps cover the following services (deductibles and coinsurance apply):

- Individual and group psychotherapy with doctors or certain other licensed professionals allowed by the state to give these services

- Family counseling if the main purpose is to help with your treatment

- Testing to find out if you are getting the services you need and/or if your current treatment is helping you

- Psychiatric evaluation

- Medication management

- Occupational therapy that's part of your mental health treatment

- Certain prescription drugs that aren't usually self-administered, like some injections

- Individual patient training and education about your condition

- Diagnostic tests

- A screening for depression during the one-time "Welcome to Medicare" physical exam (Note: This physical exam is only covered if you have it within the first 12 months you have Medicare Part B.)

- Partial hospitalization (This may be covered.)

What You Pay

After you pay your yearly Medicare Part B deductible ($155 in 2010), how much you pay for mental health services will depend on whether the purpose of your visit is to diagnose your condition or to get treatment.

For visits to a doctor or other health care provider to diagnose your condition, you pay 20% of the Medicare-approved amount.

For outpatient treatment of your condition (such as psychotherapy), you pay 45% of the Medicare-approved amount in 2010 (which is less than in 2009). Congress passed legislation that reduces how much people with Medicare pay for outpatient mental health treatment to be in line with coinsurance amounts for other medical services. How much you pay for these services will continue to decrease over the next few years.

Assignment

Getting treatment from a doctor or provider who accepts "assignment" can reduce your out-of-pocket costs. If doctors or providers accept assignment, they agree to the following conditions:

- To accept only the amounts Medicare approves for their services

- To be paid by Medicare

- To only charge you, or other insurance you may have, the Medicare deductible or coinsurance amount

Medicare May Cover Partial Hospitalization

Medicare Part B covers partial hospitalization in some cases. It's a structured program of outpatient active psychiatric treatment that's more intense than the care you get in a doctor's or therapist's office. This type of treatment is provided during the day and doesn't require an overnight stay. These programs are usually given through hospital outpatient departments and local community mental health centers.

Your doctor or therapist may think that you could benefit from a partial hospitalization program. For Medicare to cover a partial hospitalization program, a doctor must certify that you would otherwise need inpatient treatment. Your doctor and the partial hospitalization program must accept Medicare payment.

In 2010, you pay a percentage of the Medicare-approved amount for each service you get from a qualified professional. You also pay 20% of the Medicare-approved amount for each day of service when provided in a hospital outpatient department or a community mental health center.

What Original Medicare Doesn't Cover

Medicare doesn't cover the cost of the following:

- Meals

- Transportation to or from mental health care services

- Support groups that bring people together to talk and socialize (Unlike group psychotherapy, which is covered.)

- Testing or training for job skills that isn't part of your mental health treatment

Note: If you have a Medigap (Medicare Supplement Insurance) policy, an employee or retiree plan, or other health insurance coverage, be sure to tell your doctor or other health care provider so your bills get paid correctly.

Inpatient Mental Health Care

What Original Medicare Covers

If you have Original Medicare and Medicare Part A (Hospital Insurance), Medicare helps pay for mental health services given in a hospital that require you to be admitted as an inpatient. These services can be provided in a general hospital or in a psychiatric hospital that only cares for people with mental health conditions. Regardless of which type of hospital you choose, Medicare Part A will help cover mental health services.

If you're in a psychiatric hospital (instead of a general hospital), Medicare Part A only pays for up to 190 days of inpatient psychiatric hospital services during your lifetime.

What You Pay

Medicare measures your use of hospital services, including services you get in a psychiatric hospital, in benefit periods. A benefit period begins the day you go into a hospital or skilled nursing facility for either physical or mental health care. The benefit period ends after you haven't had hospital or skilled nursing care for 60 days in a row. If you go into a hospital again after 60 days, a new benefit period begins, and you must pay a new inpatient hospital deductible.

There's no limit to the number of benefit periods you can have when you get mental health care in a general hospital. You can also have multiple benefit periods when you get care in a psychiatric hospital, but remember, there's a lifetime limit of 190 days.

For each benefit period, you pay the following in 2010:

- $1,100 deductible and no coinsurance for days 1–60 of each benefit period

- $275 per day for days 61–90 of each benefit period

- $550 per "lifetime reserve day" after day 90 of each benefit period (up to 60 days over your lifetime)

Note: Medicare Part B helps cover mental health services provided by doctors and other providers if you're admitted as a hospital inpatient. You pay 20% of the Medicare-approved amount for these mental health services while you're a hospital inpatient.

What Original Medicare Doesn't Cover

Medicare doesn't cover the cost of private duty nursing, a telephone or television in your room, personal items (like toothpaste, socks, or razors), or a private room unless medically necessary.

Note: If you have Medigap (Medicare Supplement Insurance) or other health insurance coverage, be sure to tell your doctor or other health care provider so your bills get paid correctly.

Medicare Prescription Drug Coverage (Medicare Part D)

Medicare offers prescription drug coverage for everyone with Medicare. To get Medicare prescription drug coverage, you must join a Medicare drug plan. Medicare drug plans are run by insurance companies and other private companies approved by Medicare. Each Medicare drug plan can vary in cost and in the specific drugs it covers. It's important to know your plan's coverage rules and your rights as a member of a Medicare drug plan.

Chapter 42

Finding and Choosing a Therapist

These resources can help you locate and choose a therapist who is right for you.

Finding a Therapist

There are many ways to find a therapist. You can start by asking friends and family if they can recommend anyone. Make sure the therapist has skills in treating trauma survivors.

On the Phone

One way to locate a therapist is to make some phone calls. When you call, say that you are trying to find a therapist who specializes in effective treatment for depression, such as cognitive behavioral therapy (CBT).

- Contact your local mental health agency or family doctor.
- Call your state psychological association.
- Call the psychology department at a local college or university.
- Call the Anxiety Disorders Association of America at 240-485-1001 to access their referral network

---

Excerpted from "Finding and Choosing a Therapist," by the National Center for Posttraumatic Stress Disorder (NCPTSD, www.ptsd.va.gov), part of the Veterans Administration, June 1, 2011.

- Call the National Center for Victims of Crime's toll-free information and referral service at 800-FYI-CALL.

If you work for a large company, call the human resources office or employee assistance plan to see if they make referrals.

If you have health insurance, call to find out about mental health providers the insurance company will cover.

Some mental health services are listed in the phone book. In the Government pages, look in the "County Government Offices" section. In that section, look for "Health Services (Dept. of)" or "Department of Health Services." Then in that section, look under "Mental Health."

In the yellow pages, therapists are listed under "counseling," "psychologists," "social workers," "psychotherapists," "social and human services," or "mental health."

Online

Information can also be found using the Internet. Some organizations have databases that allow you to search for therapists near you. These databases include profiles of therapists with their areas of expertise and the types of therapy they provide. Search online for "find a therapist."

Websites you can try are the following:

- Anxiety Disorders Association of America [http://www.adaa.org/findatherapist]

- The Find a Therapist Service from the Association of Behavioral and Cognitive Therapies [http://www.abct.org/Members/?m=FindTherapist&fa=FT_Form&nolm=1]

- The Psychologist Locator from the American Psychological Association [http://locator.apa.org]

- *Psychology Today*'s Therapy Directory [http://therapists.psychologytoday.com/rms/prof_search.php]

- The Mental Health Services Locator from the Substance Abuse and Mental Health Services Administration [http://store.samhsa.gov/mhlocator]

Help for Veterans

All VA Medical Centers provide posttraumatic stress disorder (PTSD) care. Or you can use this online VA PTSD Program Locator [http://www2.va.gov/directory/guide/ptsd_flsh.asp] to find a VA PTSD

Treatment program at a VA facility near you. You can also go online to read more about services at Vet Centers [http://www.vetcenter .va.gov].

Other resources include:

- The 24/7 Veteran Combat Call Center: 877-927-8387 (WAR-VETS)

- VA Mental Health for Returning Veterans [http://www.mental-health.va.gov/returningservicevets.asp]

- VA Returning Service Members (OEF/OIF/OND) Page [http://www.oefoif.va.gov]

- My HealtheVet [http://www.myhealth.va.gov]

VA Medical Centers and Vet Centers are listed in the phone book. In the Government pages, look under "United States Government Offices." Then look for "Veterans Affairs, Dept of." In that section, look under "Medical Care" and "Vet Centers—Counseling and Guidance."

Finding a Support Group

- Anxiety Disorders Association of America offers a self-help group network. [http://www.adaa.org/finding-help/getting-support/support-groups]

- National Alliance for Mental Illness (NAMI) has a website with information for those with mental health problems. You may also find family support groups in a state or local affiliate of NAMI. [http://www.nami.org]

Choosing a Therapist

There are many things to consider in choosing a therapist. Some practical issues are location, cost, and what insurance the therapist accepts. Other issues include the therapist's background, training, and the way he or she works with people.

Here is a list of questions you may want to ask a possible therapist.

- What is your education? Are you licensed? How many years have you been practicing?

- What are your special areas of practice?

- Have you ever worked with people who have been through trauma? Do you have any special training in PTSD treatment?

- What kinds of PTSD treatments do you use? Have they been proven effective for dealing with my kind of problem or issue?

- What are your fees? (Fees are usually based on a 45-minute to 50-minute session.) Do you have any discounted fees? How much therapy would you recommend?

- What types of insurance do you accept? Do you file insurance claims? Do you accept Medicare or Medicaid insurance?

These questions are just guidelines. In the end, your choice of a therapist will come down to many factors. Think about your comfort with the person as well as his or her qualifications and experience treating PTSD.

Paying for Therapy

If you have health insurance, check to see what mental health services are covered. Medicare, Medicaid, and most major health plans typically cover a certain number of mental health counseling sessions per year, though you may have a small additional amount you will have to pay called a co-pay. Call your insurance company to see what they cover so you won't be surprised by a big bill.

If you don't have health insurance that will cover your therapy, you may still be able to get counseling, even if you can't afford to pay full price. Many community mental health centers have sliding scales that base your fee on what you are able to pay.

Who is available to provide therapy? There are many types of professionals who can provide therapy for mental health issues.

Clinical Psychologists

Clinical psychologists focus on mental health assessment and treatment. Licensed psychologists have doctoral degrees (PhD, PsyD, EdD). Their graduate training is in clinical, counseling, or school psychology. In addition to their graduate study, licensed psychologists must have another one to two years of supervised clinical experience. Psychologists have the title of "doctor," but in most states they cannot prescribe medicine.

Clinical Social Workers

The purpose of social work is to enhance human well-being. Social workers help meet the basic human needs of all people. They help people manage the forces around them that contribute to problems in living. Certified social workers have a master's degree or doctoral degree in social work (MSW, DSW, or PhD).

Master's Level Clinicians

Master's Level Clinicians have a master's degree in counseling, psychology, or marriage and family therapy (MA, MFT). They have at least two years of training beyond the four-year college degree. To be licensed, master's level clinicians must meet requirements that vary by state.

Psychiatrists

Psychiatrists have a Doctor of Medicine degree (MD). After they complete four years of medical school, they must have three to four years of residency training. Board certified psychiatrists have also passed written and oral exams given by the American Board of Psychiatry and Neurology. Since they are medical doctors, psychiatrists can prescribe medicine. Some also provide psychotherapy.

Chapter 43

Therapy for Depression

Chapter Contents

Section 43.1

Psychotherapy (Talk Therapy)

Everyone experiences sadness from time to time. But depression lasts
longer, interferes with daily life, and can cause physical pain. Fortunately,
depression is highly treatable, and getting effective treatment is crucial.
This text explains depression and how it can be treated successfully.

How does depression differ from occasional sadness?

While everyone occasionally feels sad or "blue," these feelings tend
to pass rather quickly.

By contrast, someone with depression experiences extreme sadness or
despair that lasts for at least two weeks or longer. Depressed individuals
tend to feel helpless and hopeless and to blame themselves for having
these feelings. Depression interferes with activities of daily living—such
as working or concentrating on tasks, or even eating and sleeping.

Other possible symptoms of depression include chronic pain, headaches, or stomach aches. Some people may feel angry or restless for
long periods.

People who are depressed may become overwhelmed and exhausted
and stop participating in certain everyday activities altogether. They
may withdraw from family and friends. Some depressed individuals
may have thoughts of death or suicide.

What causes depression?

A combination of genetic, chemical, biological, psychological, social
and environmental factors likely contributes to the disorder. Depression
is often a signal that certain mental, emotional, and physical aspects

of a person's life are out of balance. Chronic and serious illness such as heart disease or cancer may be accompanied by depression.

Significant transitions and major life stressors such as the death of a loved one or the loss of a job can help bring about depression. Other more subtle factors that lead to a loss of self-identity or self-esteem may also contribute. The causes of depression are not always immediately apparent, so the disorder requires careful evaluation and diagnosis by a trained mental health care professional.

Sometimes the circumstances involved in depression are ones over which an individual has little or no control. At other times, however, depression occurs when people are unable to see that they actually have choices and can bring about change in their lives.

Can depression be treated successfully?

Absolutely. Depression is highly treatable when an individual receives competent care. Licensed psychologists are highly trained mental health professionals with years of experience studying depression and helping patients recover from it.

There is still some stigma or reluctance associated with seeking help for emotional and mental health problems, including depression. Unfortunately, feelings of depression often are viewed as a sign of weakness rather than as a signal that something is out of balance. The fact is that people with depression cannot simply "snap out of it" and feel better spontaneously.

Persons with depression who do not seek help suffer needlessly. Unexpressed feelings and concerns accompanied by a sense of isolation can worsen a depression.

Getting quality treatment is crucial. If depression goes untreated, it can last for a long time and worsen other illnesses. Even people with severe depression benefit from treatment.

What evidence supports the use of psychotherapy for treatment?

Many research studies have demonstrated that psychotherapy, or talk therapy, is effective for treating depression and relieving symptoms experienced by individuals who suffer from depression. Psychological treatments may prevent a person with milder depression from becoming more severely depressed.

And although a past history of depression increases the risk of future episodes, there is evidence that ongoing psychotherapy may lessen the chance of recurrence.

How does psychotherapy help people recover?

There are several approaches to psychotherapy—including cognitive-behavioral, interpersonal, and other kinds of talk therapy—that help individuals recover from depression. Psychotherapy helps people identify the factors that contribute to their depression and deal effectively with the psychological, behavioral, interpersonal, and situational contributors.

Skilled health and mental health professionals such as licensed psychologists can work with individuals who are depressed to:

- pinpoint the life problems that contribute to their depression, and help them understand which aspects of those problems they may be able to solve or improve. A licensed psychologist can help depressed patients identify options for the future and set realistic goals that enable them to enhance their mental and emotional well-being. Psychotherapy also can assist individuals who have been depressed in the past with identifying how they have successfully dealt with similar feelings.

- identify negative or distorted thought patterns that contribute to feelings of hopelessness and helplessness that accompany depression.

- develop skills to relieve suffering and prevent later bouts of depression. Skills may include developing or strengthening social networks, creating new ways to cope with challenges, and crafting a personal self-care plan that includes positive lifestyle changes.

In what other ways do psychologists help individuals suffering from depression, and also help their loved ones?

Living with a depressed person can be very difficult and stressful on family members and friends. The pain of watching a loved one suffer from depression can bring about feelings of helplessness and loss.

Family or couples therapy may be beneficial in bringing together all the individuals affected by depression and helping them learn effective ways to cope together. This type of psychotherapy can also provide a good opportunity for individuals who have never experienced depression themselves to learn more about it and to identify constructive ways to support a loved one who is suffering from depression.

The support and involvement of family and friends can play a crucial role in aiding someone who is depressed.

Individuals in the "support system" can encourage a depressed loved one to stick with treatment and practice the coping techniques and problem-solving skills he or she is learning through psychotherapy.

Are medications useful for treating depression?

Medications are helpful for reducing symptoms of depression in some people, particularly when their depression is severe. Some health care professionals treating depression may favor using a combination of psychotherapy and medications. Given the side effects, any use of medication requires close monitoring.

Psychotherapy is often recommended as a first line of treatment for children and adolescents, especially those with mild to moderate depression. Further, some adults with depression may prefer psychotherapy to the use of medications if their depression is not severe.

By conducting a thorough assessment, a licensed and trained mental health professional can help make recommendations about an effective course of treatment for an individual's depression.

Depression can seriously impair a person's ability to function in everyday situations. But the prospects for recovery are good for individuals with depression who receive appropriate professional care.

Section 43.2

Cognitive Behavioral Therapy

Excerpted and adapted from "Treatment of PTSD," by the National
Center for Posttraumatic Stress Disorder (NCPTSD, www.ncptsd.va.gov),
part of the Veterans Administration, October 5, 2010.

What is cognitive therapy?

In cognitive therapy (CBT), your therapist helps you understand and
change how you think about your depression. You will learn to identify
thoughts about the world and yourself that are making you feel afraid
or upset. With the help of your therapist, you will learn to replace these
thoughts with more accurate and less distressing thoughts. You will also
learn ways to cope with feelings such as anger, guilt, and fear.

After depression or a traumatic event, you might blame yourself for
things you couldn't have changed. For example, a soldier may feel guilty
about decisions he or she had to make during war. Cognitive therapy, a type
of CBT, helps you understand that your depression was not your fault.

What is group therapy?

Many people want to talk about their depression with others who have
had similar experiences. In group therapy, you talk with a group of people
who also have been through depression. Sharing your story with others may
help you feel more comfortable talking about your depression. This can help
you cope with your symptoms, memories, and other parts of your life.

Group therapy helps you build relationships with others who understand what you've been through. You learn to deal with emotions such
as shame, guilt, anger, rage, and fear. Sharing with the group also can
help you build self-confidence and trust. You'll learn to focus on your
present life, rather than feeling overwhelmed by the past.

What is brief psychodynamic psychotherapy?

In this type of therapy, you learn ways of dealing with emotional
conflicts caused by your depression. This therapy helps you understand
how your past affects the way you feel now.

Your therapist can help you do the following:

- Identify what triggers your stressful memories and other symp-toms

- Find ways to cope with intense feelings about the past

- Become more aware of your thoughts and feelings, so you can change your reactions to them

- Raise your self-esteem

What is family therapy?

Depression can affect your whole family. Your kids or your partner may not understand why you feel depressed sometimes, or why you're under so much stress. They may feel scared, guilty, or even angry about your condition.

Family therapy is a type of counseling that involves your whole fam-ily. A therapist helps you and your family to communicate, maintain good relationships, and cope with tough emotions. Your family can learn more about depression and how it is treated.

In family therapy, each person can express his or her fears and concerns. It's important to be honest about your feelings and to listen to others.

You can talk about your depression symptoms and what triggers them. You also can discuss the important parts of your treatment and re-covery. By doing this, your family will be better prepared to help you.

You may consider having individual therapy for your depression symptoms and family therapy to help you with your relationships.

Section 43.3

Case-Managed Care Improves Outcomes for Depressed Patients

From "Case-Managed Care Improves Outcomes for Depressed Patients with Multiple Medical Conditions," by the National Institute of Mental Health (NIMH, www.nimh.nih.gov), part of the National Institutes of Health, December 30, 2010.

People with diabetes or heart disease plus depression fare better if their medical care is coordinated by a care manager who also educates patients about their condition and provides motivational support, compared to those who receive care from their primary care physician only, according to an NIMH-funded study published December 30, 2010, in the *New England Journal of Medicine*.

Background

Coexisting depression is common among patients with diabetes or heart disease, especially if their medical conditions are poorly controlled. Having depression puts these patients at higher risk for poor self-care and more medical complications, and a higher risk for death. Patients dealing with multiple chronic conditions also tend to incur higher medical costs.

Wayne Katon, MD, of the University of Washington, and colleagues at Group Health Research Institute in Seattle developed a team-based intervention approach—TEAMcare—that aimed to improve medical outcomes and ease depression symptoms among these patients. They tested the intervention in a randomized controlled trial of 214 participants in 14 primary care clinics in Washington state. The participants all had poorly controlled diabetes and/or heart disease with coexisting depression.

Half of the patients were randomized to a 12-month trial of TEAMcare, in which a medically supervised nurse care manager coordinated their care with their primary care provider (PCP) and other medical professionals. The nurse care manager also helped patients set goals for controlling their medical conditions, provided motivation and education about taking their medications correctly, consulted with patients' PCPs about changes in medications recommended by supervisors, and encouraged better self-care. The other half of the participants received usual care, in which their PCP consulted with them about depression care and medical disease control, but they did not have a nurse care manager coordinating their care.

Results of the Study

Overall, patients in the TEAMcare intervention fared better than those in usual care. Symptoms of depression eased in the TEAMcare group more so than in the usual care group. Patients in the TEAMcare intervention also showed greater improvements in blood glucose levels, blood pressure, and "bad" cholesterol levels, compared to patients in usual care. Patients in TEAMcare were also more likely to have their medications adjusted, indicating a desire to fine-tune their care to achieve better results. TEAMcare patients also reported greater satisfaction with their medical care and a higher quality of life.

Significance

Previous research suggests that patients who are more satisfied with their medical care tend to be more motivated to take better care of themselves and therefore have better outcomes. According to the researchers, TEAMcare offers a promising way of improving outcomes in patients with multiple medical illnesses and depression because it provides systematic patient support as well as assistance to PCPs.

The researchers also note that patients with multiple medical conditions tend to have high health care costs. The study results suggest that a proactive, coordinated intervention like TEAMcare may facilitate better, more efficient care of these patients in particular.

What's Next

TEAMcare was tested among a specific population enrolled in one health plan, using highly trained nurse care managers. Further study is needed to determine whether the approach can be cost-effectively applied to broader populations, and whether less experienced nurse care managers could be used without sacrificing quality of care.

Reference

Katon WJ, Lin EHB, Von Korff M, Ciechanowski P, Ludman EJ, Young B, Peterson D, Rutter CM, McGregor M, McCulloch D. Multi-condition collaborative care for chronic illnesses and depression. *New England Journal of Medicine*. Dec. 30, 2010.

Section 43.4

Telephone-Based Depression Treatment Program Effective While Cost Efficient

From "Telephone-Based Depression Treatment Program Effective While Cost Efficient," by the National Institute of Mental Health (NIMH, www.nimh.nih .gov), part of the National Institutes of Health, November 3, 2009.

Patients who receive structured, telephone-based support to manage their depression gain significant benefits with only moderate increases in health care costs compared to those who receive usual care, according to an NIMH-funded analysis published in the October 2009 issue of the *Archives of General Psychiatry*.

Background

Previous research found structured depression treatment programs in primary care to be effective, but the success of their dissemination likely will depend on whether benefits can be balanced with costs, according to researchers at Group Health Research Institute in Seattle led by Gregory Simon, MD, MPH.

Simon and colleagues conducted a randomized controlled trial of a telephone-based depression treatment program within one health care plan.

Between November 2000 and June 2004, 600 patients were randomly assigned for two years to one of three depression treatment groups:

- Telephone care management that included outreach calls for monitoring and support

- Telephone care management plus telephone-based cognitive behavioral therapy (CBT)

- Usual care, which consisted of follow-up by a primary care provider and referral to a mental health care specialist

Previously published data showed that telephone care management plus CBT yielded the most significant and sustained improvements in depression, while the care management program alone showed modest improvements.[1,2] This most recent paper examined the cost effectiveness of the program.

Results of the Study

When compared to usual care, participants who received telephone care plus CBT had 46 more depression-free days at an increased cost of $397 over usual care.

Those who received just telephone care had 29 more depression-free days at an increased cost of $676 over usual care. Costs included outpatient depression treatment as well as health care plan costs for all other outpatient services.

Although adding CBT to telephone care management required more upfront costs, it led to more significant and sustained improvements, and therefore, more modest costs overall.

Significance

The findings offer some guidance to insurers and health care systems that are considering ways to improve depression care. Both interventions led to increased spending over usual care, but the costs were balanced by improvements in depression symptoms, potentially allowing for improved worker productivity.

What's Next?

Additional research is needed to determine to what extent depression and depression treatment affect other economic factors such as work productivity and burden on families. In addition, findings may be different among health care plans that calculate mental health care costs separately from overall health care spending.

References

Simon GE, Ludman EJ, Rutter C. Incremental benefit and cost of telephone care management and telephone psychotherapy for depression in primary care. *Archives of General Psychiatry*. 2009 Oct;66(10):1081–1089.

1. Simon GA, Ludman EJ, Tutty S, Operskalski B, Van Korff M. Telephone psychotherapy and telephone care management for primary care patients starting antidepressant treatment: A randomized controlled trial. *Journal of the American Medical Association*. 2004;292(8): 935–942.

2. Ludman EJ, Simon GE, Tutty S, Von Korff M. A randomized trial of telephone psychotherapy and pharmacotherapy for depression: Continuation and durability of effects. *Journal of Consulting and Clinical Psychology.* 2007;75(2): 257–266.

Chapter 44

Mental Health Medications

Chapter Contents

Section 44.1

Understanding Psychiatric Medications

Excerpted from "Mental Health Medications," by the National
Institute of Mental Health (NIMH, www.nimh.nih.gov), part of
the National Institutes of Health, April 25, 2011.

What are psychiatric medications?

Psychiatric medications treat mental disorders. Sometimes called
psychotropic or psychotherapeutic medications, they have changed the
lives of people with mental disorders for the better. Many people with
mental disorders live fulfilling lives with the help of these medications.
Without them, people with mental disorders might suffer serious and
disabling symptoms.

How are medications used to treat mental disorders?

Medications treat the symptoms of mental disorders. They cannot cure
the disorder, but they make people feel better so they can function.

Medications work differently for different people. Some people get
great results from medications and only need them for a short time.
For example, a person with depression may feel much better after
taking a medication for a few months, and may never need it again.
People with disorders like schizophrenia or bipolar disorder, or people
who have long-term or severe depression or anxiety may need to take
medication for a much longer time.

Some people get side effects from medications and other people
don't. Doses can be small or large, depending on the medication and
the person. Factors that can affect how medications work in people
include the following:

- Type of mental disorder, such as depression, anxiety, bipolar disorder, and schizophrenia

- Age, sex, and body size

- Physical illnesses

- Habits like smoking and drinking

- Liver and kidney function

- Genetics

- Other medications and herbal/vitamin supplements

- Diet

- Whether medications are taken as prescribed

What medications are used to treat schizophrenia?

Antipsychotic medications are used to treat schizophrenia and schizophrenia-related disorders. Some of these medications have been available since the mid-1950s. They are also called conventional "typical" antipsychotics. Some of the more commonly used medications include the following (See Table 44.1):

- Chlorpromazine (Thorazine)

- Haloperidol (Haldol)

- Perphenazine (generic only)

- Fluphenazine (generic only)

In the 1990s, new antipsychotic medications were developed. These new medications are called second generation, or "atypical" antipsychotics.

One of these medications was clozapine (Clozaril). It is a very effective medication that treats psychotic symptoms, hallucinations, and breaks with reality, such as when a person believes he or she is the president. But clozapine can sometimes cause a serious problem called agranulocytosis, which is a loss of the white blood cells that help a person fight infection. Therefore, people who take clozapine must get their white blood cell counts checked every week or two. This problem and the cost of blood tests make treatment with clozapine difficult for many people. Still, clozapine is potentially helpful for people who do not respond to other antipsychotic medications.

Other atypical antipsychotics were developed. All of them are effective, and none cause agranulocytosis. These include the following:

- Risperidone (Risperdal)

- Olanzapine (Zyprexa)

- Quetiapine (Seroquel)

- Ziprasidone (Geodon)

Table 44.1. Combination Antipsychotic and Antidepressant Medications

Trade Name	Generic Name	FDA Approved Age
Combination Antipsychotic and Antidepressant Medication		
Symbyax (Prozac & Zyprexa)	fluoxetine & olanzapine	18 and older
Antipsychotic Medications		
Abilify	aripiprazole	10 and older for bipolar disorder, manic or mixed episodes; 13–17 for schizophrenia and bipolar
Clozaril	clozapine	18 and older
Fanapt	iloperidone	18 and older
fluphenazine (generic only)	fluphenazine	18 and older
Geodon	ziprasidone	18 and older
Haldol	haloperidol	3 and older
Invega	paliperidone	18 and older
Loxitane	loxapine	18 and older
Moban	molindone	18 and older
Navane	thiothixene	18 and older
Orap (for Tourette's syndrome)	pimozide	12 and older
perphenazine (generic only)	perphenazine	18 and older
Risperdal	risperidone	13 and older for schizophrenia; 10 and older for bipolar mania and mixed episodes; 5–16 for irritability associated with autism
Seroquel	quetiapine	13 and older for schizophrenia; 18 and older for bipolar disorder; 10–17 for treatment of manic and mixed episodes of bipolar disorder
Stelazine	trifluoperazine	18 and older
thioridazine (generic only)	thioridazine	2 and older
Thorazine	chlorpromazine	18 and older
Zyprexa	olanzapine	18 and older; ages 13–17 as second line treatment for manic or mixed episodes of bipolar disorder and schizophrenia

- Aripiprazole (Abilify)

- Paliperidone (Invega)

The antipsychotics listed here are some of the medications used to treat symptoms of schizophrenia.

Note: The FDA [U.S. Food and Drug Administration] issued a Public Health Advisory for atypical antipsychotic medications. The FDA determined that death rates are higher for elderly people with dementia when taking this medication. A review of data has found a risk with conventional antipsychotics as well. Antipsychotic medications are not FDA-approved for the treatment of behavioral disorders in patients with dementia.

What are the side effects?

Some people have side effects when they start taking these medications. Most side effects go away after a few days and often can be managed successfully.

People who are taking antipsychotics should not drive until they adjust to their new medication. Side effects of many antipsychotics include the following:

- Drowsiness

- Dizziness when changing positions

- Blurred vision

- Rapid heartbeat

- Sensitivity to the sun

- Skin rashes

- Menstrual problems for women

Atypical antipsychotic medications can cause major weight gain and changes in a person's metabolism. This may increase a person's risk of getting diabetes and high cholesterol. A person's weight, glucose levels, and lipid levels should be monitored regularly by a doctor while taking an atypical antipsychotic medication.

Typical antipsychotic medications can cause side effects related to physical movement, such as the following:

- Rigidity

- Persistent muscle spasms

- Tremors

- Restlessness

Long-term use of typical antipsychotic medications may lead to a condition called tardive dyskinesia (TD). TD causes muscle movements a person can't control. The movements commonly happen around the mouth. TD can range from mild to severe, and in some people the problem cannot be cured. Sometimes people with TD recover partially or fully after they stop taking the medication.

Every year, an estimated 5 percent of people taking typical antipsychotics get TD. The condition happens to fewer people who take the new, atypical antipsychotics, but some people may still get TD. People who think that they might have TD should check with their doctor before stopping their medication.

How are antipsychotics taken and how do people respond to them?

Antipsychotics are usually pills that people swallow, or liquid they can drink. Some antipsychotics are shots that are given once or twice a month. Symptoms of schizophrenia, such as feeling agitated and having hallucinations, usually go away within days. Symptoms like delusions usually go away within a few weeks. After about six weeks, many people will see a lot of improvement.

However, people respond in different ways to antipsychotic medications, and no one can tell beforehand how a person will respond. Sometimes a person needs to try several medications before finding the right one. Doctors and patients can work together to find the best medication or medication combination, and dose.

Some people may have a relapse—their symptoms come back or get worse. Usually, relapses happen when people stop taking their medication, or when they only take it sometimes. Some people stop taking the medication because they feel better or they may feel they don't need it anymore. But no one should stop taking an antipsychotic medication without talking to his or her doctor. When a doctor says it is okay to stop taking a medication, it should be gradually tapered off, never stopped suddenly.

How do antipsychotics interact with other medications?

Antipsychotics can produce unpleasant or dangerous side effects when taken with certain medications. For this reason, all doctors treating a patient need to be aware of all the medications that person is taking. Doctors need to know about prescription and over-the-counter medicine, vitamins, minerals, and herbal supplements. People also need to discuss any alcohol or other drug use with their doctor.

To find out more about how antipsychotics work, the National Institute of Mental Health (NIMH) funded a study called CATIE (Clinical Antipsychotic Trials of Intervention Effectiveness). This study compared the effectiveness and side effects of five antipsychotics used to treat people with schizophrenia. In general, the study found that the older medication perphenazine worked as well as the newer, atypical medications. But because people respond differently to different medications, it is important that treatments be designed carefully for each person. You can find more information on CATIE at www.nimh.nih.gov/trials/practical/catie/index.shtml.

What medications are used to treat depression?

Depression is commonly treated with antidepressant medications. Antidepressants work to balance some of the natural chemicals in our brains. These chemicals are called neurotransmitters, and they affect our mood and emotional responses. Antidepressants work on neurotransmitters such as serotonin, norepinephrine, and dopamine.

The most popular types of antidepressants are called selective serotonin reuptake inhibitors (SSRIs). These include the following (See Table 44.2):

- Fluoxetine (Prozac)
- Citalopram (Celexa)
- Sertraline (Zoloft)
- Paroxetine (Paxil)
- Escitalopram (Lexapro)

Other types of antidepressants are serotonin and norepinephrine reuptake inhibitors (SNRIs). SNRIs are similar to SSRIs and include venlafaxine (Effexor) and duloxetine (Cymbalta). Another antidepressant that is commonly used is bupropion (Wellbutrin). Bupropion, which works on the neurotransmitter dopamine, is unique in that it does not fit into any specific drug type.

SSRIs and SNRIs are popular because they do not cause as many side effects as older classes of antidepressants. Older antidepressant medications include tricyclics, tetracyclics, and monoamine oxidase inhibitors (MAOIs). For some people, tricyclics, tetracyclics, or MAOIs may be the best medications.

Table 44.2. Antidepressant Medications
(Also Used for Anxiety Disorders)

Trade Name	Generic Name	FDA Approved Age
Anafranil (tricyclic)	clomipramine	10 and older (for OCD only)
Asendin	amoxapine	18 and older
Aventyl (tricyclic)	nortriptyline	18 and older
Celexa (SSRI)	citalopram	18 and older
Cymbalta (SNRI)	duloxetine	18 and older
Desyrel	trazodone	18 and older
Effexor (SNRI)	venlafaxine	18 and older
Elavil (tricyclic)	amitriptyline	18 and older
Emsam	selegiline	18 and older
Lexapro (SSRI)	escitalopram	18 and older; 12–17 (for major depressive disorder)
Ludiomil (tricyclic)	maprotiline	18 and older
Luvox (SSRI)	fluvoxamine	8 and older (for OCD only)
Marplan (MAOI)	isocarboxazid	18 and older
Nardil (MAOI)	phenelzine	18 and older
Norpramin (tricyclic)	desipramine	18 and older
Pamelor (tricyclic)	nortriptyline	18 and older
Parnate (MAOI)	tranylcypromine	18 and older
Paxil (SSRI)	paroxetine	18 and older
Pexeva (SSRI)	paroxetine-mesylate	18 and older
Pristiq	desvenlafaxine (SNRI)	18 and older
Prozac (SSRI)	fluoxetine	8 and older
Remeron	mirtazapine	18 and older
Sarafem (SSRI)	fluoxetine	18 and older for premenstrual dysphoric disorder (PMDD)
Sinequan (tricyclic)	doxepin	12 and older
Surmontil (tricyclic)	trimipramine	18 and older
Tofranil (tricyclic)	imipramine	6 and older (for bedwetting)
Tofranil-PM (tricyclic)	imipramine pamoate	18 and older
Vivactil (tricyclic)	protriptyline	18 and older
Wellbutrin	bupropion	18 and older
Zoloft (SSRI)	sertraline	6 and older (for OCD only)

What are the side effects?

Antidepressants may cause mild side effects that usually do not last long. Any unusual reactions or side effects should be reported to a doctor immediately.

The most common side effects associated with SSRIs and SNRIs include the following:

- Headache, which usually goes away within a few days

- Nausea (feeling sick to your stomach), which usually goes away within a few days

- Sleeplessness or drowsiness, which may happen during the first few weeks but then goes away (Sometimes the medication dose needs to be reduced or the time of day it is taken needs to be adjusted to help lessen these side effects.)

- Agitation (feeling jittery)

- Sexual problems, which can affect both men and women and may include reduced sex drive and problems having and enjoying sex

Tricyclic antidepressants can cause side effects, including the following:

- Dry mouth

- Constipation

- Bladder problems (It may be hard to empty the bladder, or the urine stream may not be as strong as usual. Older men with enlarged prostate conditions may be more affected.)

- Sexual problems, which can affect both men and women and may include reduced sex drive and problems having and enjoying sex

- Blurred vision, which usually goes away quickly

- Drowsiness (Usually, antidepressants that make you drowsy are taken at bedtime.)

People taking MAOIs need to be careful about the foods they eat and the medicines they take. Foods and medicines that contain high levels of a chemical called tyramine are dangerous for people taking MAOIs. Tyramine is found in some cheeses, wines, and pickles. The chemical is also in some medications, including decongestants and over-the-counter cold medicine.

401

Mixing MAOIs and tyramine can cause a sharp increase in blood pressure, which can lead to stroke. People taking MAOIs should ask their doctors for a complete list of foods, medicines, and other substances to avoid. An MAOI skin patch has recently been developed and may help reduce some of these risks. A doctor can help a person figure out if a patch or a pill will work for him or her.

How should antidepressants be taken?

People taking antidepressants need to follow their doctors' directions. The medication should be taken in the right dose for the right amount of time. It can take three or four weeks until the medicine takes effect. Some people take the medications for a short time, and some people take them for much longer periods. People with long-term or severe depression may need to take medication for a long time.

Once a person is taking antidepressants, it is important not to stop taking them without the help of a doctor. Sometimes people taking antidepressants feel better and stop taking the medication too soon, and the depression may return.

When it is time to stop the medication, the doctor will help the person slowly and safely decrease the dose. It's important to give the body time to adjust to the change. People don't get addicted, or "hooked," on the medications, but stopping them abruptly can cause withdrawal symptoms.

If a medication does not work, it is helpful to be open to trying another one. A study funded by NIMH found that if a person with difficult-to-treat depression did not get better with a first medication, chances of getting better increased when the person tried a new one or added a second medication to his or her treatment. The study was called STAR*D (Sequenced Treatment Alternatives to Relieve Depression).

Are herbal medicines used to treat depression?

The herbal medicine St. John's wort has been used for centuries in many folk and herbal remedies. Today in Europe, it is used widely to treat mild-to-moderate depression. In the United States, it is one of the top-selling botanical products.

The National Institutes of Health conducted a clinical trial to determine the effectiveness of treating adults who have major depression with St. John's wort. The study included 340 people diagnosed with major depression. One-third of the people took the herbal medicine, one-third took an SSRI, and one-third took a placebo, or "sugar pill." The people did not know what they were taking. The study found that

St. John's wort was no more effective than the placebo in treating major depression. A study currently in progress is looking at the effectiveness of St. John's wort for treating mild or minor depression.

Other research has shown that St. John's wort can dangerously interact with other medications, including those used to control HIV [human immunodeficiency virus]. On February 10, 2000, the FDA issued a Public Health Advisory letter stating that the herb appears to interfere with certain medications used to treat heart disease, depression, seizures, certain cancers, and organ transplant rejection. Also, St. John's wort may interfere with oral contraceptives.

Because St. John's wort may not mix well with other medications, people should always talk with their doctors before taking it or any herbal supplement.

FDA warning on antidepressants: Antidepressants are safe and popular, but some studies have suggested that they may have unintentional effects, especially in young people. In 2004, the FDA looked at published and unpublished data on trials of antidepressants that involved nearly 4,400 children and adolescents. They found that 4 percent of those taking antidepressants thought about or tried suicide (although no suicides occurred), compared to 2 percent of those receiving placebos (sugar pill).

In 2005, the FDA decided to adopt a "black box" warning label—the most serious type of warning—on all antidepressant medications. The warning says there is an increased risk of suicidal thinking or attempts in children and adolescents taking antidepressants. In 2007, the FDA proposed that makers of all antidepressant medications extend the warning to include young adults up through age 24.

The warning also says that patients of all ages taking antidepressants should be watched closely, especially during the first few weeks of treatment. Possible side effects to look for are depression that gets worse, suicidal thinking or behavior, or any unusual changes in behavior such as trouble sleeping, agitation, or withdrawal from normal social situations. Families and caregivers should report any changes to the doctor.

Results of a comprehensive review of pediatric trials conducted between 1988 and 2006 suggested that the benefits of antidepressant medications likely outweigh their risks to children and adolescents with major depression and anxiety disorders. The study was funded in part by NIMH.

Finally, the FDA has warned that combining the newer SSRI or SNRI antidepressants with one of the commonly-used "triptan" medications used to treat migraine headaches could cause a life-threatening illness called serotonin syndrome. A person with serotonin syndrome may be agitated, have hallucinations (see or hear things that are not real), have a high temperature, or have unusual blood pressure changes. Serotonin syndrome is usually associated with the older antidepressants called MAOIs, but it can happen with the newer antidepressants as well, if they are mixed with the wrong medications.

What medications are used to treat bipolar disorder?

Bipolar disorder, also called manic-depressive illness, is commonly treated with mood stabilizers. Sometimes, antipsychotics and antidepressants are used along with a mood stabilizer. See Table 44.3.

Table 44.3. Mood Stabilizing and Anticonvulsant Medications

Trade Name	Generic Name	FDA Approved Age
Depakote	divalproex sodium (valproic acid)	2 and older (for seizures)
Eskalith	lithium carbonate	12 and older
Lamictal	lamotrigine	18 and older
lithium citrate (generic only)	lithium citrate	12 and older
Lithobid	lithium carbonate	12 and older
Neurontin	gabapentin	18 and older
Tegretol	carbamazepine	any age (for seizures)
Topamax	topiramate	18 and older
Trileptal	oxcarbazepine	4 and older

What are mood stabilizers?

People with bipolar disorder usually try mood stabilizers first. In general, people continue treatment with mood stabilizers for years. Lithium is a very effective mood stabilizer. It was the first mood stabilizer approved by the FDA in the 1970s for treating both manic and depressive episodes.

Anticonvulsant medications also are used as mood stabilizers. They were originally developed to treat seizures, but they were found to help control moods as well. One anticonvulsant commonly used as a mood stabilizer is valproic acid, also called divalproex sodium (Depakote). For some people, it may work better than lithium. Other anticonvulsants used as mood stabilizers are carbamazepine (Tegretol), lamotrigine (Lamictal), and oxcarbazepine (Trileptal).

What are atypical antipsychotics?

Atypical antipsychotic medications are sometimes used to treat symptoms of bipolar disorder. Often, antipsychotics are used along with other medications.

Antipsychotics used to treat people with bipolar disorder include the following:

- Olanzapine (Zyprexa), which helps people with severe or psychotic depression, which often is accompanied by a break with reality, hallucinations, or delusions

- Aripiprazole (Abilify), which can be taken as a pill or as a shot

- Risperidone (Risperdal)

- Ziprasidone (Geodon)

- Clozapine (Clozaril), which is often used for people who do not respond to lithium or anticonvulsants.

Are antidepressants used to treat bipolar disorder symptoms?

Antidepressants are sometimes used to treat symptoms of depression in bipolar disorder. Fluoxetine (Prozac), paroxetine (Paxil), or sertraline (Zoloft) are a few that are used. However, people with bipolar disorder should not take an antidepressant on its own. Doing so can cause the person to rapidly switch from depression to mania, which can be dangerous. To prevent this problem, doctors give patients a mood stabilizer or an antipsychotic along with an antidepressant.

Research on whether antidepressants help people with bipolar depression is mixed. An NIMH-funded study found that antidepressants were no more effective than a placebo to help treat depression in people with bipolar disorder. The people were taking mood stabilizers along with the antidepressants.

What are the side effects?

Treatments for bipolar disorder have improved over the last 10 years. But everyone responds differently to medications. If you have any side effects, tell your doctor right away. He or she may change the dose or prescribe a different medication.

Different medications for treating bipolar disorder may cause different side effects. Some medications used for treating bipolar disorder have been linked to unique and serious symptoms, which are described in the following text.

Lithium can cause several side effects, and some of them may become serious. They include the following:

- Loss of coordination

- Excessive thirst

- Frequent urination

- Blackouts

- Seizures

- Slurred speech

- Fast, slow, irregular, or pounding heartbeat

- Hallucinations (seeing things or hearing voices that do not exist)

- Changes in vision

- Itching and rash

- Swelling of the eyes, face, lips, tongue, throat, hands, feet, ankles, or lower legs

If a person with bipolar disorder is being treated with lithium, he or she should visit the doctor regularly to check the levels of lithium in the blood, and make sure the kidneys and the thyroid are working normally.

Some possible side effects linked with valproic acid/divalproex sodium include the following:

- Changes in weight

- Nausea

- Stomach pain

- Vomiting

- Anorexia

- Loss of appetite

Valproic acid may cause damage to the liver or pancreas, so people taking it should see their doctors regularly.

Valproic acid may affect young girls and women in unique ways. Sometimes, valproic acid may increase testosterone (a male hormone) levels in teenage girls and lead to a condition called polycystic ovarian syndrome (PCOS). PCOS is a disease that can affect fertility and make the menstrual cycle become irregular, but symptoms tend to go away after valproic acid is stopped. It also may cause birth defects in women who are pregnant.

Lamotrigine can cause a rare but serious skin rash that needs to be treated in a hospital. In some cases, this rash can cause permanent disability or be life-threatening.

In addition, valproic acid, lamotrigine, carbamazepine, oxcarbazepine, and other anticonvulsant medications have an FDA warning. The warning states that their use may increase the risk of suicidal thoughts and behaviors. People taking anticonvulsant medications for bipolar or other illnesses should be closely monitored for new or worsening symptoms of depression, suicidal thoughts or behavior, or any unusual changes in mood or behavior. People taking these medications should not make any changes without talking to their health care professional.

Other medications for bipolar disorder may also be linked with rare but serious side effects. Always talk with the doctor or pharmacist about any potential side effects before taking the medication.

How should medications for bipolar disorder be taken?

Medications should be taken as directed by a doctor. Sometimes a person's treatment plan needs to be changed. When changes in medicine are needed, the doctor will guide the change. A person should never stop taking a medication without asking a doctor for help.

There is no cure for bipolar disorder, but treatment works for many people. Treatment works best when it is continuous, rather than on and off. However, mood changes can happen even when there are no breaks in treatment. Patients should be open with their doctors about treatment. Talking about how treatment is working can help it be more effective.

It may be helpful for people or their family members to keep a daily chart of mood symptoms, treatments, sleep patterns, and life events. This chart can help patients and doctors track the illness. Doctors can use the chart to treat the illness most effectively.

Because medications for bipolar disorder can have serious side effects, it is important for anyone taking them to see the doctor regularly to check for possibly dangerous changes in the body.

What medications are used to treat anxiety disorders?

Antidepressants, anti-anxiety medications, and beta-blockers are the most common medications used for anxiety disorders (See Table 44.4). Anxiety disorders include the following:

- Obsessive-compulsive disorder (OCD)
- Posttraumatic stress disorder (PTSD)
- Generalized anxiety disorder (GAD)
- Panic disorder
- Social phobia

Table 44.4. Anti-Anxiety Medications

Trade Name	Generic Name	FDA Approved Age
Ativan	lorazepam	18 and older
BuSpar	buspirone	18 and older
Klonopin	clonazepam	18 and older
Librium	chlordiazepoxide	18 and older
oxazepam (generic only)	oxazepam	18 and older
Tranxene	clorazepate	18 and older
Valium	diazepam	18 and older
Xanax	alprazolam	18 and older

Note: All of these anti-anxiety medications are benzodiazepines, except BuSpar.

Are antidepressants used to treat anxiety disorder symptoms?

Antidepressants were developed to treat depression, but they also help people with anxiety disorders. SSRIs such as fluoxetine (Prozac), sertraline (Zoloft), escitalopram (Lexapro), paroxetine (Paxil), and citalopram (Celexa) are commonly prescribed for panic disorder, OCD, PTSD, and social phobia. The SNRI venlafaxine (Effexor) is commonly used to treat GAD. The antidepressant bupropion (Wellbutrin) is also sometimes used. When treating anxiety disorders, antidepressants generally are started at low doses and increased over time.

Some tricyclic antidepressants work well for anxiety. For example, imipramine (Tofranil) is prescribed for panic disorder and GAD. Clomipramine (Anafranil) is used to treat OCD. Tricyclics are also started at low doses and increased over time.

MAOIs are also used for anxiety disorders. Doctors sometimes prescribe phenelzine (Nardil), tranylcypromine (Parnate), and isocarboxazid (Marplan).

People who take MAOIs must avoid certain food and medicines that can interact with their medicine and cause dangerous increases in blood pressure.

What are benzodiazepines (anti-anxiety medications)?

The anti-anxiety medications called benzodiazepines can start working more quickly than antidepressants. The ones used to treat anxiety disorders include the following:

- Clonazepam (Klonopin), which is used for social phobia and GAD

- Lorazepam (Ativan), which is used for panic disorder

- Alprazolam (Xanax), which is used for panic disorder and GAD

Buspirone (BuSpar) is an anti-anxiety medication used to treat GAD. Unlike benzodiazepines, however, it takes at least two weeks for buspirone to begin working.

Clonazepam, listed in the preceding text, is an anticonvulsant medication.

What are beta-blockers?

Beta-blockers control some of the physical symptoms of anxiety, such as trembling and sweating. Propranolol (Inderal) is a beta-blocker usually used to treat heart conditions and high blood pressure. The medicine also helps people who have physical problems related to anxiety. For example, when a person with social phobia must face a stressful situation, such as giving a speech, or attending an important meeting, a doctor may prescribe a beta-blocker. Taking the medicine for a short period of time can help the person keep physical symptoms under control.

What are the side effects?

The most common side effects for benzodiazepines are drowsiness and dizziness. Other possible side effects include the following:

- Upset stomach

- Blurred vision

- Headache

- Confusion

- Grogginess

- Nightmares

Possible side effects from buspirone (BuSpar) include the following:

- Dizziness

- Headaches

- Nausea

- Nervousness

- Lightheadedness

- Excitement

- Trouble sleeping

Common side effects from beta-blockers include the following:

- Fatigue

- Cold hands

- Dizziness

- Weakness

In addition, beta-blockers generally are not recommended for people with asthma or diabetes because they may worsen symptoms.

How should medications for anxiety disorders be taken?

People can build a tolerance to benzodiazepines if they are taken over a long period of time and may need higher and higher doses to get the same effect. Some people may become dependent on them. To avoid these problems, doctors usually prescribe the medication for short periods, a practice that is especially helpful for people who have substance abuse problems or who become dependent on medication easily. If people suddenly stop taking benzodiazepines, they may get withdrawal symptoms, or their anxiety may return. Therefore, they should be tapered off slowly.

Buspirone and beta-blockers are similar. They are usually taken on a short-term basis for anxiety. Both should be tapered off slowly. Talk to the doctor before stopping any anti-anxiety medication.

What medications are used to treat ADHD?

Attention deficit hyperactivity disorder (ADHD) occurs in both children and adults. ADHD is commonly treated with stimulants, such as the following (See Table 44.5):

- Methylphenidate (Ritalin, Metadate, Concerta, Daytrana)
- Amphetamine (Adderall)
- Dextroamphetamine (Dexedrine, Dextrostat)

In 2002, the FDA approved the nonstimulant medication atomoxetine (Strattera) for use as a treatment for ADHD. In February 2007, the FDA approved the use of the stimulant lisdexamfetamine dimesylate (Vyvanse) for the treatment of ADHD in children ages 6 to 12 years.

Table 44.5. ADHD Medications

Trade Name	Generic Name	FDA Approved Age
Adderall	amphetamine	3 and older
Adderall XR	amphetamine (extended release)	6 and older
Concerta	methylphenidate (long acting)	6 and older
Daytrana	methylphenidate patch	6 and older
Desoxyn	methamphetamine	6 and older
Dexedrine	dextroamphetamine	3 and older
Dextrostat	dextroamphetamine	3 and older
Focalin	dexmethylphenidate	6 and older
Focalin XR	dexmethylphenidate (extended release)	6 and older
Intuniv	guanfacine	6 and older
Metadate ER	methylphenidate (extended release)	6 and older
Metadate CD	methylphenidate (extended release)	6 and older
Methylin	methylphenidate (oral solution and chewable tablets)	6 and older
Ritalin	methylphenidate	6 and older
Ritalin SR	methylphenidate (extended release)	6 and older
Ritalin LA	methylphenidate (long-acting)	6 and older
Strattera	atomoxetine	6 and older
Vyvanse	lisdexamfetamine dimesylate	6 and older

Note: All of these ADHD medications are stimulants, except Intuniv and Strattera.

What are the side effects?

Most side effects are minor and disappear when dosage levels are lowered. The most common side effects include the following:

- **Decreased appetite:** Children seem to be less hungry during the middle of the day, but they are often hungry by dinnertime as the medication wears off.

- **Sleep problems:** If a child cannot fall asleep, the doctor may prescribe a lower dose. The doctor might also suggest that parents give the medication to their child earlier in the day, or stop the afternoon or evening dose. To help ease sleeping problems, a doctor may add a prescription for a low dose of an antidepressant or a medication called clonidine.

- **Stomachaches and headaches:** These can also occur with the use of ADHD medications.

- **Less common side effects:** A few children develop sudden, repetitive movements or sounds called tics. These tics may or may not be noticeable. Changing the medication dosage may make tics go away. Some children also may appear to have a personality change, such as appearing "flat" or without emotion. Talk with your child's doctor if you see any of these side effects.

How are ADHD medications taken?

Stimulant medications can be short-acting or long-acting, and can be taken in different forms such as a pill, patch, or powder. Long-acting, sustained, and extended release forms allow children to take the medication just once a day before school. Parents and doctors should decide together which medication is best for the child and whether the child needs medication only for school hours or for evenings and weekends, too.

ADHD medications help many children and adults who are hyperactive and impulsive. They help people focus, work, and learn. Stimulant medication also may improve physical coordination. However, different people respond differently to medications, so children taking ADHD medications should be watched closely.

Are ADHD medications safe?

Stimulant medications are safe when given under a doctor's supervision. Some children taking them may feel slightly different or "funny." Some parents worry that stimulant medications may lead to drug abuse or dependence, but there is little evidence of this. Research shows that teens with ADHD who took stimulant medications were less likely to abuse drugs than those who did not take stimulant medications.

FDA warning on possible rare side effects: In 2007, the FDA required that all makers of ADHD medications develop Patient Medication Guides. The guides must alert patients to possible heart and psychiatric problems related to ADHD medicine. The FDA required the Patient Medication Guides because a review of data found that ADHD patients with heart conditions had a slightly higher risk of strokes, heart attacks, and sudden death when taking the medications. The review also found a slightly higher risk (about one in 1,000) for medication-related psychiatric problems, such as hearing voices, having hallucinations, becoming suspicious for no reason, or becoming manic. This happened to patients who had no history of psychiatric problems.

The FDA recommends that any treatment plan for ADHD include an initial health and family history examination. This exam should look for existing heart and psychiatric problems.

The non-stimulant ADHD medication called atomoxetine (Strattera) carries another warning. Studies show that children and teenagers with ADHD who take atomoxetine are more likely to have suicidal thoughts than children and teenagers with ADHD who do not take atomoxetine. If your child is taking atomoxetine, watch his or her behavior carefully. A child may develop serious symptoms suddenly, so it is important to pay attention to your child's behavior every day. Ask other people who spend a lot of time with your child, such as brothers, sisters, and teachers, to tell you if they notice changes in your child's behavior. Call a doctor right away if your child shows any of the following symptoms:

- Acting more subdued or withdrawn than usual
- Feeling helpless, hopeless, or worthless
- New or worsening depression
- Thinking or talking about hurting himself or herself
- Extreme worry
- Agitation
- Panic attacks
- Trouble sleeping
- Irritability
- Aggressive or violent behavior
- Acting without thinking

- Extreme increase in activity or talking

- Frenzied, abnormal excitement

- Any sudden or unusual changes in behavior

While taking atomoxetine, your child should see a doctor often, especially at the beginning of treatment. Be sure that your child keeps all appointments with his or her doctor.

Which groups have special needs when taking psychiatric medications?

Psychiatric medications are taken by all types of people, but some groups have special needs, including the following:

- Children and adolescents

- Older adults

- Women who are pregnant or may become pregnant

Children and adolescents: Most medications used to treat young people with mental illness are safe and effective. However, many medications have not been studied or approved for use with children. Researchers are not sure how these medications affect a child's growing body. Still, a doctor can give a young person an FDA-approved medication on an "off-label" basis. This means that the doctor prescribes the medication to help the patient even though the medicine is not approved for the specific mental disorder or age.

For these reasons, it is important to watch young people who take these medications. Young people may have different reactions and side effects than adults. Also, some medications, including antidepressants and ADHD medications, carry FDA warnings about potentially dangerous side effects for young people.

More research is needed on how these medications affect children and adolescents. NIMH has funded studies on this topic. For example, NIMH funded the Preschoolers with ADHD Treatment Study (PATS), which involved 300 preschoolers (3 to 5 years old) diagnosed with ADHD. The study found that low doses of the stimulant methylphenidate are safe and effective for preschoolers. However, children of this age are more sensitive to the side effects of the medication, including slower growth rates. Children taking methylphenidate should be watched closely.

In addition to medications, other treatments for young people with mental disorders should be considered. Psychotherapy, family therapy, educational courses, and behavior management techniques can help everyone involved cope with the disorder.

Older adults: Because older people often have more medical problems than other groups, they tend to take more medications than younger people, including prescribed, over-the-counter, and herbal medications. As a result, older people have a higher risk for experiencing bad drug interactions, missing doses, or overdosing.

Older people also tend to be more sensitive to medications. Even healthy older people react to medications differently than younger people because their bodies process it more slowly. Therefore, lower or less frequent doses may be needed.

Sometimes memory problems affect older people who take medications for mental disorders. An older adult may forget his or her regular dose and take too much or not enough. A good way to keep track of medicine is to use a seven-day pill box, which can be bought at any pharmacy. At the beginning of each week, older adults and their caregivers fill the box so that it is easy to remember what medicine to take. Many pharmacies also have pillboxes with sections for medications that must be taken more than once a day.

Women who are pregnant or may become pregnant: The research on the use of psychiatric medications during pregnancy is limited. The risks are different depending on what medication is taken, and at what point during the pregnancy the medication is taken. Research has shown that antidepressants, especially SSRIs, are safe during pregnancy. Birth defects or other problems are possible, but they are very rare.

However, antidepressant medications do cross the placental barrier and may reach the fetus. Some research suggests the use of SSRIs during pregnancy is associated with miscarriage or birth defects, but other studies do not support this. Studies have also found that fetuses exposed to SSRIs during the third trimester may be born with "withdrawal" symptoms such as breathing problems, jitteriness, irritability, trouble feeding, or hypoglycemia (low blood sugar).

Most studies have found that these symptoms in babies are generally mild and short-lived, and no deaths have been reported. On the flip side, women who stop taking their antidepressant medication during pregnancy may get depression again and may put both themselves and their infant at risk.

In 2004, the FDA issued a warning against the use of certain antidepressants in the late third trimester. The warning said that doctors may want to gradually taper pregnant women off antidepressants in the third trimester so that the baby is not affected. After a woman delivers, she should consult with her doctor to decide whether to return to a full dose during the period when she is most vulnerable to postpartum depression.

Some medications should not be taken during pregnancy. Benzodiazepines may cause birth defects or other infant problems, especially if taken during the first trimester. Mood stabilizers are known to cause birth defects. Benzodiazepines and lithium have been shown to cause "floppy baby syndrome," which is when a baby is drowsy and limp, and cannot breathe or feed well.

Research suggests that taking antipsychotic medications during pregnancy can lead to birth defects, especially if they are taken during the first trimester. But results vary widely depending on the type of antipsychotic. The conventional antipsychotic haloperidol has been studied more than others, and has been found not to cause birth defects.

After the baby is born, women and their doctors should watch for postpartum depression, especially if they stopped taking their medication during pregnancy.

In addition, women who nurse while taking psychiatric medications should know that a small amount of the medication passes into the breast milk. However, the medication may or may not affect the baby. It depends on the medication and when it is taken. Women taking psychiatric medications and who intend to breastfeed should discuss the potential risks and benefits with their doctors.

Decisions on medication should be based on each woman's needs and circumstances. Medications should be selected based on available scientific research, and they should be taken at the lowest possible dose. Pregnant women should be watched closely throughout their pregnancy and after delivery.

What should I ask my doctor if I am prescribed a psychiatric medication?

You and your family can help your doctor find the right medications for you. The doctor needs to know your medical history; family history; information about allergies; other medications, supplements or herbal remedies you take; and other details about your overall health. You or a family member should ask the following questions when a medication is prescribed:

- What is the name of the medication?

- What is the medication supposed to do?

- How and when should I take it?

- How much should I take?

- What should I do if I miss a dose?

- When and how should I stop taking it?

- Will it interact with other medications I take?

- Do I need to avoid any types of food or drink while taking the medication?

- What should I avoid?

- Should it be taken with or without food?

- Is it safe to drink alcohol while taking this medication?

- What are the side effects? What should I do if I experience them?

- Is the Patient Package Insert for the medication available?

After taking the medication for a short time, tell your doctor how you feel, if you are having side effects, and any concerns you have about the medicine.

Section 44.2

Effects on Personality May Be Mechanism of Antidepressant Effectiveness

From "Effects on Personality May Be Mechanism of Antidepressant Effectiveness," by the National Institute on Mental Health (NIMH, www .nimh.nih.gov), part of the National Institutes of Health, July 16, 2010.

Results of a study of antidepressant treatment for major depression suggest that changes in personality traits seen in patients taking the drug paroxetine (Paxil) may not be the result of the medication's lifting of mood but may instead be a direct effect of this class of drugs and part of the mechanism by which they relieve depression.

Background

People with a high level of the personality trait neuroticism—characterized by a tendency to experience negative emotions and moodiness—are more likely than others to develop depression. Neuroticism is one of five personality traits that psychologists use as an organizing scheme for understanding personality: The other four traits are extraversion, openness, conscientiousness, and agreeableness. People who take antidepressants report lower levels of neuroticism and increased extroversion, in addition to a lifting of depression. The assumption has been that these changes in personality measures were the result, not the cause, of a lifting of depression.

Studies in twins suggest that to a large degree the same genetic factors underlie both neuroticism and depression risk. Research also suggests that the neurotransmitter serotonin plays a role in the expression of both neuroticism and extraversion. The class of antidepressant drugs to which paroxetine belongs—the selective serotonin reuptake inhibitors (SSRIs)—increase the neurotransmitter's availability in the brain.

This Study

To test the relationship between SSRIs and personality, investigator Tony Tang and colleagues at Northwestern University, Evanston,

Illinois, the University of Pennsylvania in Philadelphia, and Vanderbilt University in Nashville, Tennessee, randomly assigned patients with major depressive disorder (MDD) to receive paroxetine (120 patients), placebo (60 patients), or cognitive therapy (60 patients).

After eight weeks, medication and cognitive therapy (CT) each proved more effective than placebo in reducing depression. In addition, measures of neuroticism (based on standard surveys) in the groups receiving medication or cognitive therapy dropped, while extraversion scores rose. The changes were striking; while patients receiving placebo also reported small changes in both traits, the changes in patients on paroxetine were four to eight times as large. Patients receiving paroxetine had much greater changes in personality traits than patients receiving placebo even when the degree of improvement in depression was the same. This suggested that the effects on personality traits were not the result of the drug's lifting of depression. After accounting for decreases in depression in patients receiving CT, the improvement in extraversion, but not neuroticism, remained significant.

In further comparison of paroxetine with placebo, patients who had initially taken placebo were given the option after eight weeks to take paroxetine. During the placebo phase, there were small changes in neuroticism and extraversion; much greater changes occurred after eight weeks on paroxetine. Finally, those patients on paroxetine with the greatest degree of change in neuroticism (but not extraversion) were least likely to relapse to depression; the degree of changes in personality in those receiving CT did not affect the chances of relapse.

Significance

While the neurochemical effects of SSRIs are known, how those changes act to reduce depression is not clear. These results contradict the prevailing assumption that changes seen in personality traits in patients taking SSRIs are a result of the drugs' effects on depression. SSRIs may alter personality directly—and thus lift depression—or may act on a third factor that underlies both. CT may alter personality by a different path. Continued research on how these treatments work can provide a clearer understanding of the mechanism of action of SSRIs and how treatment can be best used to reduce depression and minimize relapse.

Reference

Tang, T.Z., DeRubeis, R.J., Hollon, S.D., Amsterdam, J., Shelton, R., and Schalet, B. Personality change during depression treatment. *Archives of General Psychiatry* 2009 Dec;66(12):1322–30.

Section 44.3

Rapid Antidepressant Works by Boosting Brain's Connections

From "Rapid Antidepressant Works by Boosting Brain's Connections,"
by the National Institute on Mental Health (NIMH, www.nimh.nih.gov),
part of the National Institutes of Health, September 9, 2010.

An experimental drug that lifts depression in hours likely works by rapidly stimulating connections between brain cells, a study in rats has revealed. The drug, called ketamine, quickly generated such synapses in a brain circuit implicated in human depression by triggering a key enzyme.

"Discovery of this cellular mechanism helps point the way to development of a ketamine-like agent that could become a practical, rapid-acting treatment for depression," said NIMH grantee Dr. Ronald Duman, of Yale University, who led the research team.

Duman, Dr. George Aghajanian, and colleagues, report on their findings in the August 20, 2010 issue of the journal *Science*.

Background

Conventional antidepressants fail to help up to 40 percent of depressed patients and take at least a few weeks to begin working. Studies in both major depressive disorder and bipolar depression by NIMH intramural scientists have found that 70 percent of such treatment-resistant patients improve dramatically within a day after receiving just one dose of ketamine. Since it must be administered intravenously and risks significant side effects, ketamine itself isn't a practical treatment. So it has spurred a hunt for more suitable agents that work via the same mechanism. Until now, that mechanism was not well understood.

Commonly prescribed antidepressants work primarily through the brain's serotonin chemical messenger system, while ketamine works mainly through the glutamate system. Evidence suggests that the serotonin drugs trigger a cascade of events that stimulate the birth of new neurons, which eventually establish connections, or synapses, with other neurons, enhancing brain circuit activity. Since this process takes a few weeks, it's thought to explain the delay in response to the medications. Ketamine's speedy effects suggest that the glutamate mechanism is acting more directly—via pathways closer to the root of the problem.

It was known that ketamine blocks the binding of glutamate to a receptor protein on cell membranes called the NMDA receptor. To find out how this leads to an antidepressant effect, Duman's team explored the path of the signal triggered by the receptor blockade.

Findings

In the executive hub at the front of the brain—or prefrontal cortex—of rats, they discovered that a low dose of ketamine rapidly activates an enzyme, called the mammalian target of rapamycin (mTOR), that makes proteins forming the connections between neurons, or synapses. Neither conventional antidepressants nor ECT similarly activated mTOR.

Stress and depression produce the opposite effect of ketamine, causing synapses to shrivel. A single dose of ketamine boosted levels of synapse-associated proteins within 2 hours and increased the number of neuronal "spines"—or budding synapses—within 24 hours. It also rapidly reversed depression-like behavior that developed in rats exposed to stress. These effects lasted at least a week. Injection of rapamycin, which blocks mTOR, blocked ketamine's ability to produce such beneficial neuronal and behavioral effects. Another agent that also blocks the NMDA receptor performed similarly to ketamine in these tests.

Significance

The research identifies the key cellular signaling pathway by which ketamine works. It demonstrates that mTOR is required for ketamine to enhance synapse formation.

While the serotonin antidepressant mechanism seems to work by triggering the birth of new neurons, or neurogenesis, in the brain's hippocampus, the glutamate mechanism appears to work by stimulating connections of existing neurons, or synaptogenesis, in the brain's prefrontal cortex—a quicker, more direct, process.

"Rapid activation of the mTOR signaling pathway may be an important and novel strategy for the rational design of fast-acting antidepressants," note the authors of an accompanying editorial in the same issue of *Science*. "The exciting results also demonstrate that ketamine may be a useful tool to identify molecular mediators of rapid antidepressant effects."

What's Next?

Ketamine's effects appear to be specific to the mTOR brain pathway, according to Duman. Any new treatment targeting the same pathway would have to be similarly specific, since mTOR also makes proteins in other parts of the body, and has been implicated in some types of cancers. Duman said his lab is currently investigating how stress affects the growth of neuronal spines, where synapses form, and how ketamine affects this process.

The new findings in rats complement ongoing human studies with ketamine at the NIMH Division of Intramural Research Programs. For example, the researchers there recently identified a brain signal detectible using a MEG [magneto-encephalography] scanner that predicts whether a patient will likely respond to ketamine treatment.

"Contrary to traditional notions of drug development, examining drug effects on brain cells and molecules in animals after clinical human trials is revealing much in the unfolding ketamine story," noted Dr. Carlos Zarate, Chief of the NIMH Experimental Therapeutics & Pathophysiology Branch, who directs the intramural ketamine studies.

References

1. mTOR-dependent synapse formation underlies the rapid antidepressant effects of NMDA antagonists. Li N, Lee B, Liu RJ, Banasr M, Dwyer JM, Iwata M, Li XY, Aghajanian G, Duman RS. *Science*. 2010 Aug 20;329(5994):959–64.

2. A randomized trial of an N-methyl-D-aspartate antagonist in treatment-resistant major depression. Zarate CA Jr, Singh JB, Carlson PJ, Brutsche NE, Ameli R, Luckenbaugh DA, Charney DS, Manji HK. *Arch Gen Psychiatry*. 2006 Aug;63(8):856–64.

3. Neuroscience. A glutamate pathway to faster-acting antidepressants? Cryan JF, O'Leary OF. *Science*. 2010 Aug 20;329(5994):913–4.

Section 44.4

Smoking Cessation Medicines and Antidepressants: The Risks

From "Public Health Advisory: FDA Requires New Boxed Warnings for the Smoking Cessation Drugs Chantix and Zyban," by the U.S. Food and Drug Administration (FDA, www.fda.gov), July 1, 2009.

The U.S. Food and Drug Administration (FDA) is notifying the public that the use of Chantix (varenicline) or Zyban (bupropion hydrochloride), two prescription medicines that are used as part of smoking cessation programs, has been associated with reports of changes in behavior such as hostility, agitation, depressed mood, and suicidal thoughts or actions. The FDA is requiring the manufacturers of these products, including generic versions of Zyban (bupropion), to add a new boxed warning to the product labeling to alert healthcare professionals to this important safety information.

People who are taking Chantix or Zyban and experience any serious and unusual changes in mood or behavior or who feel like hurting themselves or someone else should stop taking the medicine and call their healthcare professional right away.

Friends or family members who notice these changes in behavior in someone who is taking Chantix or Zyban for smoking cessation should tell the person their concerns and recommend that he or she stop taking the drug and call a healthcare professional right away.

Although Chantix and Zyban are effective aids in helping people stop smoking, they have been associated with serious adverse effects. Some people who have taken Chantix or Zyban to help them quit smoking have reported experiencing unusual behavior changes, have become depressed or have had their depression worsen, or have had thoughts about suicide or dying; some have attempted suicide either while using one of these drugs or after they stopped taking them.

Since Chantix and Zyban do not contain nicotine, people who decide to use these drugs to help them stop smoking may still experience symptoms of nicotine withdrawal. It is common for people who are attempting to break their nicotine habit to experience unpleasant symptoms like depressed mood, irritability, restlessness, feeling anxious, and trouble sleeping.

Smoking is known to cause serious and potentially fatal health consequences, including lung cancer and other cancers, heart attacks, stroke, emphysema, and other breathing/lung diseases. The risks that are known to be associated with smoking must be balanced against the small, but real risk of serious adverse effects associated with medicines that can help patients quit smoking when making the decision on whether to use a medicine and/or other method to help stop smoking.

In addition to the boxed warning, FDA is also requiring the manufacturers of Chantix, Zyban, and generic versions of Zyban to describe these risks in the medication guides for these products. The medication guides are required to be provided to all patients prescribed Chantix, Zyban or generic versions of Zyban for smoking cessation.

Section 44.5

Serotonin Syndrome: A Risk of Taking Antidepressants

"Serotonin Syndrome," © 2011 A.D.A.M., Inc. Reprinted with permission.

Serotonin syndrome is a potentially life threatening drug reaction that causes the body to have too much serotonin, a chemical produced by nerve cells.

Causes

Serotonin syndrome most often occurs when two drugs that affect the body's level of serotonin are taken together at the same time. The drugs cause too much serotonin to be released or to remain in the brain area.

For example, you can develop this syndrome if you take migraine medicines called triptans together with antidepressants called selective serotonin reuptake inhibitors (SSRIs) and selective serotonin/norepinephrine reuptake inhibitors (SSNRIs). Popular SSRIs include Celexa, Zoloft, Prozac, Zoloft, Paxil, and Lexapro. SNRIs include Cymbalta and Effexor. Brand names of triptans include Imitrex, Zomig, Frova, Maxalt, Axert, Amerge, and Relpax.

The FDA [U.S. Food and Drug Administration] recently asked the manufacturers of these types of drugs to include warning labels on their products that tell you about the potential risk of serotonin syndrome. Talk to your doctor before stopping any medication.

Serotonin syndrome is more likely to occur when you first start or increase the medicine.

Older antidepressants called monoamine oxidase inhibitors (MAO-Is) can also cause serotonin syndrome with the medicines describe above, as well as meperidine (Demerol, a painkiller) or dextromethorphan (cough medicine).

Drugs of abuse, such as ecstasy and LSD [lysergic acid diethylamide], have also been associated with serotonin syndrome.

Symptoms

Symptoms occur within minutes to hours, and may include:

- agitation or restlessness;
- diarrhea;
- fast heart beat;
- hallucinations;
- increased body temperature;
- loss of coordination;
- nausea;
- overactive reflexes;
- rapid changes in blood pressure;
- vomiting.

Exams and Tests

The diagnosis is usually made by asking questions about your medical history, including the types of drugs you take.

To be diagnosed with serotonin syndrome, you must have been taking a drug that changes the body's serotonin levels (serotonergic drug) and have at least three of the following signs or symptoms:

- Agitation
- Diarrhea

425

- Heavy sweating not due to activity
- Fever
- Mental status changes such as confusion or hypomania
- Muscle spasms (myoclonus)
- Overactive reflexes (hyperreflexia)
- Shivering
- Tremor
- Uncoordinated movements (ataxia)

Serotonin syndrome is not diagnosed until all other possible causes have been ruled out, including infections, intoxications, metabolic and hormone problems, and drug withdrawal. Some symptoms of serotonin syndrome can mimic those due to an overdose of cocaine, lithium, or an MAOI.

If you have just started taking or increased the dosage of a tranquilizer (neuroleptic drug), other conditions such as neuroleptic malignant syndrome will be considered.

Tests may include:

- blood cultures (to check for infection);
- complete blood count (CBC);
- drug (toxicology) screen;
- electrolyte levels;
- electrocardiogram (ECG);
- kidney and liver function tests;
- thyroid function tests.

Treatment

Patients with serotonin syndrome should stay in the hospital for at least 24 hours for close observation.

Treatment may include:

- benzodiazepines such as diazepam (Valium) or lorazepam (Ativan) to decrease agitation, seizure-like movements, and muscle stiffness;
- cyproheptadine (Periactin), a drug that blocks serotonin production;
- fluids by IV [intravenous fluids];

- withdrawal of medicines that caused the syndrome.

In life-threatening cases, medicines that keep your muscles still (paralyze them) and a temporary breathing tube and breathing machine will be needed to prevent further muscle damage.

Outlook (Prognosis)

Patients may get slowly worse and can become severely ill if not quickly treated. Untreated serotonin syndrome can be deadly. However, with treatment, symptoms can usually go away in less than 24 hours.

Possible Complications

Uncontrolled muscle spasms can cause severe muscle breakdown. The products produced when the muscles break down are released into your blood and eventually go through the kidneys. This can cause severe kidney damage if not recognized and treated appropriately. With appropriate treatment, the condition is reversible.

When to Contact a Medical Professional

Call your health care provider right away if you have symptoms of serotonin syndrome.

Prevention

Always tell all of your healthcare providers what medicines you take. Patients who take triptans with SSRIs or SNRIs should be closely followed, especially right after starting a medicine or increasing its dosage.

Chapter 45

Combination Treatment

Chapter Contents

Section 45.1

Combination Treatment for Psychotic Depression Holds Promise

From "Combination Treatment for Psychotic Depression Holds Promise," from the National Institute of Mental Health (NIMH, www.nimh.nih.gov), part of the National Institutes of Health, June 9, 2011.

A combination of an atypical antipsychotic medication and an antidepressant known as a selective serotonin reuptake inhibitor (SSRI) may be more effective in treating psychotic depression than an atypical antipsychotic alone, according to results from an NIMH-funded clinical study.

Background

Psychotic depression is characterized by major depression accompanied by symptoms such as hallucinations, delusions, and breaks with reality. A person with psychotic depression may be unwilling or unable to care for him- or herself and often is admitted to the hospital. Typically, psychotic depression is treated with electroconvulsive therapy (ECT), known to be effective but not always acceptable to patients and their families. It is less commonly treated with an antipsychotic or an antipsychotic plus an antidepressant.

Results of the Study

In a 12-week trial, all 259 participants were required to have psychotic depression with at least one delusion or irrational belief, although not all had hallucinations. Participants were randomly assigned to one of two treatments—the atypical antipsychotic olanzapine (Zyprexa) plus the SSRI sertraline (Zoloft) (combination therapy), or to olanzapine plus a placebo, or inactive, pill (monotherapy). Barnett S. Meyers, MD, of Cornell University, and colleagues compared rates of remission and side effects among the participants. They also compared the responses of the 117 patients younger than 60 with the responses of the 142 patients older than 60 to determine if the two age groups responded differently.

The researchers conducted assessments at the beginning of the trial, weekly for the first six weeks, and then every other week until week 12. They found that 42 percent of those on combination therapy remitted compared to 24 percent of those on the monotherapy, with no significant differences in remission rates between age groups. Combination therapy's superiority became most evident between weeks eight and 12 of the trial.

Overall, the two age groups experienced comparable side effects. Both groups experienced significant increases in cholesterol and triglyceride levels, and both gained weight. However, the younger age group gained twice as much on average—about 14 pounds—compared to the older group, which gained an average of seven pounds. This finding is consistent with other reports that have found older adults tend to gain less weight with atypical antipsychotics, specifically olanzapine, the researchers said. However, older participants also tended to be on lower doses of the antipsychotic than the younger adults, which may partially explain the disparity in weight gain, according to the researchers.

Unexpectedly, older participants had no more difficulty tolerating the medications than younger participants, nor were they any more likely to experience falls, sedation, or have greater movement disorder symptoms than younger participants.

Overall, about 45 percent of participants dropped out of the study, although the drop-out rate was lower in the combination treatment group (37 percent) compared to the monotherapy group (53 percent).

Significance

Because the drop-out rate was relatively high and no follow-up data on those who discontinued were collected, the authors caution against applying the study's results to clinical practice prematurely. Still, the authors suggest that combination therapy holds promise as an alternative therapy to ECT. "Psychotic depression is difficult to treat," said NIMH Director Thomas R. Insel, MD.

"This study provides insight into one approach to treatment that may be a valid alternative for many patients who cannot or will not undergo ECT."

What's Next?

Longer-term studies are needed to evaluate side effects. "Future research must weigh the benefits of continuing atypical antipsychotic medication beyond 12 weeks against the risks of associated metabolic side effects," lead author Meyers concluded.

Reference

Meyers BS, Flint AJ, Rothschild AJ, Mulsant BH, Whyte EM, Peasley-Miklus C, Papademetriou E, Leon AC, Heo M for the STOP-PD study group. A double-blind randomized controlled trial of olanzapine plus sertraline versus olanzapine plus placebo for psychotic depression—The Study of Pharmacotherapy of Psychotic Depression (STOP-PD). *Archives of General Psychiatry.* 2009;66(3):838–847.

Section 45.2

Combination Therapy May Not Improve Odds of Remission among Chronically Depressed

From "Combination Antidepressant Therapy May Not Improve Odds of Remission Among Chronically Depressed," by the National Institute of Mental Health (NIMH, www.nimh.nih.gov), part of the National Institutes of Health, May 3, 2011.

A combination of two antidepressants may not be any more effective in treating chronic major depression than a single antidepressant, according to a study published May 2, 2011, in the *American Journal of Psychiatry.*

Background

When treating depression, doctors sometimes prescribe a second antidepressant medication if a patient does not improve after several weeks. Because some antidepressants work for some people and not others, the hope is that adding another one will increase the odds of remission. However, treatment guidelines generally do not recommend adding another medication until it is evident the first one is not working.

Madhukar H. Trivedi, MD, at the University of Texas Southwestern, and colleagues aimed to determine if combination antidepressant therapy as a first treatment step might produce a higher remission rate among people with chronic major depression. In the Combining Medications to Enhance Depression Outcomes (CO-MED) trial, 665 adult participants from several sites around the country were randomly assigned to one of three antidepressant combinations:

- Escitalopram plus placebo

- Bupropion sustained release plus escitalopram

- Venlafaxine plus mirtazapine

Although participants did not know which treatments they were receiving, clinicians were aware of their patients' treatment assignments so that they could adjust doses as necessary to manage symptoms and side effects. The measurement of primary outcome was based on a self-reporting scale called the Quick Inventory of Depressive Symptoms.

Results of the Study

After three months, remission rates among the three groups all were around 38 percent. After seven months, remission rates continued to be similar among the three treatment groups and averaged around 45 percent. However, the venlafaxine plus mirtazapine combination was associated with a higher risk for side effects and serious adverse events compared to the other treatment options.

Significance

Despite other research suggesting combination antidepressant treatment may work better than a single medication, neither of the combination therapies in this trial appeared to be more effective than the single medication plus placebo. The researchers suggest that the chronic nature of participants' major depression may be associated with lower remission rates. They also noted that dosage differences may account for the difference in outcomes compared to other studies.

What's Next?

Further evaluation is needed to determine if other drug combinations may affect remission rates differently. Results also highlight the need to evaluate biological markers as a means of personalizing treatment and possibly improving remission rates in major depression.

Reference

Rush AJ, Trivedi MH, Stewart JW, Nierenberg AA, Fava M, Kurian BT, Warden D, Morris DW, Luther JF, Husain MM, Cook IA, Shelton RC, Lesser IM, Kornstein SG, Wisniewski SR. Combining medications to enhance depression outcomes (CO-MED): Acute and long-term outcomes: a single-blind randomized study. *Journal of American Psychiatry* online ahead of print, May 2, 2011.

Chapter 46

Light Therapy for Seasonal Affective Disorder

Chapter Contents

Section 46.1

What Is Light Therapy?

What the Research Shows

Do people who feel blue as the days get shorter have to live near the equator? Thankfully not, due to the diligent inquiries of psychologists and other health-care experts. Seasonal affective disorder (SAD), a mood disorder that brings episodes of depression associated with seasonal variations of light, got its name in the early 1980s. Within a decade, researchers shed light on this mysterious disorder and developed a relatively simple treatment using very bright lights.

According the National Institute of Mental Health, the symptoms of SAD vary predictably with the seasons. Biologists believe that because living things evolved to change with the seasons, it may have become normal for people to experience some seasonal variation in biological rhythms such as for sleeping and appetite. Charmane Eastman, PhD, director of the Biological Rhythms Research Laboratory at Rush University Medical Center in Chicago, observes, "Now, if people want to sleep a lot and do nothing in the winter, society condemns it—which in my view may lead to guilt and depression."

Despite the advent of 24/7 electric light, humans may still be just as subject to changing patterns of sunlight as other animals, who mate or hibernate in rhythm with day length. With winter's late dawn and early dusk, mood can suffer. Indeed, most people with SAD feel the poorest when the days are shortest, in January and February.

People in the northern latitudes, especially young women, are more prone to the disorder.

A small share of people with SAD show the reverse pattern, being sensitive to summer's longer days. The very existence of opposite winter-summer patterns suggested to researchers that this mood disorder stems from a problem in adapting to the physical environment.

Once SAD was identified, researchers hypothesized that its typical appearance with winter had something to do with lowered exposure to sunlight. The obvious next step was to lengthen exposure to light intensity more akin to outdoor levels; it worked. By 1998, researchers were studying treatment variations.

In a key four-week study, Eastman and her colleagues randomly assigned 96 patients with winter SAD to one of three bright-light treatments that are about 10 to 20 times brighter than ordinary indoor lights. Patients either got an hour and a half of bright light in the morning, an hour and a half in the evening, or a morning placebo of two deactivated negative-ion generators.

After three weeks, significantly more people in the morning light treatment group than in the placebo group showed significantly more complete or near-complete remission of their symptoms. The response to evening light was also better than placebo, but not at a level of significance. Importantly, Eastman's group found that effective phototherapy fostered full remission of depression, a prized goal for a disorder that often seems to come back after treatment.

Additional Findings

Other studies have assessed bright-light's side effects and probed the biological bases of seasonal affective disorder. Side effects are usually mild; light therapy can make people mildly jumpy and create headache and nausea.

Other researchers report that women with SAD may be more vulnerable to the amount of light they get, because although they don't spend less time outdoors than other women, they do spend more time outside in the summer, resulting in a larger overall change between seasons. Finally, scientists continue to probe not only why some people are more vulnerable to SAD than others, but also how seasonal changes in light shape mood via its impact on the brain. Research centers around the way high-intensity light reaches the pineal gland in the middle of the brain, which secretes melatonin—the "jet lag" hormone that helps to regulate biorhythms.

How We Use the Research

For the estimated half a million people in the United States who may experience winter depression, bright light therapy, known as phototherapy, is now commonly prescribed. During phototherapy, patients sit facing a "light box" with a bank of fluorescent bulbs of up to 10,000 lux total intensity for about a half hour per session throughout their low season. They can't wear or use anything that blocks the ability of the light to pass through the retina and stimulate the brain's suprachiasmatic nucleus (SCN), its circadian clock. Light goes there first and then on to the pineal gland.

For people whose symptoms are mild, outdoor time—perhaps an hour's walk under the winter sun—or greater indoor exposure to sunlight can help.

As a result of ongoing research into SAD, psychologists diagnosing patients with depression can take into account whether the symptoms come and go with the seasons. If they do, phototherapy is a validated treatment for brightening things up.

Sources and Further Reading

Eastman, Ch. I.; Young, M. A., Fogg, L. F., Liu, L., & Meaden, P. M. (1998). Bright light treatment of winter depression: A placebo-controlled trial. *Archives of General Psychiatry*, 55, 883–889.

Graw, P., Recker, S., Sand, L., Kraeuchi, K., & Wirz-Justice, A. (1999). Winter and summer outdoor light exposure in women with and without seasonal affective disorder. *Journal of Affective Disorders*, 56, 163–169.

National Institute of Mental Health. (2006, May 1). Properly timed light, melatonin lift winter depression by syncing rhythms. Available: http://www.nimh.nih.gov.

Papolos, D. F. (1991). Serotonin, seasonality, and mood disorders. In Brown, S-L., & Herman, M., Eds., *The Role of Serotonin in Psychiatric Disorders*, 260–283. New York: Brunner/Mazel, Inc.

Terman, M., & Terman, J. S. (1999). Bright light therapy: Side effects and benefits across the symptom spectrum. *Journal of Clinical Psychiatry*, 60, 799–808.

Wehr, T. A., & Rosenthal, N. E. (1989). Seasonality and affective illness. *American Journal of Psychiatry*, 146, 829–839.

Health Reference Series Medical Advisor's Notes and Updates

Evidence for the use of light therapy for seasonal affective disorder continues to accumulate. A considerable amount of research is now focused on whether some types of light therapy are superior to others. For example, some data suggest that blue light may be more effective than white light, and there are conflicting results regarding whether dim light therapy may be as effective as bright light therapy. Limited evidence also suggests that LED-generated lights might be more effective than fluorescent lights. The ideal type, intensity, and duration of light therapy for seasonal affective disorder is still being determined.

Section 46.2

Properly Timed Light and Melatonin Lift Winter Depression by Syncing Rhythms

From "Properly Timed Light, Melatonin Lift Winter Depression by Syncing Rhythms," by the National Institute of Mental Health (NIMH, www.nimh.nih.gov), part of the National Institutes of Health, May 1, 2006. Reviewed by David A. Cooke, MD, FACP, November 13, 2011.

Most seasonal affective disorder (SAD) symptoms stem from daily body rhythms that have gone out of sync with the sun, a NIMH-funded study has found. The researchers propose that most patients will respond best to a low dose of the light-sensitive hormone melatonin in the afternoon in addition to bright light in the morning. Rhythms that have lost their bearings due to winter's late dawn and early dusk accounted for 65 percent of SAD symptoms; realigning them explained 35 percent of melatonin's antidepressant effect in patients with delayed rhythms, the most common form of SAD, report NIMH grantee Alfred Lewy, MD, PhD, and colleagues at the Oregon Health & Science University, online, April 28, 2006, in the *Proceedings of the National Academy of Sciences*.

SAD affects many people in northern latitudes in winter, especially young women, and is usually treated with bright light in the morning. The pineal gland, located in the middle of the brain, responds to darkness by secreting melatonin, which resets the brain's central clock and helps the light/dark cycle reset the sleep/wake cycle and other daily rhythms. Lewy and colleagues pinpointed how rhythms go astray in SAD and how they can be reset by taking melatonin supplements at the right time of day. The findings strengthen the case for daily rhythm mismatches as the cause of SAD.

The researchers tracked sleep, activity levels, melatonin rhythms, and depression symptoms of 68 SAD patients who took either low doses of melatonin or a placebo in the morning or afternoon for a winter month when they were most symptomatic.

They had determined from healthy subjects that a person's rhythms are synchronized when the interval between the time the pineal gland begins secreting melatonin and the middle of sleep is about six hours.

Seventy-one percent of the SAD patients had intervals shorter than six hours, indicating that their rhythms were delayed due to the later winter dawn. Taking melatonin capsules in the afternoon lengthened their intervals, bringing their rhythms back toward normal. The closer their intervals approached the ideal six hours, the more their mood improved on depression rating scales, supporting the hypothesized link between out-of-sync rhythms and SAD.

"SAD may be the first psychiatric disorder in which a physiological marker correlates with symptom severity before, and in the course of, treatment in the same patients," explained Lewy, referring to patients' rhythm shifts towards the six-hour interval in response to melatonin.

Taking melatonin at the correct time of day—afternoon for patients with short intervals and morning for the 29 percent of patients with long intervals—more than doubled their improvement in depression scores, compared to taking a placebo or the hormone at the incorrect time. While the study was not designed to test the efficacy of melatonin treatment, the researchers suggest that its clinical benefit "appears to be substantial, although not as robust as light treatment." They propose that the six-hour interval index may be useful for analyzing the circadian components of non-seasonal depression and other sleep and psychiatric disorders.

Lewy AJ, Lefler BJ, Emens JS, Bauer VK. The circadian basis of winter depression. *Proc Natl Acad Sci USA.* 2006 Apr 28.

Chapter 47

Alternative and Complementary Therapies Used for Depression

Chapter Contents

Section 47.1

Acupuncture May Aid Depression during Pregnancy

From "Acupuncture Helps with Depression during Pregnancy," by the Agency for Healthcare Research and Quality (AHRQ, www.ahrq.gov), August 2010.

For women who become depressed during pregnancy, acupuncture may offer a way to reduce symptoms in a safe and effective manner, suggested a March 2010 study. It found that women receiving 12 sessions of acupuncture treatment had good response rates and decreased severity of symptoms. The researchers enrolled 150 pregnant women who were diagnosed with major depressive disorder. The women were randomized to one of three groups. One group received acupuncture treatment specific for depression, while a second group received acupuncture that was not designed for depression. A third group received Swedish massage therapy. All groups received two 25-minute sessions each week for four weeks, followed by one session a week for another four weeks. All of the women were assessed for depressive symptoms at baseline and then after four and eight weeks of treatment.

Women receiving acupuncture specific for depression had a significantly greater reduction in symptoms compared with the other two groups combined. The group who received eight weeks of depression-specific acupuncture had a 53 percent reduction in depression scores and a 29 percent remission rate. This compares well with one study that reported a 52 percent reduction rate and a 19 percent remission rate after 16 weeks of psychotherapy. Women receiving acupuncture specific for depression also had a significantly greater response rate (63 percent), defined as at least 50 percent reduction in depressive symptom severity, compared with the other two groups combined (44.3 percent) or the non-depression-specific acupuncture group (37.5 percent).

There were no significant differences in symptom reduction or response rates between the massage and nonspecific acupuncture groups. The acupuncture treatment was well tolerated with relatively few side effects that were mild and transient. The study was supported in part by the Agency for Healthcare Research and Quality.

Source: Acupuncture for depression during pregnancy, by Rachel Manber, PhD, Rosa N. Schnyer, DAOM, Deirdre Lyell, MD, and others in the March 2010 *Obstetrics & Gynecology* 115(3), pp. 511–520.

Section 47.2

Mindfulness Practice May Increase Ability to Cope with Difficult Emotions

From "Mindfulness Practice in the Treatment of Traumatic Stress," by the National Center for Posttraumatic Stress Disorder (NCPTSD, www .ptsd.va.gov), part of the Veterans Administration, September 28, 2010.

What Is Mindfulness?

Mindfulness is a way of thinking and focusing that can help you become more aware of your present experiences. Practicing mindfulness can be as simple as noticing the taste of a mint on your tongue. There are some things you might do every day without even thinking about them, like brushing your teeth in the morning. Mindfulness involves paying attention to the feelings and sensations of these experiences.

Research has shown mindfulness to be helpful with other anxiety problems. It has also been shown to help with symptoms of posttraumatic stress disorder (PTSD) such as avoidance and hyperarousal. If you have gone through trauma, you may want to learn what mindfulness is and how it might be helpful to you.

Mindfulness practice has two key parts:

- Paying attention to and being aware of the present moment

- Accepting or being willing to experience your thoughts and feelings without judging them

For example, focusing on the inhale and exhale of your breathing is one way to concentrate on the present moment. Mindfulness involves allowing your thoughts and feelings to pass without either clinging to them or pushing them away. You just let them take their natural course. While practicing mindfulness, you may become distracted by your thoughts and that is okay. The process is about being willing to notice where your thoughts take you, and then bringing your attention back to the present.

How Mindfulness Can Help

Mindfulness might increase your ability to cope with difficult emotions, such as anxiety and depression. Practicing mindfulness can help you to be more focused and aware of the present moment while also being more willing to experience the difficult emotions that sometimes come up after trauma.

For example, mindfulness practice might help you to notice your thoughts and feelings more and to be able to just let them go, without labeling them as "good" or "bad" and without acting on them by avoiding or behaving impulsively.

Mindfulness is a practice, a continual process. Although it may be hard to do at first, regular mindfulness practice can help you notice your thoughts and learn to take a step back from them. Mindfulness practice can also help you develop more compassion toward yourself and others. You may be less likely to sit in judgment of your thoughts, feelings, and actions.

You may become less critical of yourself. Using mindfulness can help you become more aware and gentle in response to your trauma reactions. This is an important step in recovery.

Cognitive processing therapy and prolonged exposure have been shown to be the most effective treatments for PTSD. In both of these treatments, you are asked to write or talk about trauma with the guidance of your therapist. Mindfulness can prepare you for these treatments by giving you skills and confidence that you can handle your feelings. As you learn to be mindful, you learn to observe what is happening in your body and your mind. You can learn to be more willing to cope with difficult thoughts and feelings in a healthy way. This will help you keep going when you are asked to think and talk about your trauma in treatment. In this way you may get even more out of the PTSD treatment.

There are several types of therapy that use mindfulness practices. These therapies have been used to treat problems that often affect people with PTSD, such as anxiety, depression, and substance use. The therapies may target specific problems such as:

- difficult feelings and stress in daily living;

- the stress of physical health problems, such as chronic pain;

- negative thinking patterns that can lead to repeated episodes of depression;

- trouble working toward your goals in life; or

- urges to use drugs or alcohol.

Section 47.3

St. John's Wort and Depression

Excerpted from "St. John's Wort and Depression," by the National Center for Complementary and Alternative Medicine (NCCAM, www.nccam .nih.gov), part of the National Institutes of Health, December 2007.

St. John's wort (*Hypericum perforatum*) is a long-living plant with yellow flowers whose medicinal uses were first recorded in ancient Greece. It contains many chemical compounds. Some are believed to be the active ingredients that produce the herb's effects, including the compounds hypericin and hyperforin.

How these compounds actually work is not yet fully understood, but several theories have been suggested. Preliminary studies suggest that St. John's wort might work by preventing nerve cells in the brain from reabsorbing the chemical messenger serotonin, or by reducing levels of a protein involved in the body's immune system functioning.

St. John's wort has been used over the centuries for mental conditions, nerve pain, and a wide variety of other health conditions. Today, St. John's wort is used for anxiety, mild to moderate depression, and sleep disorders.

In Europe, St. John's wort is widely prescribed for depression. In the United States, there is public interest in St. John's wort as a treatment for depression, but it is not a prescription medicine.

In the United States, St. John's wort products are sold as the following:

- Capsules and tablets

- Teas (The dried herb is added to boiling water and steeped.)

- Liquid extracts (Specific types of chemicals are removed from the herb, leaving the desired chemicals in a concentrated form.)

About Depression

Depression is a medical condition that affects nearly 21 million American adults each year, according to the National Institute of Mental Health. Mood, thoughts, physical health, and behavior all may be affected.

Depression comes in several forms and its symptoms and severity can vary from person to person. Depression can be treated effectively with conventional medicine including antidepressants and certain types of psychotherapy.

What the Science Says about St. John's Wort for Depression

Scientific evidence regarding the effectiveness of St. John's wort for depression is inconsistent. An analysis of the results of 37 clinical trials concluded that St. John's wort may have only minimal beneficial effects on major depression. However, the analysis also found that St. John's wort may benefit people with minor depression; these benefits may be similar to those from standard antidepressants. Overall, St. John's wort appeared to produce fewer side effects than some standard antidepressants.

One of the studies included in the analysis was cofunded by NCCAM and two other components of the National Institutes of Health (NIH)— the National Institute of Mental Health and the Office of Dietary Supplements. This study found that St. John's wort was no more effective than placebo in treating major depression of moderate severity. However, the antidepressant sertraline, used in one arm of the study, also showed little difference from placebo.

Side Effects and Risks

The most common side effects of St. John's wort include dry mouth, dizziness, diarrhea, nausea, increased sensitivity to sunlight, and fatigue.

Research has shown that taking St. John's wort can limit the effectiveness of some prescription medicines, including the following:

- Antidepressant medicines

- Birth control pills

- Cyclosporine, a medicine that helps prevent the body from rejecting transplanted organs

- Digoxin, a medicine used to strengthen heart muscle contractions

- Indinavir and other medicines used to control HIV [human immunodeficiency virus] infection

- Irinotecan and other anticancer medicines

- Warfarin and related medicines used to thin the blood (known as anticoagulants)

When combined with certain antidepressants, St. John's wort also may increase side effects such as nausea, anxiety, headache, and confusion.

Herbal Products: Issues to Consider

Herbal products such as St. John's wort are classified as dietary supplements by the U.S. Food and Drug Administration (FDA). The FDA's requirements for testing and obtaining approval to sell dietary supplements are different from its requirements for drugs. Unlike drugs, herbal products can be sold without requiring studies on dosage, safety, or effectiveness.

The strength and quality of herbal products are often unpredictable. Products can differ in content not only from brand to brand, but from batch to batch. Information on labels may be misleading or inaccurate.

In addition, "natural" does not necessarily mean "safe." Many natural substances can have harmful effects—especially if they are taken in large quantities or if they interact with other supplements or with prescription medicines.

Tell your health care providers about any complementary and alternative practices you use. Give them a full picture of what you do to manage your health. This will help ensure coordinated and safe care.

Research on St. John's Wort

Recent projects supported by NCCAM include studies of the following:

- Safety and effectiveness of St. John's wort for the treatment of minor depression

- Safety of St. John's wort for the treatment of social anxiety disorder

- Effectiveness of St. John's wort for the treatment of obsessive-compulsive disorder

- Effects of St. John's wort on how well birth control pills work

- Possible adverse interactions of St. John's wort and narcotic pain medicines

- Safety and effectiveness of St. John's wort for attention deficit hyperactivity disorder

Section 47.4

Transcendental Meditation for Depression

Two new studies show the benefit of using the Transcendental Meditation technique for reducing symptoms of depression.

The studies included African Americans and Native Hawaiians, 55 years and older, who were at risk for cardiovascular disease.

Researchers randomly placed participants in the Transcendental Meditation program or a health education control group.

Study members were then assessed with a standard test for depression—the Center for Epidemiological Studies-Depression (CES-D) inventory—over 9 to 12 months.

"Clinically meaningful reductions in depressive symptoms were associated with practice of the Transcendental Meditation program," said Sanford Nidich, EdD, lead author and senior researcher at the Institute for Natural Medicine and Prevention at Maharishi University of Management (MUM).

"The findings of these studies have important implications for improving mental health and reducing the risk of cardiovascular morbidity and mortality," said Dr. Nidich.

Participants in both studies who practiced the Transcendental Meditation program showed significant reductions in depressive symptoms compared to health education controls.

The largest decreases were found in those participants who had indications of clinically significant depression, with those practicing

Transcendental Meditation showing an average reduction in depressive symptoms of 48 percent.

"These results are encouraging and provide support for testing the efficacy of Transcendental Meditation as a therapeutic adjunct in the treatment of clinical depression," said Hector Myers, PhD, study co-author and professor and director of Clinical Training in the Department of Psychology at UCLA.

The results of these studies are timely. For older Americans, depression is a particularly debilitating disease, with approximately 20 percent suffering from some form of depression. Overall, 18 million men and women suffer from depression in the United States.

Depression is a major risk factor for cardiovascular disease, with even a moderate level of depressive symptoms associated with increased cardiac events.

"The clinically significant reductions in depression without drugs or psychotherapy in these studies suggest the Transcendental Meditation program may improve mental and associated physical health in older high risk subjects," said Robert Schneider, MD, FACC, director of MUM's Institute for Natural Medicine and Prevention.

"The importance of reducing depression in the elderly at risk for heart disease cannot be overestimated," said Gary P. Kaplan, MD, PhD, clinical associate professor of neurology at New York University School of Medicine.

"Any technique not involving extra medication in this population is a welcome addition. I look forward to further research on the Transcendental Meditation technique and prevention of depression in other at-risk elderly populations, including those with stroke and other chronic diseases."

Source: Maharishi University of Management

Section 47.5

Valerian

From "Valerian," by the National Center for Complementary and Alternative Medicine (NCCAM, www.nccam.nih.gov), part of the National Institutes of Health, July 2010.

Valerian (common names—valerian, all-heal, garden heliotrope; Latin name—*Valeriana officinalis*) is a plant native to Europe and Asia; it is also found in North America. Valerian has been used as a medicinal herb since at least the time of ancient Greece and Rome. Its therapeutic uses were described by Hippocrates, and in the 2nd century, Galen prescribed valerian for insomnia.

What Valerian Is Used For

Valerian has long been used for sleep disorders and anxiety. Valerian has also been used for other conditions, such as headaches, depression, irregular heartbeat, and trembling.

How Valerian Is Used

The roots and rhizomes (underground stems) of valerian are typically used to make supplements, including capsules, tablets, and liquid extracts, as well as teas.

What the Science Says

Research suggests that valerian may be helpful for insomnia, but there is not enough evidence from well-designed studies to confirm this.

There is not enough scientific evidence to determine whether valerian works for other conditions, such as anxiety or depression.

NCCAM-funded research on valerian includes studies on the herb's effects on sleep in healthy older adults and in people with Parkinson disease.

NCCAM-funded researchers are also studying the potential of valerian and other herbal products to relieve menopausal symptoms.

Side Effects and Cautions

Studies suggest that valerian is generally safe to use for short periods of time (for example, four to six weeks).

No information is available about the long-term safety of valerian.

Valerian can cause mild side effects, such as headaches, dizziness, upset stomach, and tiredness the morning after its use.

Tell all your health care providers about any complementary and alternative practices you use. Give them a full picture of what you do to manage your health. This will help ensure coordinated and safe care.

Section 47.6

Yoga Might Improve
Mood and Sense of Well-Being

Excerpted from "Yoga for Health: An Introduction," by the National Center for Complementary and Alternative Medicine (NCCAM, www .nccam.nih.gov), part of the National Institutes of Health, June 2009.

Yoga is a mind-body practice in complementary and alternative medicine (CAM) with origins in ancient Indian philosophy. The various styles of yoga that people use for health purposes typically combine physical postures, breathing techniques, and meditation or relaxation. This text provides a general overview of yoga and suggests sources for more information.

Key Points

People use yoga for a variety of health conditions and to achieve fitness and relaxation.

It is not fully known what changes occur in the body during yoga; whether they influence health; and if so, how. There is, however, growing evidence to suggest that yoga works to enhance stress-coping mechanisms and mind-body awareness. Research is under way to find out more about yoga's effects, and the diseases and conditions for which it may be most helpful.

Tell your health care providers about any complementary and alternative practices you use. Give them a full picture of what you do to manage your health. This will help ensure coordinated and safe care.

Overview

Yoga in its full form combines physical postures, breathing exercises, meditation, and a distinct philosophy. Yoga is intended to increase relaxation and balance the mind, body, and the spirit.

Early written descriptions of yoga are in Sanskrit, the classical language of India. The word yoga comes from the Sanskrit word *yuj*, which means "yoke or union." It is believed that this describes the union between the mind and the body. The first known text, *The Yoga Sutras,* was written more than 2,000 years ago, although yoga may have been practiced as early as 5,000 years ago. Yoga was originally developed as a method of discipline and attitudes to help people reach spiritual enlightenment. The *Sutras* outline eight limbs or foundations of yoga practice that serve as spiritual guidelines:

1. Yama (moral behavior)

2. Niyama (healthy habits)

3. Asana (physical postures)

4. Pranayama (breathing exercises)

5. Pratyahara (sense withdrawal)

6. Dharana (concentration)

7. Dhyana (contemplation)

8. Samadhi (higher consciousness)

The numerous schools of yoga incorporate these eight limbs in varying proportions. Hatha yoga, the most commonly practiced in the United States and Europe, emphasizes two of the eight limbs: Postures (asanas) and breathing exercises (pranayama). Some of the major styles of hatha yoga include Ananda, Anusara, Ashtanga, Bikram, Iyengar, Kripalu, Kundalini, and Viniyoga.

Use of Yoga for Health in the United States

According to the 2007 National Health Interview Survey (NHIS), which included a comprehensive survey of CAM use by Americans, yoga is one of the top 10 CAM modalities used. More than 13 million adults had used yoga in the previous year, and between the 2002 and 2007 NHIS, use of yoga among adults increased by 1 percent (or approximately 3 million people). The 2007 survey also found that more than 1.5 million children used yoga in the previous year.

People use yoga for a variety of health conditions including anxiety disorders or stress, asthma, high blood pressure, and depression. People also use yoga as part of a general health regimen—to achieve physical fitness and to relax.

The Status of Yoga Research

Research suggests that yoga might help with the following:

- Improve mood and sense of well-being

- Counteract stress

- Reduce heart rate and blood pressure

- Increase lung capacity

- Improve muscle relaxation and body composition

- Help with conditions such as anxiety, depression, and insomnia

- Improve overall physical fitness, strength, and flexibility

- Positively affect levels of certain brain or blood chemicals

More well-designed studies are needed before definitive conclusions can be drawn about yoga's use for specific health conditions.

Side Effects and Risks

Yoga is generally considered to be safe in healthy people when practiced appropriately. Studies have found it to be well tolerated, with few side effects.

People with certain medical conditions should not use some yoga practices. For example, people with disk disease of the spine, extremely high or low blood pressure, glaucoma, retinal detachment, fragile or atherosclerotic arteries, a risk of blood clots, ear problems, severe osteoporosis, or cervical spondylitis should avoid some inverted poses.

Although yoga during pregnancy is safe if practiced under expert guidance, pregnant women should avoid certain poses that may be problematic.

Training, Licensing, and Certification

There are many training programs for yoga teachers throughout the country. These programs range from a few days to more than 2 years. Standards for teacher training and certification differ depending on the style of yoga.

There are organizations that register yoga teachers and training programs that have complied with minimum educational standards. For example, one nonprofit group requires at least 200 hours of training, with a specified number of hours in areas including techniques, teaching methodology, anatomy, physiology, and philosophy. However, there are currently no official or well-accepted licensing requirements for yoga teachers in the United States.

If You Are Thinking about Yoga

- Do not use yoga as a replacement for conventional care or to postpone seeing a doctor about a medical problem.

- If you have a medical condition, consult with your health care provider before starting yoga.

- Ask about the physical demands of the type of yoga in which you are interested, as well as the training and experience of the yoga teacher you are considering.

- Look for published research studies on yoga for the health condition you are interested in.

- Tell your health care providers about any complementary and alternative practices you use. Give them a full picture of what you do to manage your health. This will help ensure coordinated and safe care.

Chapter 48

Treating Depression in Children and Adolescents

Chapter Contents

Section 48.1

Nearly Two Thirds of America's Adolescents with Depression Do Not Get Treatment

From "Nearly Two-Thirds of America's 2 Million Adolescents Suffering from Major Depressive Episodes in the Past Year Did Not Receive Treatment," by the Substance Abuse and Mental Health Services Administration (SAMHSA, www.samhsa.gov), part of the U.S. Department of Health and Human Services, April 28, 2011.

A national report indicates that 8.1 percent of America's adolescents aged 12 to 17 (2 million youth) experienced at least one major depressive episode (MDE) in the past year. The report by the Substance Abuse and Mental Health Services Administration (SAMHSA) also shows that only 34.7 percent of these adolescents suffering from major depressive episodes received treatment during this period.

An MDE is defined as a period of two weeks or longer during which there is either depressed mood or loss of interest or pleasure and at least four other symptoms that reflect a change in functioning, including problems with sleep, eating, energy, concentration, and self-image.

"Depression among adolescents is a serious public health problem that is all too often overlooked and the consequences can be devastating," said SAMHSA Administrator, Pamela S. Hyde, J.D. "If depression among young people is identified and treated early we can turn a life around and reduce the impact of mental illness and substance abuse on America's communities."

One of the study's most notable findings was that adolescents who had suffered from an MDE in the past year were more than three times as likely as those without a past year MDE to have had a substance use disorder in the past year (18.9 percent versus 6 percent).

The study also found significant differences in the rates of past year MDE experiences among subgroups of adolescents. For example, adolescent females were twice as likely as their male counterparts to have experienced a past year MDE (11.7 percent versus 4.7 percent). Rates of past year MDE experience also rose as adolescents grew older with rates increasing from 3.6 percent of adolescents aged 12 to 10.4 percent of adolescents aged 15.

Among the nearly 700,000 adolescents who suffered from MDE and received treatment, more than half (58.5 percent) saw or met with a medical doctor or other health professional only—without being prescribed medication.

The next largest segment of adolescents receiving treatment—34.7 percent—met with a medical doctor or other heath professional and were also prescribed medication. The remaining 6.7 percent receiving treatment used prescription medication only.

Section 48.2

Taking Your Child to a Therapist

Sometimes kids, like adults, can benefit from therapy. Therapy can help kids develop problem-solving skills and also teach them the value of seeking help. Therapists can help kids and families cope with stress and a variety of emotional and behavioral issues.

Many kids need help dealing with school stress, such as homework, test anxiety, bullying, or peer pressure. Others need help to discuss their feelings about family issues, particularly if there's a major transition, such as a divorce, move, or serious illness.

Should My Child See a Therapist?

Significant life events—such as the death of a family member, friend, or pet; divorce or a move; abuse; trauma; a parent leaving on military deployment; or a major illness in the family—can cause stress that might lead to problems with behavior, mood, sleep, appetite, and academic or social functioning.

In some cases, it's not as clear what's caused a child to suddenly seem withdrawn, worried, stressed, sulky, or tearful. But if you feel your child might have an emotional or behavioral problem or needs help coping with a difficult life event, trust your instincts.

Signs that a child may benefit from seeing a psychologist or licensed therapist include:

- developmental delay in speech, language, or toilet training;
- learning or attention problems (such as ADHD [attention deficit hyperactivity disorder]);
- behavioral problems (such as excessive anger, acting out, bed-wetting, or eating disorders);
- maintains high grades;
- episodes of sadness, tearfulness, or depression;
- social withdrawal or isolation;
- being the victim of bullying or bullying other children;
- decreased interest in previously enjoyed activities;
- overly aggressive behavior (such as biting, kicking, or hitting);
- sudden changes in appetite (particularly in adolescents);
- insomnia or increased sleepiness;
- excessive school absenteeism or tardiness;
- mood swings (e.g., happy one minute, upset the next);
- development of or an increase in physical complaints (such as headache, stomachache, or not feeling well) despite a normal physical exam by your doctor;
- management of a serious, acute, or chronic illness;
- signs of alcohol, drug, or other substance use (such as solvents or prescription drug abuse);
- problems in transitions (following separation, divorce, or reloca-tion);
- bereavement issues;
- custody evaluations;
- following sexual, physical, or emotional abuse or other events.

Kids who aren't yet school-age could benefit from seeing a developmental or clinical psychologist if there's a significant delay in achieving developmental milestones such as walking, talking, and potty training, and if there are concerns regarding autism or other developmental disorders.

Talk to Caregivers, Teachers, and the Doctor

It's also helpful to speak to caregivers and teachers who interact regularly with your child. Is your child paying attention in class and turning in assignments on time? What's his or her behavior like at recess and with peers? Gather as much information as possible to determine the best course of action.

Discuss your concerns with your child's doctor, who can offer perspective and evaluate your child to rule out any medical conditions that could be having an effect. The doctor also may be able to refer you to a qualified therapist for the help your child needs.

Finding the Right Therapist

How do you find a qualified clinician who has experience working with kids and teens? While experience and education are important, it's also important to find a counselor your child feels comfortable talking to. Look for one who not only has the right experience, but also the best approach to help your child in the current circumstances.

Your doctor can be a good source of a referral. Most doctors have working relationships with mental health specialists such as child psychologists or clinical social workers. Friends, colleagues, or family members might also be able to recommend someone.

Consider a number of factors when searching for the right therapist for your child. A good first step is to ask if the therapist is willing to meet with you for a brief consultation or to talk with you during a phone interview before you commit to regular visits. Not all therapists are able to do this, given their busy schedules. Most therapists charge a fee for this type of service; others consider it a complimentary visit.

Factors to Consider

Consider the following factors when evaluating a potential therapist:

- Is the therapist licensed to practice in your state? (You can check with the state board for that profession or check to see if the license is displayed in the office.)

- Is the therapist covered by your health insurance plan's mental health benefits? If so, how many sessions are covered by your plan? What will your co-pay be?

- What are his or her credentials?

- What type of experience does the therapist have?

- How long has the therapist worked with children and adolescents?

- Would your child find the therapist friendly?

- What is the cancellation policy if you're unable to keep an appointment?

- Is the therapist available by phone during an emergency?

- Who will be available to your child during the therapist's vacation or illness or during off-hours?

- What types of therapy does the therapist specialize in?

- Is the therapist willing to meet with you in addition to working with your child?

The right therapist-client match is critical, so you might need to meet with a few before you find one who clicks with both you and your child.

As with other medical professionals, therapists may have a variety of credentials and specific degrees. As a general rule, your child's therapist should hold a professional degree in the field of mental health (psychology, social work, or psychiatry) and be licensed by your state. Psychologists, social workers, and psychiatrists all diagnose and treat mental health disorders.

It's also a good idea to know what those letters that follow a therapist's name mean:

Psychiatrists

Psychiatrists (MDs or DOs) are medical doctors who have advanced training and experience in psychotherapy and pharmacology. They can also prescribe medications.

Clinical Psychologists

Clinical psychologists (PhDs, PsyDs, or EdDs) are therapists who have a doctorate degree that includes advanced training in the practice of psychology, and many specialize in treating children and teens and their families. Psychologists may help clients manage medications but do not prescribe medication.

Clinical Social Workers

A licensed clinical social worker (LCSW) has a master's degree, specializes in clinical social work, and is licensed in the state in which he or she practices. An LICSW is also a licensed clinical social worker. A CSW is a certified social worker. Many social workers are trained in psychotherapy, but the credentials vary from state to state. Likewise, the designations (i.e., LCSW, LICSW, CSW) can vary from state to state.

Different Types of Therapy

There are many types of therapy. Therapists choose the strategies that are most appropriate for a particular problem and for the individual child and family. Therapists will often spend a portion of each session with the parents alone, with the child alone, and with the family together.

Any one therapist may use a variety of strategies, including Cognitive Behavioral Therapy (CBT). This type of therapy is often helpful with kids and teens who are depressed, anxious, or having problems coping with stress.

Cognitive behavioral therapy restructures negative thoughts into more positive, effective ways of thinking. It can include work on stress management strategies, relaxation training, practicing coping skills, and other forms of treatment.

Psychoanalytic therapy is less commonly used with children but can be used with older kids and teens who may benefit from more in-depth analysis of their problems. This is the quintessential "talk therapy" and does not focus on short-term problem-solving in the same way as CBT and behavioral therapies.

In some cases, kids benefit from individual therapy, one-on-one work with the therapist on issues they need guidance on, such as depression, social difficulties, or worry. In other cases, the right option is group therapy, where kids meet in groups of six to 12 to solve problems and learn new skills (such as social skills or anger management).

Family therapy can be helpful in many cases, such as when family members aren't getting along; disagree or argue often; or when a child or teen is having behavior problems. Family therapy involves counseling sessions with some, or all, family members, helping to improve communication skills among them. Treatment focuses on problem-solving techniques and can help parents re-establish their role as authority figures.

Preparing for the First Visit

You may be concerned that your child will become upset when told of an upcoming visit with a therapist. Although this is sometimes the case, it's essential to be honest about the session and why your child (or family) will be going. The issue will come up during the session, but it's important for you to prepare your child for it.

Explain to young kids that this type of visit to the doctor doesn't involve a physical exam or shots. You may also want to stress that this type of doctor talks and plays with kids and families to help them solve problems and feel better. Kids might feel reassured to learn that the therapist will be helping the parents and other family members too.

Older kids and teens may be reassured to hear that anything they say to the therapist is confidential and cannot be shared with anyone else, including parents or other doctors, without their permission—the exception is if they indicate that they're having thoughts of suicide or otherwise hurting themselves or others.

Giving kids this kind of information before the first appointment can help set the tone, prevent your child from feeling singled out or isolated, and provide reassurance that the family will be working together on the problem.

Providing Additional Support

While your child copes with emotional issues, be there to listen and care, and offer support without judgment. Patience is critical, too, as many young children are unable to verbalize their fears and emotions.

Try to set aside some time to discuss your child's worries or concerns. To minimize distractions, turn off the TV and let voice mail answer your phone calls. This will let your child know that he or she is your first priority.

Other ways to communicate openly and problem-solve include:

- Talk openly and as frequently with your child as you can.

- Show love and affection to your child, especially during troubled times.

- Set a good example by taking care of your own physical and emotional needs.

- Enlist the support of your partner, immediate family members, your child's doctor, and teachers.

- Improve communication at home by having family meetings that end with a fun activity (e.g., playing a game, making ice-cream sundaes).

- No matter how hard it is, set limits on inappropriate or problematic behaviors. Ask the therapist for some strategies to encourage your child's cooperation.

- Communicate frequently with the therapist.

- Be open to all types of feedback from your child and from the therapist.

- Respect the relationship between your child and the therapist. If you feel threatened by it, discuss this with the therapist (it's nothing to be embarrassed about).

- Enjoy favorite activities or hobbies with your child.

By recognizing problems and seeking help early on, you can help your child—and your entire family—move through the tough times toward happier, healthier times ahead.

Section 48.3

Antidepressant Medications for Children and Adolescents: Information for Parents

Excerpted from "Antidepressant Medications for Children and Adolescents: Information for Parents and Caregivers," by the National Institute of Mental Health (NIMH, www.nimh.nih.gov), part of the National Institutes of Health, June 13, 2011.

Depression is a serious disorder that can cause significant problems in mood, thinking, and behavior at home, in school, and with peers. It is estimated that major depressive disorder (MDD) affects about 5 percent of adolescents.

Research has shown that, as in adults, depression in children and adolescents is treatable. Certain antidepressant medications, called selective serotonin reuptake inhibitors (SSRIs), can be beneficial to children and adolescents with MDD. Certain types of psychological therapies also have been shown to be effective. However, our knowledge of antidepressant treatments in youth, though growing substantially, is limited compared to what we know about treating depression in adults.

Recently, there has been some concern that the use of antidepressant medications themselves may induce suicidal behavior in youths. Following a thorough and comprehensive review of all the available published and unpublished controlled clinical trials of antidepressants in children and adolescents, the U.S. Food and Drug Administration (FDA) issued a public warning in October 2004 about an increased risk of suicidal thoughts or behavior (suicidality) in children and adolescents treated with SSRI antidepressant medications. In 2006, an advisory committee to the FDA recommended that the agency extend the warning to include young adults up to age 25.

More recently, results of a comprehensive review of pediatric trials conducted between 1988 and 2006 suggested that the benefits of antidepressant medications likely outweigh their risks to children and adolescents with major depression and anxiety disorders. The study, partially funded by NIMH, was published in the April 18, 2007, issue of the *Journal of the American Medical Association.*

What did the FDA review find?

In the FDA review, no completed suicides occurred among nearly 2,200 children treated with SSRI medications. However, about 4 percent of those taking SSRI medications experienced suicidal thinking or behavior, including actual suicide attempts—twice the rate of those taking placebo, or sugar pills.

In response, the FDA adopted a "black box" label warning indicating that antidepressants may increase the risk of suicidal thinking and behavior in some children and adolescents with MDD. A black-box warning is the most serious type of warning in prescription drug labeling.

The warning also notes that children and adolescents taking SSRI medications should be closely monitored for any worsening in depression, emergence of suicidal thinking or behavior, or unusual changes in behavior, such as sleeplessness, agitation, or withdrawal from normal social situations. Close monitoring is especially important during the first 4 weeks of treatment. SSRI medications usually have few side effects in children and adolescents, but for unknown reasons, they may trigger agitation and abnormal behavior in certain individuals.

What do we know about antidepressant medications?

The SSRIs include:

- fluoxetine (Prozac);

- sertraline (Zoloft);

- paroxetine (Paxil);

- citalopram (Celexa);

- escitalopram (Lexapro);

- fluvoxamine (Luvox).

Another antidepressant medication, venlafaxine (Effexor), is not an SSRI but is closely related.

SSRI medications are considered an improvement over older antidepressant medications because they have fewer side effects and are less likely to be harmful if taken in an overdose, which is an issue for patients with depression already at risk for suicide. They have been shown to be safe and effective for adults.

However, use of SSRI medications among children and adolescents ages 10 to 19 has risen dramatically in the past several years. Fluoxetine (Prozac) is the only medication approved by the FDA for use in treating depression in children ages eight and older. The other SSRI medications and the SSRI-related antidepressant venlafaxine have not been approved for treatment of depression in children or adolescents, but doctors still sometimes prescribe them to children on an "off-label" basis. In June 2003, however, the FDA recommended that paroxetine not be used in children and adolescents for treating MDD.

Fluoxetine can be helpful in treating childhood depression, and can lead to significant improvement of depression overall. However, it may increase the risk for suicidal behaviors in a small subset of adolescents. As with all medical decisions, doctors and families should weigh the risks and benefits of treatment for each individual patient.

What should you do for a child with depression?

A child or adolescent with MDD should be carefully and thoroughly evaluated by a doctor to determine if medication is appropriate. Psychotherapy often is tried as an initial treatment for mild depression. Psychotherapy may help to determine the severity and persistence of the depression and whether antidepressant medications may be warranted. Types of psychotherapies include cognitive behavioral therapy, which helps people learn new ways of thinking and behaving, and interpersonal therapy, which helps people understand and work through troubled personal relationships.

Those who are prescribed an SSRI medication should receive ongoing medical monitoring. Children already taking an SSRI medication should remain on the medication if it has been helpful, but should be carefully monitored by a doctor for side effects. Parents should promptly seek medical advice and evaluation if their child or adolescent experiences suicidal thinking or behavior, nervousness, agitation, irritability, mood instability, or sleeplessness that either emerges or worsens during treatment with SSRI medications.

Once started, treatment with these medications should not be abruptly stopped. Although they are not habit-forming or addictive, abruptly ending an antidepressant can cause withdrawal symptoms or lead to a relapse. Families should not discontinue treatment without consulting their doctor.

All treatments can be associated with side effects. Families and doctors should carefully weigh the risks and benefits, and maintain appropriate follow-up and monitoring to help control for the risks.

Section 48.4

Substance Use Associated with Low Response to Depression Treatment among Teens

From "Substance Use Associated with Low Response to Depression Treatment Among Teens," by the National Institute of Mental Health (NIMH, www.nimh.nih.gov), part of the National Institutes of Health, December 9, 2009.

Depressed teens who report low levels of impairment related to drug or alcohol use tended to respond better to depression treatment than depressed teens with higher levels of substance-related impairment, according to an analysis of data from the NIMH-funded Treatment of SSRI-Resistant Depression in Adolescents (TORDIA) study. However, it is unclear whether less substance-related impairment allowed for better response to depression treatment, or if better treatment response led to less substance-related impairment. The study was published in the December 2009 issue of the *Journal of the American Academy of Child and Adolescent Psychiatry*.

Background

Substance use is more common among teens with depression than among those without depression. Researchers have also found that depression can inhibit teens' response to treatment of substance abuse, and substance abuse is associated with a poorer response to treatment of depression. Still, few trials have examined how coexisting depression and substance use among teens may affect treatment outcomes for both.

In the TORDIA study, 334 teens who did not respond to a type of antidepressant called a selective serotonin reuptake inhibitor (SSRI) before the trial were randomly assigned to one of four treatments for 12 weeks:

- Switch to another SSRI

- Switch to venlafaxine (Effexor), a different type of antidepressant

- Switch to another SSRI and add cognitive behavioral therapy (CBT), a type of psychotherapy

- Switch to venlafaxine and add CBT

Results of the trial were previously reported in February 2008. They showed that teens who received combination therapy, with either type of antidepressant, were more likely to improve than those on medication alone.

In this new analysis, Benjamin Goldstein, MD, of the University of Toronto, and colleagues examined TORDIA data to determine the relationship, if any, between substance use, major depression, and response to depression treatment.

Substance use was defined as using alcohol or drugs without meeting criteria for having a full-blown substance abuse disorder. Teens who were diagnosed with a substance abuse disorder were excluded from the TORDIA study.

Results of the Study

Substance use was fairly common among TORDIA participants. At baseline, about 28 percent reported experimenting with drugs or alcohol. Those who showed more substance-related impairment were older, felt more hopeless, had greater family conflict, developed depression at an earlier age, were more likely to have a history of physical or sexual abuse, and were more likely to have coexisting oppositional defiant disorder (ODD) or conduct disorder (CD). Substance-related impairment included certain attitudes and behaviors such as craving the substance, feeling hooked on it, accidentally hurting oneself or others while using it, and other similar effects.

Participants with low levels of substance use and substance-related impairment throughout the study tended to respond better to depression treatment than those who showed persistently high or increasing levels of substance-related impairment. There were no significant differences in rates of substance use and impairment among the treatment groups.

Significance

This study is one of the first to examine the association between substance use and depression treatment among depressed teens. The findings are consistent with other studies that found depression severity to be associated with a history of physical or sexual abuse, coexisting

ODD or CD, and substance-related impairment. However, the direction of the association is uncertain. The data could not determine whether low substance-related impairment facilitates improvement in depression symptoms, or whether improvement in depressed mood leads to a decrease in substance-related impairment.

What's Next?

The authors caution that the study does not provide definitive conclusions about depression treatment and substance use. However, they do suggest that clinicians treating teens for depression screen for signs of substance use and address those issues as well, even if the teen does not meet criteria for a full-blown substance abuse disorder.

Reference

Goldstein BI, Shamseddeen W, Spirito A, Emslie G, Clarke G, Wagner KD, Asarnow JR, Vitiello B, Ryan N, Birmaher B, Mayes T, Onorato M, Zelazny J, Brent D. Substance use and the treatment of resistant depression in adolescents. *Journal of the American Academy of Child and Adolescent Psychiatry*. 2009 Dec. 48(12):1182–1192.

Section 48.5

Teens Who Recover from Hard-to-Treat Depression Still at Risk for Relapse

From the National Institute of Mental Health (NIMH, www.nimh.nih .gov), part of the National Institutes of Health, December 3, 2010.

Teens with hard-to-treat depression who reach remission after 24 weeks of treatment are still at a significant risk for relapse, according to long-term, follow-up data from an NIMH-funded study published online November 16, 2010, in the *Journal of Clinical Psychiatry*. The long-term data reiterate the need for aggressive treatment decisions for teens with stubborn depression.

Background

In the Treatment of Resistant Depression in Adolescents (TORDIA) study, teens whose depression had not improved after an initial course of selective serotonin reuptake inhibitor (SSRI) antidepressant treatment were randomly assigned to one of four interventions for 12 weeks:

- Switch to another SSRI-paroxetine (Paxil), citalopram (Celexa), or fluoxetine (Prozac)

- Switch to a different SSRI plus cognitive behavioral therapy (CBT), a type of psychotherapy that emphasizes problem-solving and behavior change

- Switch to venlafaxine (Effexor), a different type of antidepressant called a serotonin and norepinephrine reuptake inhibitor (SNRI)

- Switch to venlafaxine plus CBT

As reported in May 2010, nearly 40 percent of those who completed 24 weeks of treatment achieved remission, regardless of the treatment to which they had initially been assigned. However, those who achieved remission were more likely to have responded to treatment early—during the first 12 weeks.

After 24 weeks of treatment, the participants were discharged from the study and urged to continue care within their community. They were then asked to return for an assessment at 72 weeks.

Results of the Study

Of the 334 original TORDIA participants, about 61 percent had reached remission by week 72. Symptoms of depression steadily decreased after the initial 24 weeks of treatment. But at 72 weeks, many participants still reported having residual symptoms of depression, such as irritability, fatigue, and low self-esteem.

Those with more severe depression at baseline were less likely to reach remission. Those who responded early to treatment—within the first six weeks of treatment—were more likely to reach remission. Initial treatment assignment during the study did not appear to influence the remission rate or time to remission.

However, of the 130 participants who had remitted by week 24, 25 percent had relapsed by week 72. Ethnic minorities tended to have a higher risk for relapse than whites.

Significance

Because more than one-third of the teens did not recover and the relapse rate was high, the authors conclude that more effective interventions early in the treatment process are needed. In addition, the higher risk of relapse for ethnic minorities suggests that cultural factors may influence the long-term course of depression and recovery, but it is unclear what those factors may be.

What's Next?

The findings indicate that new methods are needed to accurately identify those who may not respond early in treatment so that patients unlikely to reach remission using a particular treatment may be offered alternative treatments earlier in the process. More data is needed, however, to be able to predict who might be more likely to remit and who may not.

Reference

Vitiello B, Emslie G, Clarke G, Wagner K, Asarnow JR, Keller M, Birmaher B, Ryan N, Kennard B, Mayes T, DeBar L, Lynch F, Dickerson

J, Strober M, Suddath R, McCraken JT, Spirito A, Onorato M, Zelazny J, Porta G, Iyengar S, Brent D. Long-term outcome of adolescent depression initially resistant to SSRI treatment. *Journal of Clinical Psychiatry,* online November 16, 2010.

Chapter 49

Treatment-Resistant or Relapsed Depression

Chapter Contents

Section 49.1

What Is Treatment-Resistant Depression?

Excerpted from "Nonpharmacologic Interventions for Treatment-Resistant Depression in Adults: Executive Summary," by the Agency for Healthcare Research and Quality (AHRQ, www.ahrq.gov), September 2011.

Major depressive disorder (MDD) is common and costly. Over the course of a year, between 13.1 million and 14.2 million people will experience MDD.

Approximately half of these people seek help for this condition, and only 20 percent of those receive adequate treatment. For those who do initiate treatment for their depression, approximately 50 percent will not adequately respond following acute phase treatment; this refractory group has considerable clinical and research interest.

Patients with only one prior treatment failure are sometimes included in this group, but patients with two or more prior treatment failures are a particularly important and poorly understood group and are considered to have treatment-resistant depression (TRD). These TRD patients represent a complex population with a disease that is difficult to manage.

Patients with TRD incur the highest direct and indirect medical costs among those with MDD. These costs increase with the severity of TRD. Treatment-resistant patients are twice as likely to be hospitalized, and their cost of hospitalization is more than six times the mean total costs of depressed patients who are not treatment resistant. After considering both medical and disability claims from an employer's perspective, one study found that TRD employees cost $14,490 per employee per year, whereas the cost for non-TRD employees was $6,665 per employee per year.

Given the burden of TRD generally, the uncertain prognosis of the disorder, and the high costs of therapy, clinicians and patients alike need clear evidence to guide their treatment decisions. The choices are wide ranging, include both pharmacologic and nonpharmacologic interventions, and are fraught with incomplete, potentially conflicting evidence. Somatic treatments, which may involve use of a pharmacologic intervention or a device, are commonly considered for patients with TRD. Antidepressant medications, which are the most commonly used intervention, have decreasing efficacy for producing remission after patients have experienced two treatment failures. Such drugs also often have side effects, sometimes minor but sometimes quite serious. For these reasons, clinicians often look for alternative strategies for their TRD patients.

This review from the RTI International–University of North Carolina at Chapel Hill Evidence-based Practice Center (EPC) provides a comprehensive summary of the available data addressing the comparative effectiveness of four nonpharmacologic treatments as therapies for patients with TRD: Electroconvulsive therapy (ECT), repetitive transcranial magnetic stimulation (rTMS), vagus nerve stimulation (VNS), and cognitive behavioral therapy or interpersonal psychotherapy (CBT or IPT).

The core patient population of interest was patients with MDD who met our definition of TRD: Failure to respond following two or more adequate antidepressant treatments. We also included TRD studies in which the patient population could include a "mix" of up to 20 percent of patients with bipolar disorder (i.e., 80 percent or more of patients had only MDD), assuming that this small mix would not substantially alter outcomes seen with MDD-only populations.

Conclusion

Our review suggests that comparative clinical research on nonpharmacologic interventions in a TRD population is early in its infancy, and many clinical questions about efficacy and effectiveness remain unanswered.

Interpretation of the data is substantially hindered by varying definitions of TRD and the paucity of relevant studies. The greatest volume of evidence is for ECT and rTMS. However, even for the few comparisons of treatments that are supported by some evidence, the strength of evidence is low for benefits, reflecting low confidence that the evidence reflects the true effect and indicating that further research is likely to change our confidence in these findings. This finding of low strength is most notable in two cases: ECT and rTMS did not produce different clinical outcomes in TRD, and ECT produced better outcomes than pharmacotherapy.

No trials directly compared the likelihood of maintaining remission for nonpharmacologic interventions. The few trials addressing adverse events, subpopulations, subtypes, and health-related outcomes provided low or insufficient evidence of differences between nonpharmacologic interventions. The most urgent next steps for research are to apply a consistent definition of TRD, to conduct more head-to-head clinical trials comparing nonpharmacologic interventions with themselves and with pharmacologic treatments, and to delineate carefully the number of treatment failures following a treatment attempt of adequate dose and duration in the current episode.

Section 49.2

Causes of Depression Relapse

Causes of Relapse

- Failure to take medication
- Use of alcohol or drugs
- Increased stress (once a person becomes schizophrenic it is a stress-related disorder)
- Family chaos

People with schizophrenia or bipolar disorder have over-stimulated brains and thus, have less tolerance for stress. Environmental stigma causes stress. The effort to appear normal and behave normally takes great effort. A person with a brain disorder is emotionally or mentally frail the same way an elderly person is frail. Both should avoid overexertion.

Symptoms

The most frequent symptoms of relapse are paranoia, insomnia, and agitation.

Other signs can be hostility, outbursts, hallucinations, fear, agitation, restlessness, anxiety, depression, withdrawal, decrease in grooming, eating, and increase in obsession with religious fixations. Predictable stages of relapse or hospitalization can begin simply with your relative feeling overwhelmed.

Rehospitalizations

Most patients see a clear sign of impending hospitalization before it occurs. They notice more difficulty sleeping, or "the voices were bothering me much more," or they feel more agitated. Seventy percent of mentally ill people can recognize their symptoms.

Five Main Types of Responses That Are Helpful in Relapse

- "Brace" your relative with additional support, i.e., temporary meds increase until they feel stable, change the focus of his/her activities.

- Decrease the amount of stress in their lives anyway you can.

- Don't shout, don't squabble, don't threaten or criticize, and don't bait the ill person.

- Give your relative an opportunity to describe what is happening to them, but do not engage their voices. Mirror back to your relative that you know this is difficult for him/her. It can be very helpful if they feel validated and understood.

- Seek additional help from other resources. See if there are other people who can help reduce the load. Three main sources: Professionals such as psychiatrists, therapists, and family friends; secondly, peers and self-help groups.

Stress and Relapse

Asking your ill relative to work all day may not be a reasonable request. Try to avoid stressful situations.

Holidays are really stressful for ill people. Members of extended family may have a new job or a new baby. They involve unfavorable comparisons for the person with mental illness.

You might need to change family holidays to reduce stress. Sometimes an environment that is stimulating for a normal person can be overwhelming for a schizophrenic. Reduce the number of people attending an event and the length of time of any event.

Parties are stressful. They would like to drink like anyone else. To feel rejected can send them off the deep end; they may not feel like taking their meds.

Your relative's feeling that their food, shelter, or clothing is threatened can be very stressful, especially if they have to move or they don't have SSI [Supplemental Security Income], or have to reapply annually. The ill are vulnerable to losing their income and being evicted.

A change in living arrangements or attending different groups or a different doctor may be stressful. All of these can trigger psychoses.

A change in success is also stressful.

Teach the person to leave the stressful situation. Give them a mantra to say over and over (i.e. "This is distressing, but not dangerous," "Calm begets calm" or "Let go and let God" or "Change focus."). This may make their internal perception of the situation less threatening. Help the mentally ill person actively manage the situation. Discuss choices with them: "You are getting too excited, why don't you take a walk," or "If you are frightened of these people, you stay with me for 10 minutes."

Relapse Recognition

When your relative can recognize their own signals of relapse, they are less likely to become hospitalized; this is primarily due to the ability to increase appropriate medication within 48 hours of symptoms appearing.

Section 49.3

Brain Stimulation Therapies for Severe Depression: Electroconvulsive Therapy, Vagus Nerve Stimulation, and Transcranial Magnetic Stimulation

From "Brain Stimulation Therapies," by the National Institute of Mental Health (NIMH, www.nimh.nih.gov), part of the National Institutes of Health, November 17, 2009.

What are brain stimulation therapies?

Brain stimulation therapies involve activating or touching the brain directly with electricity, magnets, or implants to treat depression and other disorders.

Electroconvulsive therapy is the most researched stimulation therapy and has the longest history of use. Other stimulation therapies discussed here—vagus nerve stimulation, repetitive transcranial magnetic stimulation, magnetic seizure therapy, and deep brain stimulation—are newer, more experimental methods.

What is electroconvulsive therapy?

First developed in 1938, electroconvulsive therapy (ECT) for years had a poor reputation with many negative depictions in popular culture. However, the procedure has improved significantly since its initial use and is safe and effective. People who undergo ECT do not feel any pain or discomfort during the procedure.

ECT is usually considered only after a patient's illness has not improved after other treatment options, such as antidepressant medication or psychotherapy, are tried. It is most often used to treat severe, treatment-resistant depression, but occasionally it is used to treat other mental disorders, such as bipolar disorder or schizophrenia. It also may be used in life-threatening circumstances, such as when a patient is unable to move or respond to the outside world (e.g., catatonia), is suicidal, or is malnourished as a result of severe depression.

479

One study, the Consortium for Research in ECT study, found an 86 percent remission rate for those with severe major depression. The same study found it to be effective in reducing chances of relapse when the patients underwent follow-up treatments.

How does it work?

Before ECT is administered, a person is sedated with general anesthesia and given a medication called a muscle relaxant to prevent movement during the procedure. An anesthesiologist monitors breathing, heart rate, and blood pressure during the entire procedure, which is conducted by a trained physician. Electrodes are placed at precise locations on the head. Through the electrodes, an electric current passes through the brain, causing a seizure that lasts generally less than one minute.

Scientists are unsure how the treatment works to relieve depression, but it appears to produce many changes in the chemistry and functioning of the brain. Because the patient is under anesthesia and has taken a muscle relaxant, the patient's body shows no signs of seizure, nor does he or she feel any pain, other than the discomfort associated with inserting an intravenous line.

Five to 10 minutes after the procedure ends, the patient awakens. He or she may feel groggy at first as the anesthesia wears off. But after about an hour, the patient usually is alert and can resume normal activities.

A typical course of ECT is administered about three times a week until the patient's depression lifts (usually within six to 12 treatments). After that, maintenance ECT treatment is sometimes needed to reduce the chance that symptoms will return. ECT maintenance treatment varies depending on the needs of the individual, and may range from one session per week to one session every few months. Frequently, a person who underwent ECT will take antidepressant medication or a mood stabilizing medication as well.

What are the side effects?

The most common side effects associated with ECT are headache, upset stomach, and muscle aches. Some people may experience memory problems, especially of memories around the time of the treatment. People may also have trouble remembering information learned shortly after the procedure, but this difficulty usually disappears over the days and weeks following the end of an ECT course. It is possible that a person may have gaps in memory over the weeks during which he or she receives treatment.

Research has found that memory problems seem to be more associated with the traditional type of ECT called bilateral ECT, in which the electrodes are placed on both sides of the head. Unilateral ECT, in which the electrodes are placed on just one side of the head—typically the right side because it is opposite the brain's learning and memory areas—appears less likely to cause memory problems and therefore is preferred by many doctors. In the past, a "sine wave" was used to administer electricity in a constant, high dose. However, studies have found that a "brief pulse" of electricity administered in several short bursts is less likely to cause memory loss, and therefore is most commonly used today.

What is vagus nerve stimulation?

Vagus nerve stimulation (VNS) works through a device implanted under the skin that sends electrical pulses through the left vagus nerve, half of a prominent pair of nerves that run from the brainstem through the neck and down to each side of the chest and abdomen. The vagus nerves carry messages from the brain to the body's major organs like the heart, lungs, and intestines, and to areas of the brain that control mood, sleep, and other functions.

VNS was originally developed as a treatment for epilepsy. However, it became evident that it also had effects on mood, especially depressive symptoms. Using brain scans, scientists found that the device affected areas of the brain that are also involved in mood regulation. The pulses also appeared to alter certain neurotransmitters (brain chemicals) associated with mood, including serotonin, norepinephrine, GABA [gamma-aminobutyric acid], and glutamate.

In 2005, the U.S. Food and Drug Administration (FDA) approved VNS for use in treating major depression in certain circumstances—if the illness has lasted two years or more, if it is severe or recurrent, and if the depression has not eased after trying at least four other treatments. Despite FDA approval, VNS remains a controversial treatment for depression because results of studies testing its effectiveness in treating major depression have been mixed.

How does it work?

A device called a pulse generator, about the size of a stopwatch, is surgically implanted in the upper left side of the chest. Connected to the pulse generator is a lead wire, which is guided under the skin up to the neck, where it is attached to the left-side vagus nerve.

Typically, electrical pulses that last about 30 seconds are sent about every five minutes from the generator to the vagus nerve. The duration and frequency of the pulses may vary depending on how the generator is programmed. The vagus nerve, in turn, delivers those signals to the brain. The pulse generator, which operates continuously, is powered by a battery that lasts around 10 years, after which it must be replaced. Normally, a person does not feel any sensation in the body as the device works, but it may cause coughing or the voice may become hoarse while the nerve is being stimulated.

The device also can be temporarily deactivated by placing a magnet over the chest where the pulse generator is implanted. A person may want to deactivate it if side effects become intolerable, or before engaging in strenuous activity or exercise because it may interfere with breathing. The device reactivates when the magnet is removed.

What are the side effects?

VNS is not without risk. There may be complications such as infection from the implant surgery, or the device may come loose, move around, or malfunction, which may require additional surgery to correct. Long-term side effects are unknown.

Other potential side effects include the following:

- Voice changes or hoarseness

- Cough or sore throat

- Neck pain

- Discomfort or tingling in the area where the device is implanted

- Breathing problems, especially during exercise

- Difficulty swallowing

What is repetitive transcranial magnetic stimulation?

Repetitive transcranial magnetic stimulation (rTMS) uses a magnet instead of an electrical current to activate the brain. First developed in 1985, rTMS has been studied as a possible treatment for depression, psychosis, and other disorders since the mid-1990s.

Clinical trials studying the effectiveness of rTMS reveal mixed results. When compared to a placebo or inactive (sham) treatment, some studies have found that rTMS is more effective in treating patients with major depression. But other studies have found no difference in response compared to inactive treatment.

In October 2008, rTMS was approved for use by the FDA as a treatment for major depression for patients who have not responded to at least one antidepressant medication. It is also used in countries such as in Canada and Israel as a treatment for depression for patients who have not responded to medications and who might otherwise be considered for ECT.

How does it work?

Unlike ECT, in which electrical stimulation is more generalized, rTMS can be targeted to a specific site in the brain. Scientists believe that focusing on a specific spot in the brain reduces the chance for the type of side effects that are associated with ECT. But opinions vary as to what spot is best.

A typical rTMS session lasts 30 to 60 minutes and does not require anesthesia. An electromagnetic coil is held against the forehead near an area of the brain that is thought to be involved in mood regulation. Then, short electromagnetic pulses are administered through the coil. The magnetic pulse easily passes through the skull, and causes small electrical currents that stimulate nerve cells in the targeted brain region. And because this type of pulse generally does not reach further than 2 inches into the brain, scientists can select which parts of the brain will be affected and which will not be. The magnetic field is about the same strength as that of a magnetic resonance imaging (MRI) scan. Generally, the person will feel a slight knocking or tapping on the head as the pulses are administered.

Not all scientists agree on the best way to position the magnet on the patient's head or give the electromagnetic pulses. They also do not yet know if rTMS works best when given as a single treatment or combined with medication. More research, including a large NIMH-funded trial, is underway to determine the safest and most effective use of rTMS.

What are the side effects?

Sometimes a person may have discomfort at the site on the head where the magnet is placed. The muscles of the scalp, jaw, or face may contract or tingle during the procedure. Mild headache or brief lightheadedness may result. It is also possible that the procedure could cause a seizure, although documented incidences of this are uncommon. A recent large-scale study on the safety of rTMS found that most side effects, such as headaches or scalp discomfort, were mild or moderate, and no seizures occurred. Because the treatment is new, however, long-term side effects are unknown.

What is magnetic seizure therapy?

Magnetic seizure therapy (MST) borrows certain aspects from both ECT and rTMS. Like rTMS, it uses a magnetic pulse instead of electricity to stimulate a precise target in the brain. However, unlike rTMS, MST aims to induce a seizure like ECT. So the pulse is given at a higher frequency than that used in rTMS. Therefore, like ECT, the patient must be anesthetized and given a muscle relaxant to prevent movement. The goal of MST is to retain the effectiveness of ECT while reducing the cognitive side effects usually associated with it.

MST is currently in the early stages of testing, but initial results are promising. Studies on both animals and humans have found that MST produces fewer memory side effects, shorter seizures, and allows for a shorter recovery time than ECT. However, its effect on treatment-resistant depression is not yet established. Studies are underway to determine its antidepressant effects.

What is deep brain stimulation?

Deep brain stimulation (DBS) was first developed as a treatment for Parkinson disease to reduce tremor, stiffness, walking problems, and uncontrollable movements. In DBS, a pair of electrodes is implanted in the brain and controlled by a generator that is implanted in the chest. Stimulation is continuous and its frequency and level is customized to the individual.

DBS has only recently been studied as a treatment for depression or obsessive compulsive disorder (OCD). Currently, it is available on an experimental basis only. So far, very little research has been conducted to test DBS for depression treatment, but the few studies that have been conducted show that the treatment may be promising. One small trial involving people with severe, treatment-resistant depression found that four out of six participants showed marked improvement in their symptoms either immediately after the procedure, or soon after. Another study involving 10 people with OCD found continued improvement among the majority three years after the surgery.

How does it work?

DBS requires brain surgery. The head is shaved and then attached with screws to a sturdy frame that prevents the head from moving during the surgery. Scans of the head and brain using MRI are taken. The surgeon uses these images as guides during the surgery. Patients are awake during the procedure to provide the surgeon with feedback, but they feel no pain because the head is numbed with a local anesthetic.

Once ready for surgery, two holes are drilled into the head. From there, the surgeon threads a slender tube down into the brain to place electrodes on each side of a specific part of the brain. In the case of depression, the part of the brain targeted is called Area 25. This area has been found to be overactive in depression and other mood disorders. In the case of OCD, the electrodes are placed in a different part of the brain believed to be associated with the disorder.

After the electrodes are implanted and the patient provides feedback about the placement of the electrodes, the patient is put under general anesthesia. The electrodes are then attached to wires that are run inside the body from the head down to the chest, where a pair of battery-operated generators are implanted.

From here, electrical pulses are continuously delivered over the wires to the electrodes in the brain. Although it is unclear exactly how the device works to reduce depression or OCD, scientists believe that the pulses help to "reset" the area of the brain that is malfunctioning so that it works normally again.

What are the side effects?

DBS carries risks associated with any type of brain surgery. For example, the procedure may lead to the following:

- Bleeding in the brain or stroke

- Infection

- Disorientation or confusion

- Unwanted mood changes

- Movement disorders

- Lightheadedness

- Trouble sleeping

Because the procedure is still experimental, other side effects that are not yet identified may be possible. Long-term benefits and side effects are unknown.

What research is underway on brain stimulation therapies?

Brain stimulation therapies hold promise for treating certain mental disorders that do not respond to more conventional treatments. Therefore, they are of high interest and are the subject of many studies.

For example, researchers continue to look for ways to reduce the side effects of ECT while retaining the benefits.

Studies on rTMS are ongoing and include a trial in which the procedure is being tested for safety and effectiveness for the treatment of major depression in 240 participants. Similar studies are being conducted using MST.

Other researchers are studying how the brain responds to VNS by using imaging techniques such as PET scans. Finally, although DBS as a depression treatment is still very new, researchers are beginning to conduct studies with people to determine its effectiveness and safety in treating depression, OCD, and other mental disorders.

Section 49.4

Hospital Stays Related to Depression

Excerpted from Russo, C. A. (Thomson Healthcare), Hambrick, M. M. (AHRQ), and Owens, P. L. (AHRQ). Hospital Stays Related to Depression, 2005. HCUP Statistical Brief #40. November 2007. Agency for Healthcare Research and Quality, Rockville, MD. http://www.hcup-us.ahrq.gov/reports/statbriefs/sb40.pdf

Introduction

Approximately 9.5 percent of the adult population in the United States suffers from depression. Depression is characterized by a persistent low mood, profound sadness, and lack of interest in enjoyable activities. Although many individuals with depression do not seek treatment, among those who do receive care, the treatment settings are varied. The majority will seek care in outpatient or ambulatory settings, but others will need more intense treatment in an inpatient setting such as community hospitals or long-term, residential facilities. With the declining availability of psychiatric beds in specialty facilities, community hospitals have become the primary source of short-term inpatient care for mental health disorders such as depression.

This text presents data from the Healthcare Cost and Utilization Project (HCUP) on hospital stays related to depression in 2005.

Characteristics of these stays, including associated diagnoses, are compared to stays with no mention of depression. Additionally, trends in the number of hospitalizations for depression as a principal diagnosis and as a secondary diagnosis from 1995 to 2005 are discussed. Finally, utilization is examined by region and expected primary payer. All differences between estimates noted in the text are statistically significant at the 0.05 level or better.

Findings

In 2005, nearly one in 10 hospitalizations—2.9 million—occurred among patients with depression (i.e., depression was a principal and/or coexisting condition). For about 15 percent (423,300) of these hospitalizations, depression was listed as the principal reason for admission. Although the number of stays principally for depression remained relatively stable between 1995 and 2005, the number of stays with depression as a secondary diagnosis rose by 166 percent over the same time period. In 2005, hospital stays among patients principally admitted for depression cost $1.9 billion, while stays with depression as a secondary diagnosis totaled $19.9 billion. In total, 8 percent ($21.8 billion) of hospital costs in the United States were associated with a diagnosis of depression.

General Characteristics of Hospital Stays among Patients with Depression

Compared to stays with no mention of depression, depression-related stays were more likely to occur among younger patients and among females. On average, patients hospitalized principally for depression were about 16 years younger than patients without depression (41.8 years versus 58.0 years). In fact, patients aged 18 to 44 years, accounted for nearly half of all hospitalizations in which depression was the principal reason for admission. Females accounted for 58.8 percent of all hospitalizations with a principal diagnosis of depression, and 68.3 percent of stays with depression as a secondary condition. In comparison, females accounted for 53.5 percent of hospitalizations with no mention of depression.

In 2005, the hospital resources associated with depression as a secondary diagnosis and with stays unrelated to depression were similar. For example, stays with a secondary diagnosis of depression and stays with no mention of depression averaged approximately 5 days in length—1.5 days shorter than the mean length of stay for hospitalizations principally for depression (6.6 days). Similarly, the average hospital cost per stay was $8,100 for stays with a secondary diagnosis of depression and $9,600 for stays unrelated to depression, while average hospital costs were $4,500 among stays principally for depression. As a result, hospitalizations with a principal diagnosis of depression had an average cost per day that was 63.2 percent lower than the cost per day for stays unrelated to depression ($700 versus $1,900). The average cost per day of hospitalizations with depression listed as a secondary condition was $1,600, which is comparable to stays unrelated to depression. This pattern is likely a result of more resource intensive procedures and treatments related to the principal diagnoses in stays with depression as a coexisting condition.

Differences in Hospital Stays among Patients with Depression, by Region

When adjusted for the population of each region, hospitalizations related to depression were most likely to occur in the Midwest and Northeast. Although the overall hospitalization rates for stays unrelated to depression were relatively similar in the Northeast, Midwest, and South (about 975 hospital stays per 10,000 people in each region), hospitalizations principally for depression in the Midwest (19.5 stays per 10,000 people) and Northeast (17.3 stays per 10,000 people) occurred more frequently than in the South (12.6 stays per 10,000 people). A similar pattern of hospitalization rates across regions was noted among stays with a secondary diagnosis of depression. The West had the lowest regional rate of hospitalizations related to depression (9.4 stays per 10,000 people with a principal diagnosis of depression and 62.2 stays per 10,000 people with depression as a secondary diagnosis), but also had a lower overall rate of hospitalization than the other regions (714.0 stays per 10,000 people).

Differences in Hospital Stays among Patients with Depression, by Primary Payer

Although the distribution of expected primary payer among stays with no mention of depression and stays with depression as a secondary condition was similar, stays principally for depression were more likely to be covered by Medicaid or be uninsured. In 2005, Medicaid was the expected primary payer for nearly one in four hospitalizations (24.8 percent) principally for depression. In comparison, 14.2 percent of stays with depression as a secondary diagnosis and 12.1 percent of hospitalizations unrelated to depression were covered by Medicaid.

Uninsured stays accounted for 9.8 percent of hospital stays principally for depression—about twice the percentage seen among stays with depression as a secondary diagnosis (4.9 percent) and stays with no mention of depression (5.7 percent). Medicare was the expected primary payer for only 24.8 percent of stays principally for depression, compared to nearly half of stays with a secondary diagnosis of depression and stays with no mention of depression (49.0 percent and 48.7 percent, respectively).

Most Common Principal Conditions Associated with Depression

In approximately 85 percent of all hospital stays involving a diagnosis of depression, the patient was admitted principally for another condition. One in 10 depression-related stays was principally for cardio- and cerebrovascular conditions such as nonspecific chest pain, congestive heart failure, coronary atherosclerosis, cardiac dysrhythmias, and stroke. Common respiratory conditions such as pneumonia, chronic obstructive pulmonary disease, and asthma were the principal reason for admission in 7.8 percent of stays with a secondary diagnosis of depression.

Alcohol and substance abuse was 3.5 times more likely to be a principal reason for admission among patients with depression than those without depression. Similarly, poisoning by psychotropic agents was nine times more likely to be a principal reason for admission, and poisoning by other medications and drugs was five times more likely to be a principal reason for admission among patients with depression than among those without depression.

Part Seven

Strategies for Managing Depression

Chapter 50

Understanding Mental Illness Stigma and Depression Triggers

Chapter Contents

Section 50.1

Stigmas about Mental Illness Contribute to Depression

Excerpted from *The Science of Mental Illness*. Copyright © 2005 by
BSCS. All rights reserved. Reprinted with permission. Reviewed by
David A. Cooke, MD, FACP, November 13, 2011.

"Mentally ill people are nuts, crazy, wacko." "Mentally ill people
are morally bad." "Mentally ill people are dangerous and should be
locked in an asylum forever." "Mentally ill people need somebody to
take care of them." How often have we heard comments like these or
seen these types of portrayals in movies, television shows, or books?
We may even be guilty of making comments like them ourselves. Is
there any truth behind these portrayals, or is that negative view based
on our ignorance and fear?

Stigmas are negative stereotypes about groups of people. Common
stigmas about people who are mentally ill are:

- Individuals who have a mental illness are dangerous.

- Individuals who have a mental illness are irresponsible and
  can't make life decisions for themselves.

- People who have a mental illness are childlike and must be tak-
  en care of by parents or guardians.

- People who have a mental illness should just get over it.

Each of those preconceptions about people who have a mental illness
is based on false information. Very few people who have a mental illness
are dangerous to society. Most can hold jobs, attend school, and live in-
dependently. A person who has a mental illness cannot simply decide to
get over it any more than someone who has a different chronic disease
such as diabetes, asthma, or heart disease can. A mental illness, like
those other diseases, is caused by a physical problem in the body.

Stigmas against individuals who have a mental illness lead to in-
justices, including discriminatory decisions regarding housing, employment, and education. Overcoming the stigmas commonly associated

with mental illness is yet one more challenge that people who have a mental illness must face. Indeed, many people who successfully manage their mental illness report that the stigma they face is in many ways more disabling than the illness itself. The stigmatizing attitudes toward mental illness held by both the public and those who have a mental illness lead to feelings of shame and guilt, loss of self-esteem, social dependence, and a sense of isolation and hopelessness. One of the worst consequences of stigma is that people who are struggling with a mental illness may be reluctant to seek treatment that, in most cases, would significantly relieve their symptoms.

Providing accurate information is one way to reduce stigmas about mental illness. Advocacy groups protest stereotypes imposed upon those who are mentally ill. They demand that the media stop presenting inaccurate views of mental illness and that the public stops believing these negative views. A powerful way of countering stereotypes about mental illness occurs when members of the public meet people who are effectively managing a serious mental illness: Holding jobs, providing for themselves, and living as good neighbors in a community. Interaction with people who have mental illnesses challenges a person's assumptions and changes a person's attitudes about mental illness.

Attitudes about mental illness are changing, although there is a long way to go before people accept that mental illness is a disease with a biological basis. A survey by the National Mental Health Association found that 55 percent of people who have never been diagnosed with depression recognize that depression is a disease and not something people should "snap out of." This is a substantial increase over the 38 percent of survey respondents in 1991 who recognized depression as a disease.

Section 50.2

Depression Triggers: How to Prevent Them

It's downright scary: More than 20 million Americans can expect to suffer from depression in the coming year. But you don't have to be one of them if you're alert to the events and situations that can turn the blues into something more serious. Here, the 10 most common depression triggers—and what to do to prevent them from dragging you down.

Depression Trigger #1: Losing a Job

Why: In addition to causing financial stress, losing a job can jeopardize your sense of identity and feelings of self-worth. Unemployment and financial stress also strain marriages and relationships, bringing conflict that compounds stress and unhappiness.

Who's most vulnerable: Statistics show that the older you are or the higher you were paid, the longer it's likely to take to find work again. Also, those employed in downsized industries and fields, such as the auto industry, may have to retrain or start over in a new field, which can be frightening and can undermine self-confidence.

What helps: Connect with others in the same situation, whether it's through a job skills class, training program, or job-search support group. Also, if you can afford it, use a career counselor or coach to help you create a plan, stay accountable, and feel supported. Experts also recommend building a support network by reaching out to friends and colleagues and setting up regular events throughout the week. The more you can structure your time with lunches, walks, and other get-togethers, the better. Try signing up for a morning exercise class or schedule regular morning walks to get you going each day.

If time goes by and it doesn't look like you're going to find a replacement job quickly, consider volunteering. It's not only a way to boost your self-esteem and get out of the house but it's also great for learning new skills and making new connections.

Depression Trigger #2: Sexual Issues

Why: According to sexual health expert Beverly Whipple, professor at Rutgers University and author of *The Science of Orgasm* (Johns Hopkins University Press, 2006), depression and sexual problems are interrelated in a vicious cycle. Sexual problems and sexual health issues can trigger depression by removing one of the most effective outlets we use to feel good. But many of the most common antidepressant medications, particularly the group of drugs known as SSRIs (selective serotonin reuptake inhibitors; brand names Prozac, Zoloft, Celexa) can sabotage your sex drive and make it harder to achieve orgasm.

Who's most affected: Loss of an active sex life due to age- or health-related issues can trigger depression in both men and women, but men may feel the loss more acutely. That's because sexuality is more central to a man's sense of identity, says Whipple: "When a man experiences a loss of libido or sexual dysfunction, his entire sense of self may be affected."

What helps: In a nutshell, get medical or professional help. While talking about sex and the health of our "equipment" isn't easy for any of us, it's essential to breaking the cycle before it leads to depression. If you're experiencing physical changes that are contributing to a loss of interest in sex or to performance issues, it's essential to bring them up with your doctor. And if the problem stems from relationship or other emotional issues, make use of a couples counselor or sex therapist.

If you let embarrassment or shame prevents you from speaking up, you're denying yourself one of the most effective weapons against depression. Recent studies show that having regular orgasms relieves stress, prevents prostate cancer, and releases feel-good brain chemicals that protect against depression. One of Whipple's many studies even shows that regular sex increases your pain-tolerance threshold, reducing chronic pain.

Depression Trigger #3: "Empty Nest" Syndrome

Why: Two of the hardest things to deal with are loss and change, and when a child leaves home you're suddenly hit with both, all at once. "Your entire routine changes, from the minute you wake up in the morning to the moment you go to bed at night," says Celestino Limos, dean of students at Lewis & Clark College in Portland, Oregon. "Parents tend to focus on all the practical details of getting a child ready for college, but they're unprepared for how much the rhythm of their own lives changes from day to day."

Who's most vulnerable: Women seem to suffer more acutely than men, perhaps because their self-identity is more closely associated with being parents, experts say. But men can suffer an acute sense of loss as well, and they may be less prepared for the onslaught of emotions. Those who are divorced or otherwise single are much more likely to be lonely once the kids are gone, but married couples may also find themselves struggling, particularly if the marriage is rocky or they've developed a tag-team approach to family life and don't share many activities and interests. Parents of only children are also more vulnerable.

What helps: Plan in advance. Parenting experts suggest that parents begin exploring independent interests during their child's last year of high school. Sign up for a class one night a week, or subscribe to a travel magazine and think about trips you might want to take.

When your child leaves home, give yourself a few weeks of quiet time to grieve, but don't spend too much time alone. Set up regular events you can look forward to. Organize weekly walks with friends, join a book group, or sign up for a yoga, Pilates, or dance class. Plan your weekends ahead of time, so you're not caught off guard with time heavy on your hands. Try something completely new, such as a cooking or language class. When you discover a new interest or passion, having more time available becomes a good thing rather than a liability.

Depression Trigger #4: Alcohol Abuse

Why: Recent research backs up what addiction and depression experts have long argued: Alcohol abuse and depression are often linked in what's called a "dual diagnosis" or, colloquially, "double trouble." The reason for this complicated interaction is the effect alcohol has on mood. When you stop into your local tavern for a cold one, you might think you're staving off the blues with some camaraderie and relaxation. But alcohol acts as a depressant in the central nervous system, triggering depression in those who are susceptible.

Who's most vulnerable: Those already prone to depression or those prone to overusing alcohol are at greatest risk. In either group, the combination of alcohol abuse and depression is dangerous. According to studies, between 30 and 50 percent of alcoholics suffer from major depression. And the relationship works the other way too: Studies have found that alcohol use causes relapse in people with depression, and that when people with depression drink they're more prone to suicide.

What helps: Cut back on drinking and seek help for alcohol abuse or addiction. "There's a reason we've got the stereotype of the weepy drunk," says Liliane Desjardins of Pavillion International, a treatment center in Texas. "Alcohol triggers a mood crash." But people who drink too much rarely attribute their misery to drinking, she adds. Instead they blame it on other people and factors.

There's only one solution: Cut back and see if, over time, you feel better. If you repeatedly promise yourself or others not to drink and your efforts fail or your drinking brings other negative consequences into your life, you may need help to stop. Alcoholics Anonymous and other 12-step programs are effective for some people. Others need the physical restriction and concentrated services of a residential alcohol rehabilitation facility or the supervised medical detox of an inpatient program. No matter what type of alcohol treatment program works for you, you'll find it has the additional benefit of preventing depression.

Depression Trigger #5: Illness

Why: When you're diagnosed with a serious illness, it changes your sense of what's possible in the present and affects your outlook for the future. Finding out you have diabetes, cancer, or another condition can set in motion a chain of events that profoundly alters your sense of yourself, your relationships, and your expectations for what life may hold in store.

"People call diagnosis of a serious illness a 'wake-up call,' but often it's more like a slap in the face," says Gloria Nelson, a senior oncology social worker at Montefiore-Einstein Medical Center in New York. "Nothing is as it seemed even a few days ago, which can be disorienting and terrifying." Pain and fatigue are physical symptoms, but they take an enormous emotional toll as well.

Who's most vulnerable: At highest risk are those diagnosed with cancer, Alzheimer's, COPD [chronic obstructive pulmonary disease], multiple sclerosis, Parkinson's, chronic pain, or any other debilitating condition.

What helps: A support group. "I can't say it strongly enough—no one is going to understand what you're going through like your fellow patients," says Nelson. "Your spouse, your friends, your family—they all love you and support you, but they can't really 'get it' like others going through the same thing."

Advocating for yourself to obtain effective treatment is important, too. If you aren't getting the answers or help you need from your doctor, ask for a second opinion or referral to a specialist. For many conditions, such as cancer, a social worker can be a valuable addition to your team, offering access to additional resources the doctor may not tell you about. In some circumstances, a patient advocate can be valuable in helping you pursue aggressive or experimental treatment.

Depression Trigger #6: Divorce

Why: Although every divorce is different, they all have in common one thing: A huge, sudden change in social status. You were part of a social unit, and now you're not. Loneliness and fear—how can I make it on my own?—are common reactions after divorce or separation. Divorce can also bring with it added financial strain. And if there are children involved, custody arrangements and coparenting decisions can cause ongoing conflict and stress.

Who's most vulnerable: Everyone involved in the divorce is vulnerable. A common myth is that the person who initiates a divorce or separation is better off than the person who gets left, but this isn't true, at least not over time, experts say. Even if you were the one who initially asked for the divorce or separation, it's likely the decision came after a long period of pain and unhappiness. And both parties are likely to feel a complicated mix of anger, sadness, resentment, guilt, and a pervasive sense of failure.

What helps: Therapy can be extremely beneficial while going through a divorce or separation. Individual therapy can help you work through the complicated emotions you're feeling and take concrete steps to move forward. Couples therapy, sometimes known as divorce therapy, can help you and your ex resolve your issues with a minimum of anger, bitterness, and recrimination. And family therapy is invaluable in helping kids express their emotions; studies show that kids tend to blame themselves for divorce, which can result in depression for them as well. Family therapy has also been shown to more quickly and successfully resolve custody issues and help divorced parents coparent effectively. Divorced-parent or single-parent support groups are also a great place to find support.

Depression Trigger #7: Debt and Financial Stress

Why: Worrying about how to pay the bills causes an ongoing "buzz" of stress that, over time, sabotages your mood and self-esteem and can lead to depression.

Who's most vulnerable: Those who feel alone dealing with their financial problems are at most risk. Not knowing where to turn is scary, and feelings of shame and secrecy can compound the fear and anxiety.

What helps: Sit down with your bills and a calculator and take stock. Look at what's coming and what's going out. Buy a book or two on financial management and set up a step-by-step plan for yourself. If you're not good with money or feel unable to come up with a plan of action on your own, look for a reputable financial counselor or debt advisor. Many communities offer free financial services, particularly around tax preparation time, and your bank or financial services provider may also have free services you can take advantage of.

Just don't let yourself stay "stuck" in denial while panic builds under the surface. Taking any action, even just talking to a friend or family member about your situation, will help you move forward and formulate a plan.

Depression Trigger #8: Infertility

Why: Wanting to have a baby and not being able to can be a powerful depression trigger, particularly in women. Having a miscarriage or multiple miscarriages often sends a women spiraling into depression. Going into early menopause as a result of surgery, chemotherapy for cancer treatment, or illness can also lead to depression when a woman realizes her window of fertility has closed.

Who's most vulnerable: Women with age- or health-related fertility issues, women who've suffered multiple miscarriages, and women who've had a surgically induced menopause are most prone to distress over infertility issues.

What helps: Advance planning and exploring all options for parenthood can help you if you're nearing the end of your fertile years. Look into the services available for preserving your eggs; whether or not you choose to do so, simply researching the option makes some women feel less vulnerable and powerless, one study has shown. If you're a single woman and lack of a partner is leading you to despair, look into the option of single parenthood by choice via a sperm donor. Whether or not you choose to take this route, investigating what's involved can make you feel more in charge of your choices, experts say. Exploring adoption and familiarizing yourself with the options available there can also be empowering.

Depression Trigger #9: Being a Hands-On Caregiver to Someone with a Debilitating Disease, Such as Alzheimer's or Cancer

Why: Taking on a caregiver role places enormous demands on your time and energy, adds the stress of constant decision making, and often forces you to choose between conflicting obligations, which can result in resentment, guilt, and feelings of inadequacy.

Who's most vulnerable: At greatest risk are women in their 30s and older who are juggling multiple pressures, such as being a caregiver along with working or raising children. Men assume the role of caregiver less commonly, but when they do they may be particularly prone to depression because they're less likely to have strong social bonds and to seek support from their family and community.

What helps: For starters, set boundaries around your caregiving responsibilities. Do what you can, and be clear with the person you're caring for and with other family members about what you can't do and need others to do. This is key to preventing guilt and feeling overwhelmed, both of which are major setups for depression.

Set up a support system for yourself: Schedule respite care, so you get occasional breaks; delegate tasks to others or outsource tasks in your own home. If you're spending many hours on the upkeep of your parent's home, for example, consider paying someone to clean yours, so you don't walk in the door to face more cleaning tasks. If you have siblings in a less active caregiving role, tell them the thank-you gift you'd most appreciate is a cleaning service for your home or gift certificates to restaurants, so you don't have to cook.

And don't neglect your own health and well-being. No matter how tough and strong you are, you won't be able to be an effective caregiver if you don't care for yourself first. Clear time each day to do something for yourself, whether it's to take a walk, cut a few flowers in the garden, meditate, or have a cup of tea with a friend. You need to replenish your inner resources or you won't have anything left for the others who need you.

Depression Trigger #10: Menopause and "Male Menopause"

Why: The hormonal fluctuations that accompany aging can cause levels of key hormones to drop, setting off a cluster of symptoms that can include depression and other problems, such as fatigue, low libido, and anxiety that in turn contribute to depression.

Who's most vulnerable: Women ages 40 to 55 are the most likely to suffer the wide-ranging symptoms of perimenopause—the period leading up to menopause—and menopause itself. Less well known, though, is that men go through their own midlife decline in energy and mood, a phase popularly known as "male menopause." In some men, this is caused by a drop in testosterone levels, but other men experience symptoms even when their testosterone levels remain within the normal range. Experts believe other age-related symptoms such as prostate problems, weight gain, and decline in muscle mass and fitness may be at fault when this happens. In younger women, early-onset menopause caused by surgery or cancer treatment can trigger extreme hormonal symptoms.

What helps: Talk to your doctor, and be prepared to be extremely specific about the symptoms you're experiencing. Keep an ongoing written record of your moods and physical symptoms so you can document what's happening when, and how frequently.

If a hormonal imbalance is the problem, treating the imbalance is key to an overall solution. This doesn't necessarily mean taking hormone replacement therapy, although—despite negative publicity—that's one option that's effective for many women and that appears to pose little risk to most. For men, testosterone supplementation has been shown to treat sexual dysfunction and other symptoms of male menopause if done carefully and correctly.

Many men and women can also stabilize hormones and combat midlife depression by using vitamins, herbs, and other supplements, or by using stress-management techniques such as meditation and yoga. Interestingly, studies show that stress itself inhibits testosterone release, says sexual health expert Beverly Whipple. In men, stress can be a direct cause of sexual issues and depression. Treating underlying conditions such as thyroid disorders can also get hormone levels back on track.

Chapter 51

Improving Your Quality of Life: Exercise, Nutrition, and Lifestyle Changes to Combat Depression

Every aspect of your life—the place you live, the people you live with, your friends and acquaintances, the things you do or don't do, the things you own, your work, even things like pets, music, and color affect how you feel. If you are concerned about your mental health or the quality of your life, you can do many things and make changes in your life that will help you to feel much better. This text will help you think about those areas of your life that may need to be changed and possible changes you could make.

Creating Change—Taking Action

It is not always easy to take the action necessary to create change. However, without taking some action, you cannot make changes in your life that may be necessary to help you feel better. Every time you take a positive step in creating change in your life, give yourself a pat on the back or reward yourself by doing something nice for yourself like taking a warm bath, going for a walk, or spending some time with a friend. You also may want to keep a written record of the change you are creating in your life in a notebook or journal.

Change takes time and may be difficult. You may have to overcome many obstacles. Take small steps. Don't give up. Be persistent. Keep

From "Recovery and Wellness Lifestyle: A Self-Help Guide," by the Substance Abuse and Mental Health Services Administration (SAMHSA, www.samhsa.gov), part of the U.S. Department of Health and Human Services, November 2002. Reviewed by David A. Cooke, MD, FACP, November 19, 2011.

working toward whatever it is that will help you to feel better and enjoy your life more. Making change is being able to see beyond yourself to what the solution might be.

Creating change is something you need to do for yourself. No one else can do it for you. Others can help you and support you as you create change but it is up to you to do what needs to be done. You will be the one that benefits from successful change.

Taking Charge—Regaining Control of Your Life

If you feel you have control over your own life, you have gotten over the first hurdle to creating change in your circumstances. If you don't feel you have control over your life, it is important that you take back control. It is very difficult to feel well when you are not in charge of your own life. Answering the following questions and making the suggested lists could help you figure out how to regain control of your life.

- Do you feel that you have control over your own life?

- Or do you feel other people control your life and you can't do anything about the way your life is?

- What controls your life? List things such as your children, your spouse, a disability, lack of money, etc.

- List things you could do to take back control over your life. For instance, you could do the following:

  - Talk with your spouse about issues related to control.

  - Perhaps the two of you could see a counselor together.

  - Ask your children to take care of some of their own needs and help out with chores.

  - Get a part- or full-time job doing something you enjoy.

  - Attend a class on money management.

  - Learn sign language.

- List what you think is keeping you from doing the things you need to do to take back control over your life. For instance, you might list the following:

  - Have lack of motivation

  - Have low self-esteem

  - Feel like it's too much trouble

- Feel scared
- Do not want to upset others
- Want to avoid the anger of family members
- List the benefits of taking back control over your life. For instance, you would do the following:
  - Feel better physically and emotionally
  - Have less stress
  - Have more time to do the things you enjoy
  - Have time to take good care of yourself
  - Feel more fulfilled
  - Improve the quality of your life

Getting Good Health Care

You deserve good health care. If you have a good health insurance plan, this won't be a problem. If you don't, or your access to health care is limited, see what is available in your community that is free or has sliding scale fees you could afford. Call your local department of health, health care agencies, or your local hospital to check on available options. While it may be hard for you to access good health care, it is worth making the effort to get what you need and deserve for yourself.

- Do you get good health care for yourself?
- Do you have a general health care practitioner or a team of health care professionals who know you and your life circumstances? Can they provide you with valuable assistance in monitoring your health—giving you advice on treatment, providing treatment when necessary, and referring you to other health care providers when necessary?
- What could you do to ensure that you get good health care for yourself?
- Do you get a complete physical checkup every year?
- If not, what could you do to make this happen?

Go to your checkup with a list of all the medications and health care preparations you are using, a history of your illnesses and surgeries and those of close family members, and any symptoms that have you concerned. Don't think anything is too trivial. The mildest symptoms may give your health care provider the needed clues to provide you with good treatment. See your health care provider if your condition changes or worsens.

Don't be satisfied with the outcome of your visit until all your questions have been answered and you feel comfortable with the answers and with suggested treatment strategies. If necessary, arrange follow-up visits. If treatment is recommended, especially if the situation is serious or requires surgery, get a second opinion.

Lifestyle

- Think about your lifestyle. Do you try to do too much every day?

- Do you take on more than you should?

- Do you often find yourself rushing from one thing to another and not enjoying anything?

- If you answered yes to some or all of these questions, what makes your life this way?

- What could you do to make your life more peaceful and calm (for example, take a relaxation course, take two days off every week, save time for yourself in the evening, ask others to take over your responsibilities from time to time, set aside time every day to do things you enjoy)?

- You can't take good care of someone else until you first take good care of yourself. However, you may be like people who focus their attention on others and don't take very good care of themselves. You may find that you are so busy taking care of others that you don't have time to address your own issues. You may be so busy taking care of others that you neglect personal hygiene tasks that would make you feel better—things like a regular shower or bath, washing and styling your hair, trimming your nails, brushing and flossing your teeth, changing your clothes, or even getting dressed (you may feel so badly about yourself some days that you never get out of your night clothes). Are you always taking care of others and not taking care of yourself?

- If so, why?

- What could you do to be sure that you take good care of yourself (for example, say no from time to time, ask others to take over your care-taking responsibilities from time to time, put yourself first, make a list of things you need to do for yourself every day and do the things on the list)?

- You may have more things than you need. All these things may make your life difficult to manage. If you have too many things, you will lose things more easily, your space will be cluttered, and maintaining these things may take time and energy that you would prefer to use in other ways. Do you have so many things that it makes your life difficult to manage?

- If so, describe the problem.

- What could you do to resolve this problem (for example, throw things away, give things away, have a tag sale, clean out one space at a time keeping only what you need, enlist the help of other people you live with, have a moratorium on getting new things)?

- There may be people in your life, at home, at work, or in the community, who make your life difficult—who seem to rob you of your serenity. For instance, when they are around everything feels hectic and chaotic, or very loud. Do you have people in your life who make your life difficult in some way? If so, who are they?

- What could you do to change this situation?

- Like everyone else, you need time alone to do the things you want to do and be the way you want to be. Do you have enough time alone to just be and to do the things you enjoy doing by yourself?

- If not, how could you arrange to get some time alone?

- Doing things that are fun and creative will improve the quality of your life and enhance your sense of well-being. These are the kinds of things you get lost in—like reading a good book, doing a craft project, or playing with your children. What kinds of things do you enjoy doing?

- Do you spend enough time doing these things you enjoy?

- If not, how could you arrange to spend more time doing these things?

- You need time to relax and to relieve stress. Sometimes the events and circumstances of our lives make it hard to do this. If you are unable to relax, you may notice that you feel badly. This can cause physical and emotional health problems. Do you take time to relax every day?

- If not, what could you do to relax (for example, listen to a relaxation tape, take a relaxation and stress reduction course, read a book on relaxation and do some of the exercises, set aside time each day to sit quietly and think about pleasant things)?

Home

The space where you live, your home, can affect how you feel. Perhaps you need to make some changes in your living space or living arrangement or find a different place to call home. The following questions may help you decide if you need to make some changes in living space.

- Do you look forward to going home and do you feel comfortable in your home?

- If not, why not? For instance, you may not like your living space because it is cluttered and messy. Or it may be too noisy.

- What could you change about your home that would make you want to go there and feel comfortable there?

- Do you feel safe and secure when you are at home?

- If not, why not?

- What could you do that would make you feel safe and secure when you are at home (for example, get new locks, move to a safer neighborhood)?

- You deserve private space in your own home for your own things, a place where you can go and know you will not be disturbed. Do you have private space in your home that others respect?

- If not, why not?

- What could you do to have private space in your home that is respected by others (for example, collaborate with the people you live with to arrange private space for everyone, or divide off a section of a room with furniture and make it your space)?

- The people you live with should treat you well and help you feel better. You should be supportive of each other. If you live with others, do they treat you well and help you to feel better?

- If not, why not?

- What could you do so the people you live with treat you well and help you feel better (for example, discuss it with them, telling them how you want and need to be treated, move out, ask others to move)?

- You may need access to health care providers and other services that are necessary for your recovery and wellness. Is your home easily accessible to these services?

- If not, why not?

- What could you do to make it easier for you to access needed services (for example, move, check out public transportation options, learn to drive, get a car, carpool with others)?

- Some people prefer to live in the city or in a neighborhood, whereas others are not comfortable unless they are living in a rural area. In what kind of area would you prefer to live? If you don't live in such an area now, how could you make it happen?

- Some homes require lots of upkeep while others practically take care of themselves. If your home requires lots of upkeep, it may be difficult for you to keep up when you are having a hard time. The stress of not taking care of things that need attention can cause or worsen difficult symptoms. Is your home easy to take care of? If not, why not? What could you do to resolve this problem (for example, move, hire someone to do some of the upkeep, ask for help from family members or friends, trade tasks with others)?

Employment or Career

You may not have a job and wish you had one; or you may have a job or a career. You may enjoy this work. It may help you to understand your value and provide you with needed income. This work, or parts of it, may cause you stress and make your life more difficult. While there are difficult aspects of every job or career, overall you should have a job or career that you enjoy, one that increases your enjoyment of life rather than detracting from it. The following questions may help you decide if you need to make some changes in your employment situation:

- Does your job or career enhance your life and wellness?

- If it doesn't, what needs to change in order to make it a good job for you?

- What can you do to make these things happen?

- If you don't have a job, would you like one?

- If so, how could you make that happen?

- Would you rather work for someone else or work for yourself?

- If this is not your current situation, how could you make this happen?

- Do you have interests, skills, and talents that you could use to develop your own job or career?

- If so, what are they?

- What steps could you take to make this happen?

- Various resources in your area can assist you with work-related issues. They may be agencies for employment and training, vocational rehabilitation, protection and advocacy, social security, mental health agencies, or schools, colleges, and universities. You can begin this process by reaching out to one of these places and asking them who else they would suggest. As you reach out to an agency they suggest, ask for other referrals. If you feel you need to reach out for assistance on work-related issues, who are you going to reach out to first?

- You may know or find that you need more education and/or training to get the job of your choice. How are you going to find out if you need more education and/or training?

- If you already know that you need more education or training, how are you going to work toward getting it?

Diet

The foods and other substances you put in your body may be affecting the way you feel. Many people have found that they feel much better when they pay close attention to what they put in their body, eliminating some things and adding others. If you feel your diet might be affecting the way you feel, try to become more aware of what you eat and drink. Notice how you feel half an hour or more after you have eaten that food or had that drink. If you notice you don't feel very good, try eliminating it from your diet for a short time. If you feel better not eating this particular food, you may want to avoid it as much as possible. Do you notice that you feel badly after you have eaten certain foods or drunk certain beverages like sugar, caffeine, heavily salted, or fatty foods?

You may find that you feel much better when your diet consists mostly of foods that are wholesome and natural. While it may seem that these foods are more expensive, when you choose them instead of junk foods the increase in your food bill will be hardly noticeable.

- Do you feel you have a good diet? If not, how are you going to improve it?

- Do you often overeat or avoid eating? This can cause you to feel badly. Make it a habit to eat three healthy meals a day with several healthy between-meal snacks if desired. Don't skip any meals.

Exercise

If you are exercising regularly, you will enjoy the following benefits:

- An overall feeling of well-being
- Enhanced ability to sleep with more restful sleep
- Improved memory and ability to concentrate
- A decrease in some uncomfortable symptoms
- Decreased irritability and anxiety
- Improved self-esteem
- Weight loss
- Improved muscle tone
- Increased endurance
- Increased mobility
- Do you exercise regularly to help reduce unpleasant symptoms and improve your overall stamina and health while reducing stress?
- If not, how could you make that happen?
- With some illnesses or disabilities your ability to exercise may be limited or restricted in some way. You may be able to exercise for only short periods of time. You may need to avoid strenuous activities. You may be able to exercise only some parts of your body. You may need to avoid moving some parts of your body. You can do the same kind of exercise every day or vary it according to the weather, what you feel like, and what things you need to get done. Is your exercise tailored to meet your specific needs?
- If not, what do you need to do to make sure your exercise protocol is the right one for you? If you haven't exercised recently or have health problems that may affect your ability to exercise, check with your physician before beginning an exercise program.

Light

You may notice that you have less energy than usual, feel less productive and creative, need more sleep, feel sad, down, or depressed, and have less control over your appetite as the daylight time gets shorter in the fall or when there is a series of cloudy days. If so, you may have seasonal affective disorder (more commonly known as SAD). If you think this may be an issue for you, spending more time outdoors, or near windows when you are indoors, can relieve this problem, which tends to be worse for people who live in the north and in places where it is cloudy much of the time. You can supplement your light with bright or full spectrum light indoors or by using a specially manufactured light box. You may want to plan ahead, knowing that the fall and winter are hard times for you and that you need to take very good care of yourself and get as much outdoor light as possible. If you increase the light in your life, you may notice changes in the way you feel right away, or after four or five days.

- Do you think you have SAD?
- If so, what are you going to do about it?

Sleep

You will feel better if you sleep well. Your body needs time every day to rest and heal. If you often have trouble sleeping—either falling asleep, or waking during the night and being unable to get back to sleep—one or several of the following ideas might be helpful to you:

- Go to bed at the same time every night and get up at the same time every morning. Avoid sleeping in (sleeping much later than your usual time for getting up). It will make you feel worse.

- Establish a bedtime ritual by doing the same things every night for an hour or two before bedtime so your body knows when it is time to go to sleep.

- Avoid caffeine, nicotine, and alcohol.

- Eat on a regular schedule and avoid a heavy meal prior to going to bed. Don't skip any meals.

- Eat plenty of dairy foods and dark green leafy vegetables.

- Exercise daily, but avoid strenuous or invigorating activity before going to bed.

- Play soothing music on a tape or CD that shuts off automatically after you are in bed.

- Try a turkey sandwich and a glass of milk before bedtime to make you feel drowsy.

- Try having a small snack before you go to bed, something like a piece of fruit and a piece of cheese or some cottage cheese so you don't wake up hungry in the middle of the night. Have a similar small snack if you awaken in the middle of the night.

- Take a warm bath or shower before going to bed.

- Place a drop of lavender oil on your pillow.

- Drink a cup of herbal chamomile tea or take several chamomile capsules before going to bed.

You need to see your doctor if:

- you often have difficulty sleeping and the solutions listed in the preceding text are not working for you;

- you awaken during the night gasping for breath;

- your partner reports that your breathing is interrupted when you are sleeping;

- you snore loudly;

- you wake up feeling like you haven't been asleep;

- you fall asleep often during the day.

Simple Things You Can Do to Improve the Quality of Your Life

You can do many simple things to improve the quality of your life—things that are free or that would not cost very much—things that would make you feel better. Check off which of the following ideas appeals to you. Then note how you could make it happen.

- Increase your exposure to colors you enjoy (for example, change the colors in your home, wear clothes of color you enjoy). If you feel it would be helpful to increase your exposure to colors you enjoy, how could you make this happen?

- Arrange to have more music in your life (for example, go to concerts, listen to the radio, CDs, or tapes, learn to play an instrument). How could you make this happen?

- Increase your exposure to art (for example, go to museums and art galleries, hang posters and paintings in your home, take an art course). How could you make this happen?

- Increase your exposure to the water (for example, live near water, swim, spend time near water, use a hot tub). How could you make this happen?

As you read through this text and answered the questions, you may have felt overwhelmed with all the things you need to do to help yourself feel better and improve the quality of your life. Review the booklet and draw a circle around one or two things you want to work on right away. Then, begin working on them. When you feel you have made some good progress on those issues, review the booklet again and choose something else to work on. Keep doing this until you have made your life the way you want it to be. Do it at your own pace. Take small steps—gradually they create big change.

Chapter 52

Building Resilience

Chapter Contents

Section 52.1

The Road to Resilience

How do people deal with difficult events that change their lives?
The death of a loved one, loss of a job, serious illness, terrorist attacks
and other traumatic events: These are all examples of very challenging
life experiences. Many people react to such circumstances with a flood
of strong emotions and a sense of uncertainty.

Yet people generally adapt well over time to life-changing situations
and stressful conditions. What enables them to do so? It involves resilience, an ongoing process that requires time and effort and engages
people in taking a number of steps.

This text is intended to help readers with taking their own road
to resilience. The information within describes resilience and some
factors that affect how people deal with hardship. Much of the text
focuses on developing and using a personal strategy for enhancing
resilience.

What Is Resilience?

Resilience is the process of adapting well in the face of adversity,
trauma, tragedy, threats, or even significant sources of stress—such as
family and relationship problems, serious health problems, or workplace and financial stressors. It means bouncing back from difficult
experiences.

Research has shown that resilience is ordinary, not extraordinary.
People commonly demonstrate resilience. One example is the response
of many Americans to the September 11, 2001 terrorist attacks and
individuals' efforts to rebuild their lives.

Being resilient does not mean that a person doesn't experience difficulty or distress. Emotional pain and sadness are common in people who have suffered major adversity or trauma in their lives. In fact, the road to resilience is likely to involve considerable emotional distress.

Resilience is not a trait that people either have or do not have. It involves behaviors, thoughts, and actions that can be learned and developed in anyone.

Resilience Factors and Strategies

Factors in Resilience

A combination of factors contributes to resilience. Many studies show that the primary factor in resilience is having caring and supportive relationships within and outside the family. Relationships that create love and trust, provide role models, and offer encouragement and reassurance help bolster a person's resilience.

Several additional factors are associated with resilience, including:

- the capacity to make realistic plans and take steps to carry them out;

- a positive view of yourself and confidence in your strengths and abilities;

- skills in communication and problem solving;

- the capacity to manage strong feelings and impulses;

- all of these are factors that people can develop in themselves.

Strategies for Building Resilience

Developing resilience is a personal journey. People do not all react the same to traumatic and stressful life events. An approach to building resilience that works for one person might not work for another. People use varying strategies.

Some variation may reflect cultural differences. A person's culture might have an impact on how he or she communicates feelings and deals with adversity—for example, whether and how a person connects with significant others, including extended family members and community resources. With growing cultural diversity, the public has greater access to a number of different approaches to building resilience.

Some or many of the ways to build resilience in the following text may be appropriate to consider in developing your personal strategy.

Ten Ways to Build Resilience

- **Make connections.** Good relationships with close family members, friends, or others are important. Accepting help and support from those who care about you and will listen to you strengthens resilience. Some people find that being active in civic groups, faith-based organizations, or other local groups provides social support and can help with reclaiming hope. Assisting others in their time of need also can benefit the helper.

- **Avoid seeing crises as insurmountable problems.** You can't change the fact that highly stressful events happen, but you can change how you interpret and respond to these events. Try looking beyond the present to how future circumstances may be a little better. Note any subtle ways in which you might already feel somewhat better as you deal with difficult situations.

- **Accept that change is a part of living.** Certain goals may no longer be attainable as a result of adverse situations. Accepting circumstances that cannot be changed can help you focus on circumstances that you can alter.

- **Move toward your goals.** Develop some realistic goals. Do something regularly—even if it seems like a small accomplishment—that enables you to move toward your goals. Instead of focusing on tasks that seem unachievable, ask yourself, "What's one thing I know I can accomplish today that helps me move in the direction I want to go?"

- **Take decisive actions.** Act on adverse situations as much as you can. Take decisive actions, rather than detaching completely from problems and stresses and wishing they would just go away.

- **Look for opportunities for self-discovery.** People often learn something about themselves and may find that they have grown in some respect as a result of their struggle with loss. Many people who have experienced tragedies and hardship have reported better relationships, greater sense of strength even while feeling vulnerable, increased sense of self-worth, a more developed spirituality, and heightened appreciation for life.

- **Nurture a positive view of yourself.** Developing confidence in your ability to solve problems and trusting your instincts helps build resilience.

- **Keep things in perspective.** Even when facing very painful events, try to consider the stressful situation in a broader context and keep a long-term perspective. Avoid blowing the event out of proportion.

- **Maintain a hopeful outlook.** An optimistic outlook enables you to expect that good things will happen in your life. Try visualizing what you want, rather than worrying about what you fear.

- **Take care of yourself.** Pay attention to your own needs and feelings. Engage in activities that you enjoy and find relaxing. Exercise regularly. Taking care of yourself helps to keep your mind and body primed to deal with situations that require resilience.

Additional ways of strengthening resilience may be helpful. For example, some people write about their deepest thoughts and feelings related to trauma or other stressful events in their life. Meditation and spiritual practices help some people build connections and restore hope. The key is to identify ways that are likely to work well for you as part of your own personal strategy for fostering resilience.

Learning from Your Past

Some Questions to Ask Yourself

Focusing on past experiences and sources of personal strength can help you learn about what strategies for building resilience might work for you. By exploring answers to the following questions about yourself and your reactions to challenging life events, you may discover how you can respond effectively to difficult situations in your life.

Consider the following:

- What kinds of events have been most stressful for me?

- How have those events typically affected me?

- Have I found it helpful to think of important people in my life when I am distressed?

- To whom have I reached out for support in working through a traumatic or stressful experience?

- What have I learned about myself and my interactions with others during difficult times?

- Has it been helpful for me to assist someone else going through a similar experience?

- Have I been able to overcome obstacles, and if so, how?

- What has helped make me feel more hopeful about the future?

Staying Flexible

Resilience involves maintaining flexibility and balance in your life as you deal with stressful circumstances and traumatic events. This happens in several ways, including:

- letting yourself experience strong emotions, and also realizing when you may need to avoid experiencing them at times in order to continue functioning;

- stepping forward and taking action to deal with your problems and meet the demands of daily living, and also stepping back to rest and reenergize yourself;

- spending time with loved ones to gain support and encouragement, and also nurturing yourself;

- relying on others, and also relying on yourself.

Places to Look for Help

Getting help when you need it is crucial in building your resilience. Beyond caring family members and friends, people often find it helpful to turn to:

- **Self-help and support groups:** Such community groups can aid people struggling with hardships such as the death of a loved one. By sharing information, ideas, and emotions, group participants can assist one another and find comfort in knowing that they are not alone in experiencing difficulty.

- **Books and other publications by people who have successfully managed adverse situations such as surviving cancer:** These stories can motivate readers to find a strategy that might work for them personally.

- **Online resources:** Information on the web can be a helpful source of ideas, though the quality of information varies among sources.

For many people, using their own resources and the kinds of help listed in the preceding text may be sufficient for building resilience. At times, however, an individual might get stuck or have difficulty making progress on the road to resilience.

A licensed mental health professional such as a psychologist can assist people in developing an appropriate strategy for moving forward. It is important to get professional help if you feel like you are unable to function or perform basic activities of daily living as a result of a traumatic or other stressful life experience.

Different people tend to be comfortable with somewhat different styles of interaction. A person should feel at ease and have good rapport in working with a mental health professional or participating in a support group.

Continuing on Your Journey

To help summarize several of the main points in this text, think of resilience as similar to taking a raft trip down a river. On a river, you may encounter rapids, turns, slow water, and shallows. As in life, the changes you experience affect you differently along the way.

In traveling the river, it helps to have knowledge about it and past experience in dealing with it. Your journey should be guided by a plan, a strategy that you consider likely to work well for you.

Perseverance and trust in your ability to work your way around boulders and other obstacles are important. You can gain courage and insight by successfully navigating your way through white water. Trusted companions who accompany you on the journey can be especially helpful for dealing with rapids, upstream currents, and other difficult stretches of the river.

You can climb out to rest alongside the river. But to get to the end of your journey, you need to get back in the raft and continue.

Section 52.2

Building Resilience in Children and Youth Dealing with Trauma

From "Building Resilience in Children and Youth Dealing with Trauma," by the Substance Abuse and Mental Health Services Administration (SAMHSA, www.samhsa.gov), April 2011.

Even from as young as 18 months, children can be affected by traumatic events and have serious problems later in childhood and adulthood. But the great news is that, with help from families, providers, and the community, children and youth can demonstrate resilience when dealing with trauma.

Traumatic experiences can range from a one-time incident, such as a sudden death of a loved one or a natural disaster, to ongoing exposure to experiences, such as bullying or family violence. Identifying that a child has experienced trauma is not always easy because emotional and behavioral responses to trauma vary depending on a child's age, personality, the type and severity of the incident, and availability of adult support.

Studies on stress response in children show that there can be physiological and structural changes in the brain and neurological systems and can, without intervention, result in enduring problems such as depression, anxiety, aggression, impulsiveness, delinquency, hyperactivity, and substance abuse.

- More than 60% of youth age 17 and younger have been exposed to crime, violence, and abuse either directly or indirectly.

- Young children exposed to five or more significant adversities in the first 3 years of childhood face a 76 percent likelihood of having one or more delays in their cognitive, language, or emotional development.

- As the number of traumatic events experienced during childhood increases, the risk for the following health problems in adulthood increases: Depression; alcoholism; drug abuse; suicide attempts; heart and liver diseases; pregnancy problems; high stress; uncontrollable anger; and family, financial, and job problems.

There is a range of behaviors that could be signs that a child is having difficulty dealing with a traumatic event, such as, but not limited to the following:

- Separation anxiety or clinginess towards teachers or caregivers
- Changes in appetite
- Decreased interest in and/or withdrawal from friends or family and normal activities
- Over- or under-reaction to physical contact, sudden movements, and sounds
- Angry outbursts and/or aggression
- More frequent complaints of headaches, stomachaches, or fatigue
- Repeatedly recreating the event through comments, drawings, or activity
- Emotional numbing, or expressing no feelings at all about the event
- Drop in school performance

What can teachers, caregivers, and other adults do to help a child who has experienced trauma? The U.S. Substance Abuse and Mental Health Services Administration (SAMHSA) offers these suggestions:

- Maintain usual routines.
- Make sure that the child is not being isolated.
- Provide a safe place where the child can talk about the incident.
- Be sensitive to potential environmental cues that may cause a reaction (e.g., an approaching storm or the anniversary of an event).
- Prepare the child in advance of a change in routine or other event that could be unsettling.
- Monitor what information the child shares with other children to prevent excessive curiosity from peers.
- Nurture the child's positive self-view.
- Draw on cultural and familiar assets.

With the support of caring adults, children can recover from traumatic events, reestablish a sense of well-being, and obtain treatment and other services if needed. The more you know about trauma and children, the more you can do to help them.

Chapter 53

Building Self-Esteem and Self-Image

Most people feel bad about themselves from time to time. Feelings of low self-esteem may be triggered by being treated poorly by someone else recently or in the past, or by a person's own judgments of him or herself. This is normal. However, low self-esteem is a constant companion for too many people, especially those who experience depression, anxiety, phobias, psychosis, delusional thinking, or who have an illness or a disability. If you are one of these people, you may go through life feeling bad about yourself needlessly. Low self-esteem keeps you from enjoying life, doing the things you want to do, and working toward personal goals.

You have a right to feel good about yourself. However, it can be very difficult to feel good about yourself when you are under the stress of having symptoms that are hard to manage, when you are dealing with a disability, when you are having a difficult time, or when others are treating you badly. At these times, it is easy to be drawn into a downward spiral of lower and lower self-esteem. For instance, you may begin feeling bad about yourself when someone insults you, you are under a lot of pressure at work, or you are having a difficult time getting along with someone in your family. Then you begin to give yourself negative self-talk, like "I'm no good." That may make you feel so bad about yourself that you do something to hurt yourself or someone else, such as getting drunk or yelling at your children. By using

Excerpted from "Building Self-Esteem: A Self-Help Guide," by the Substance Abuse and Mental Health Services Administration (SAMHSA, www.samhsa.gov), part of the U.S. Department of Health and Human Services, 2002. Reviewed by David A. Cooke, MD, FACP, November 23, 2011.

the ideas and activities in this text, you can avoid doing things that make you feel even worse and do those things that will make you feel better about yourself.

This text will give you ideas on things you can do to feel better about yourself—to raise your self-esteem. The ideas have come from people like yourself, people who realize they have low self-esteem and are working to improve it.

As you begin to use the methods in this text and other methods that you may think of to improve your self-esteem, you may notice that you have some feelings of resistance to positive feelings about yourself. This is normal. Don't let these feelings stop you from feeling good about yourself. They will diminish as you feel better and better about yourself. To help relieve these feelings, let your friends know what you are going through. Have a good cry if you can. Do things to relax, such as meditating or taking a nice warm bath.

As you read this text and work on the exercises, keep the following statement in mind—"I am a very special, unique, and valuable person. I deserve to feel good about myself."

Self-Esteem, Depression, and Other Illnesses

Before you begin to consider strategies and activities to help raise your self-esteem, it is important to remember that low self-esteem may be due to depression. Low self-esteem is a symptom of depression. To make things even more complicated, the depression may be a symptom of some other illness.

Have you felt sad consistently for several weeks but don't know why you are feeling so sad, i.e., nothing terribly bad has happened, or maybe something bad has happened but you haven't been able to get rid of the feelings of sadness? Is this accompanied by other changes, like wanting to eat all the time or having no appetite, wanting to sleep all the time or waking up very early and not being able to get back to sleep?

If you answered yes to either question, there are two things you need to do:

- See your doctor for a physical examination to determine the cause of your depression and to discuss treatment choices.

- Do some things that will help you to feel better right away like eating well, getting plenty of exercise and outdoor light, spending time with good friends, and doing fun things like going to a movie, painting a picture, playing a musical instrument, or reading a good book.

Things You Can Do Right Away—Every Day—to Raise Your Self-Esteem

Pay attention to your own needs and wants. Listen to what your body, your mind, and your heart are telling you. For instance, if your body is telling you that you have been sitting down too long, stand up and stretch. If your heart is longing to spend more time with a special friend, do it. If your mind is telling you to clean up your basement, listen to your favorite music, or stop thinking bad thoughts about yourself, take those thoughts seriously.

Take very good care of yourself. As you were growing up you may not have learned how to take good care of yourself. In fact, much of your attention may have been on taking care of others, on just getting by, or on behaving well. Begin today to take good care of yourself. Treat yourself as a wonderful parent would treat a small child or as one very best friend might treat another. If you work at taking good care of yourself, you will find that you feel better about yourself. Here are some ways to take good care of yourself:

- Eat healthy foods and avoid junk foods (foods containing a lot of sugar, salt, or fat).

- Exercise. Moving your body helps you to feel better and improves your self-esteem. Arrange a time every day or as often as possible when you can get some exercise, preferably outdoors. You can do many different things. Taking a walk is the most common. You could run, ride a bicycle, play a sport, climb up and down stairs several times, put on a tape, or play the radio and dance to the music—anything that feels good to you. If you have a health problem that may restrict your ability to exercise, check with your doctor before beginning or changing your exercise habits.

- Do personal hygiene tasks that make you feel better about yourself—things like taking a regular shower or bath, washing and styling your hair, trimming your nails, and brushing and flossing your teeth.

- Have a physical examination every year to make sure you are in good health.

- Plan fun activities for yourself. Learn new things every day.

- Take time to do things you enjoy. You may be so busy, or feel so badly about yourself, that you spend little or no time doing things you enjoy—things like playing a musical instrument, doing a craft project, flying a kite, or going fishing. Make a list of things you

529

enjoy doing. Then do something from that list every day. Add to the list anything new that you discover you enjoy doing.

- Get something done that you have been putting off. Clean out that drawer. Wash that window. Write that letter. Pay that bill.

- Do things that make use of your own special talents and abilities. For instance, if you are good with your hands, then make things for yourself, family, and friends. If you like animals, consider having a pet or at least playing with friends' pets.

- Dress in clothes that make you feel good about yourself. If you have little money to spend on new clothes, check out thrift stores in your area.

- Give yourself rewards—you are a great person. Listen to a CD or tape.

- Spend time with people who make you feel good about yourself—people who treat you well. Avoid people who treat you badly.

- Make your living space a place that honors the person you are. Whether you live in a single room, a small apartment, or a large home, make that space comfortable and attractive for you. If you share your living space with others, have some space that is just for you—a place where you can keep your things and know that they will not be disturbed and that you can decorate any way you choose.

- Display items that you find attractive or that remind you of your achievements or of special times or people in your life. If cost is a factor, use your creativity to think of inexpensive or free ways that you can add to the comfort and enjoyment of your space.

- Make your meals a special time. Turn off the television, radio, and stereo. Set the table, even if you are eating alone. Light a candle or put some flowers or an attractive object in the center of the table. Arrange your food in an attractive way on your plate. If you eat with others, encourage discussion of pleasant topics. Avoid discussing difficult issues at meals.

- Take advantage of opportunities to learn something new or improve your skills. Take a class or go to a seminar. Many adult education programs are free or very inexpensive. For those that are more costly, ask about a possible scholarship or fee reduction.

- Begin doing those things that you know will make you feel better about yourself—like going on a diet, beginning an exercise program, or keeping your living space clean.

- Do something nice for another person. Smile at someone who looks sad. Say a few kind words to the check-out cashier. Help your spouse with an unpleasant chore. Take a meal to a friend who is sick. Send a card to an acquaintance. Volunteer for a worthy organization.

- Make it a point to treat yourself well every day. Before you go to bed each night, write about how you treated yourself well during the day.

You may be doing some of these things now. There will be others you need to work on. You will find that you will continue to learn new and better ways to take care of yourself. As you incorporate these changes into your life, your self-esteem will continue to improve.

Changing Negative Thoughts about Yourself to Positive Ones

You may be giving yourself negative messages about yourself. Many people do. These are messages that you learned when you were young. You learned from many different sources including other children, your teachers, family members, caregivers, even from the media, and from prejudice and stigma in our society.

Once you have learned them, you may have repeated these negative messages over and over to yourself, especially when you were not feeling well or when you were having a hard time. You may have come to believe them. You may have even worsened the problem by making up some negative messages or thoughts of your own. These negative thoughts or messages make you feel bad about yourself and lower your self-esteem.

Some examples of common negative messages that people repeat over and over to themselves include: "I am a jerk," "I am a loser," "I never do anything right," "No one would ever like me," I am a klutz." Most people believe these messages, no matter how untrue or unreal they are. They come up immediately in the right circumstance, for instance if you get a wrong answer you think "I am so stupid." They may include words like should, ought, or must. The messages tend to imagine the worst in everything, especially you, and they are hard to turn off or unlearn.

You may think these thoughts or give yourself these negative messages so often that you are hardly aware of them. Pay attention to them. Carry a small pad with you as you go about your daily routine for several days and jot down negative thoughts about yourself whenever you notice them. Some people say they notice more negative thinking when they are tired, sick, or dealing with a lot of stress. As you become aware of your negative thoughts, you may notice more and more of them.

It helps to take a closer look at your negative thought patterns to check out whether or not they are true. You may want a close friend or counselor to help you with this. When you are in a good mood and when you have a positive attitude about yourself, ask yourself the following questions about each negative thought you have noticed:

- Is this message really true?

- Would a person say this to another person? If not, why am I saying it to myself?

- What do I get out of thinking this thought? If it makes me feel badly about myself, why not stop thinking it?

You could also ask someone else—someone who likes you and who you trust—if you should believe this thought about yourself. Often, just looking at a thought or situation in a new light helps.

The next step in this process is to develop positive statements you can say to yourself to replace these negative thoughts whenever you notice yourself thinking them. You can't think two thoughts at the same time. When you are thinking a positive thought about yourself, you can't be thinking a negative one. In developing these thoughts, use positive words like happy, peaceful, loving, enthusiastic, warm.

Avoid using negative words such as worried, frightened, upset, tired, bored, not, never, can't. Don't make a statement like "I am not going to worry anymore." Instead say "I focus on the positive" or whatever feels right to you. Substitute "it would be nice if" for "should." Always use the present tense, e.g., "I am healthy, I am well, I am happy, I have a good job," as if the condition already exists. Use I, me, or your own name.

You can do this by folding a piece of paper in half the long way to make two columns. In one column write your negative thought and in the other column write a positive thought that contradicts the negative thought as shown on the next page.

You can work on changing your negative thoughts to positive ones by doing the following:

- Replacing the negative thought with the positive one every time you realize you are thinking the negative thought.

- Repeating your positive thought over and over to yourself, out loud whenever you get a chance, and even sharing them with another person if possible.

- Writing them over and over.

- Making signs that say the positive thought, hanging them in places where you would see them often—like on your refrigerator door or on the mirror in your bathroom-and repeating the thought to yourself several times when you see it.

It helps to reinforce the positive thought if you repeat it over and over to yourself when you are deeply relaxed, like when you are doing a deep-breathing or relaxation exercise, or when you are just falling asleep or waking up.

Changing the negative thoughts you have about yourself to positive ones takes time and persistence. If you use the following techniques consistently for 4 to 6 weeks, you will notice that you don't think these negative thoughts about yourself as much. If they recur at some other time, you can repeat these activities. Don't give up. You deserve to think good thoughts about yourself.

Activities That Will Help You Feel Good about Yourself

Any of the following activities will help you feel better about yourself and reinforce your self-esteem over the long term. Read through them. Do those that seem most comfortable to you. You may want to do some of the other activities at another time. You may find it helpful to repeat some of these activities again and again.

Make Affirming Lists

Making lists, rereading them often, and rewriting them from time to time will help you to feel better about yourself. If you have a journal, you can write your lists there. If you don't, any piece of paper will do. Make a list of the following:

- At least five of your strengths, for example, persistence, courage, friendliness, creativity

- At least five things you admire about yourself, for example the way you have raised your children, your good relationship with your brother, or your spirituality

- The five greatest achievements in your life so far, like recovering from a serious illness, graduating from high school, or learning to use a computer

- At least 20 accomplishments—they can be as simple as learning to tie your shoes, to getting an advanced college degree

- Ten ways you can treat or reward yourself that don't include food and that don't cost anything, such as walking in woods, window shopping, watching children playing on a playground, gazing at a baby's face or at a beautiful flower, or chatting with a friend
- Ten things you can do to make yourself laugh
- Ten things you could do to help someone else
- Ten things that you do that make you feel good about yourself

Reinforcing a Positive Self-Image

To do this exercise you will need a piece of paper, a pencil or pen, and a timer or clock. Any kind of paper will do, but if you have paper and pen you really like, that will be even better.

Set a timer for 10 minutes or note the time on your watch or a clock. Write your name across the top of the paper. Then write everything positive and good you can think of about yourself. Include special attributes, talents, and achievements. You can use single words or sentences, whichever you prefer. You can write the same things over and over if you want to emphasize them.

Don't worry about spelling or grammar. Your ideas don't have to be organized. Write down whatever comes to mind. You are the only one who will see this paper. Avoid making any negative statements or using any negative words—only positive ones. When the 10 minutes are up, read the paper over to yourself. You may feel sad when you read it over because it is a new, different, and positive way of thinking about yourself—a way that contradicts some of the negative thoughts you may have had about yourself. Those feelings will diminish as your reread this paper. Read the paper over again several times. Put it in a convenient place—your pocket, purse, wallet, or the table beside your bed. Read it over to yourself at least several times a day to keep reminding yourself of how great you are. Find a private space and read it aloud. If you can, read it to a good friend or family member who is supportive.

Developing Positive Affirmations

Affirmations are positive statements that you can make about yourself that make you feel better about yourself. They describe ways you would like to feel about yourself all the time. They may not, however, describe how you feel about yourself right now. The following examples of affirmations will help you in making your own list of affirmations:

- I feel good about myself.

- I take good care of myself. I eat right, get plenty of exercise, do things I enjoy, get good health care, and attend to my personal hygiene needs.

- I spend my time with people who are nice to me and make me feel good about myself.

- I am a good person.

- I deserve to be alive.

- Many people like me.

Make a list of your own affirmations: Keep this list in a handy place, like your pocket or purse. You may want to make copies of your list so you can have them in several different places of easy access. Read the affirmations over and over to yourself—aloud whenever you can. Share them with others when you feel like it. Write them down from time to time. As you do this, the affirmations tend to gradually become true for you.

Make a personal celebratory scrapbook and place to honor yourself: Develop a scrapbook that celebrates you and the wonderful person you are. Include pictures of yourself at different ages, writings you enjoy, mementos of things you have done and places you have been, cards you have received, etc. Or set up a place in your home that celebrates you. It could be on a bureau, shelf, or table. Decorate the space with objects that remind you of the special person you are. If you don't have a private space that you can leave set up, put the objects in a special bag, box, or your purse and set them up in the space whenever you do this work. Take them out and look at them whenever you need to bolster your self-esteem.

Try this appreciation exercise: At the top of a sheet of paper write "I like _____ (your name) because: . . . ." Have friends, acquaintances, family members, etc., write an appreciative statement about you on it. When you read it, don't deny it or don't argue with what has been written, just accept it. Read this paper over and over. Keep it in a place where you will see it often.

Make a self-esteem calendar: Get a calendar with large blank spaces for each day. Schedule into each day some small thing you would enjoy doing, such as "go into a flower shop and smell the flowers," "call my sister," "draw a sketch of my cat," "buy a new CD," "tell my daughter

I love her," "bake brownies," "lie in the sun for 20 minutes," "wear my favorite scent," etc. Now make a commitment to check your "enjoy life" calendar every day and do whatever you have scheduled for yourself.

Try this mutual complimenting exercise: Get together for 10 minutes with a person you like and trust. Set a timer for 5 minutes or note the time on a watch or clock. One of you begins by complimenting the other person—saying everything positive about the other person— for the first five minutes. Then the other person does the same thing to that person for the next five minutes. Notice how you feel about yourself before and after this exercise. Repeat it often.

Use self-esteem resources: Go to your library. Look up books on self-esteem. Read one or several of them. Try some of the suggested activities.

In Conclusion

This text is just the beginning of the journey. As you work on building your self-esteem you will notice that you feel better more and more often, that you are enjoying your life more than you did before, and that you are doing more of the things you have always wanted to do.

Chapter 54

Dealing with Workplace Depression

In his classic, *The Prophet,* Kahlil Gibran writes: "Always you have been told that work is a curse. But I say to you that when you work you fulfill a part of earth's furthest dream, assigned to you when that dream was born."

Unfortunately Kahlil's words don't jibe with a new Australian study that found almost one in six cases of depression among working people caused by job stress, that nearly one in five (17 percent) working women suffering depression attribute their condition to job stress and more than one in eight (13 percent) working men. In the last decade, the number of American workers that say job stress is a major problem in their lives has doubled. In fact, the U.S. Department of Health reported that 70 percent of physical and mental complaints at work are related to stress.

What do we do? Bring our Kleenex to work and hope we don't get caught crying, or give our notice with no other job in reach? Thankfully, we have a few steps between these two extremes. Here are techniques that have helped me manage the work blues.

1. Don't quit yet.

Let me just say this first. Chances are higher that you will feel worse if you quit than if you keep on showing up to a job that you hate. Why? If you're not working, you will have even more time to think about how much you hated your job. On top of the acute anxiety you feel when you think about how you are going to pay off your next phone, electric, and mortgage bill without the regular paycheck being deposited automatically into your bank account. And then there's the isolation of having no one to talk to during the day, because—one small detail—everyone else is working. So just sit tight until you read through these before you gladly give your notice, okay?

2. Learn some calming techniques.

You know what's cool about most relaxation techniques? You can do them as you are listening to your boss give you your next assignment. Let's say, as he is telling you that he hired a nice woman half your age that you now report to, that you suddenly feel lots of tight pressure in your shoulders—naturally, because you have the desire to slug him. You relax your shoulders in a way that relieves some of that tension and tells your body that slugging him isn't an option (right now, anyway).

Then, as you walk back to your desk, where the kid right out of college hands you five assignments due by the end of the day, you can take 10 deep breaths: Counting to four as you inhale and to four million as you exhale. If you are allowed to listen to music or noise at work (or if you work from your home as I do), you might want to invest in a CD of ocean waves. Whenever I listen to mine, I take a few seconds to visualize myself on the sandy beach of Siesta Key, Florida, hunting for sea shells, a short moment to catch my sanity.

3. Turn the thing off.

I'm not talking about your sex drive, although if you're depressed, chances are that that's off, too. I mean your BlackBerry or iPhone, or at least the "ding" noise alerting you to every new (urgent) e-mail that you don't think drives you crazy but does. Trust me. When you turn it off for a day—even commit to a weekend without it—you will see that it is responsible for a sizable chunk of your madness.

It's ironic that very technological advances that were supposed to free us end up imprisoning us to our work, argues integrative doctor Roberta Lee in her astute book The *Superstress Solution*. In her introduction, she cites a recent survey commissioned by Support.com: Forty percent of 18- to 25-year-olds said they couldn't cope without their cell phone, yet the same students reported less stress and had lower heart rates and blood pressure when they stopped using them for three days. You need not join the monastery. Just try turning the thing off for a few evenings and see how you feel.

4. Make a schedule, and stick to it.

Yes, I'm a tad obsessive-compulsive, but I can feel the stress in me rise and want to explode if I don't have a handy dandy schedule in front of me that I can follow. No one gives it to me. I make it up, and therein lies its power—I am taking control back in to my own anxious hands! So, upon getting five assignments due the same week from a supervisor, I do the panic dance for 15 or 20 minutes. Then I take out my work calendar and start nailing down my deadlines. Assignment One needs to be done by lunchtime on Tuesday. Assignment Two needs to be done by Thursday morning, so that I have two full days to complete Assignment Three before the week is over. Get it? Things don't run that smoothly, of course, but by breaking down the goals or tasks into manageable bites, I stress less and produce more.

5. Improve your working conditions.

As a highly sensitive person, I can't work in certain atmospheres. I need a window—and proper lighting—and an assistant who will fetch me iced tea whenever I want, with lemon and not too much ice (kidding on that). But there are simple ways you can improve even the most sterile and miserable working conditions: Putting a nice plant in your cubicle, hanging or framing personal photos (a recent study say that looking at pictures of loved ones reduces pain), using a 10,000 lux daylight balanced light (a lamp used for seasonal affective disorder, but doesn't look any differently than an average desk light). Keeping a clean desk will also help you feel less overwhelmed. I'm not going to say anything further on that. If you've ever seen my desk you know why.

6. Get a life. Outside of work.

If I were to name the single most important lesson I learned inside the psych ward, it would be this: To get a life outside of work. You see, pre-psych ward, I invested all of my self-esteem into my profession. Thus, each career flop set me back a considerable chunk. If a book bombed, so too did my self-confidence. My goal leaving the inpatient psych program in 2006 was to get a life and to sustain that life.

I'm doing better today. I swim in a master's program. I joined a book group. I'm involved with a moms' group at the kids' school. None of these things are related to my job. I have met a whole other set of friends aside from my fellow bloggers, editors, and writers. This gives me some cushion and insurance for the days I get crappy traffic numbers and red royalty statements, as well as inviting me to join the human race on the days I can't produce a single thing.

7. *Get into the (right) zone.*

No doubt you're behind at work and feel like no matter how much you get done the day before, you always begin the next day at the foot of a mountain. You may very well have more work than is humanly possible for one person to accomplish. However, according to Elisha Goldstein, psychologist and author of the meditative CD "Mindful Solutions for Success and Stress Reduction at Work," identifying the four zones of your work day can help you do your job in less time, which will lower your stress.

This "Attention Zones Model" was developed by Rand Stagen of the Stagen's Leadership Academy, who maintains that during our day, we are in one of four zones: A reactive zone, a proactive zone, a distracted zone, or a waste zone. The goal is to stay out of the distracted and waste zones: Responding to unimportant calls and emails or killing time by surfing the web, etc. Explains Goldstein: "The cultivation of mindful awareness allows you to nonjudgmentally name what is happening right now, and turn your attention to your top priorities in the moment."

Chapter 55

Getting Through Tough Economic Times

Economic turmoil (e.g., increased unemployment, foreclosures, loss of investments, and other financial distress) can result in a whole host of negative health effects—both physical and mental. It can be particularly devastating to your emotional and mental well-being. Although each of us is affected differently by economic troubles, these problems can add tremendous stress, which in turn can substantially increase the risk for developing such problems as the following:

- Depression

- Anxiety

- Compulsive behaviors (overeating, excessive gambling, spending, etc.)

- Substance abuse

Warning Signs

It is important to be aware of signs that financial problems may be adversely affecting your emotional or mental well-being—or that of someone you care about. These signs include the following:

- Persistent sadness/crying

- Excessive anxiety

From "Getting Through Tough Economic Times," by the Substance Abuse and Mental Health Services (SAMHSA, www.samhsa.gov), March 31, 2009.

- Lack of sleep/constant fatigue
- Excessive irritability/anger
- Increased drinking
- Illicit drug use, including misuse of medications
- Difficulty paying attention or staying focused
- Apathy—not caring about things that are usually important to you
- Not being able to function as well at work, school, or home

Managing Stress

If you or someone you care about is experiencing these symptoms, you are not alone. These are common reactions to stress, and there are coping techniques that you can use to help manage it. They include the following:

- Trying to keep things in perspective, recognizing the good aspects of life, and retaining hope for the future
- Strengthening connections with family and friends who can provide important emotional support
- Engaging in activities such as physical exercise, sports, or hobbies that can relieve stress and anxiety
- Developing new employment skills that can provide a practical and highly effective means of coping and directly address financial difficulties

Getting Help

Even with these coping techniques, however, sometimes these problems can seem overwhelming and you may need additional help to get through rough patches. Fortunately, there are many people and services that can provide help. These include the following:

- Your healthcare provider
- Your spiritual leader
- Your school counselor
- Your community health clinic

If you need help finding treatment services you can access the Mental Health Services Locator at http://store.samhsa.gov/mhlocator for information and mental health resources near you. Similarly, if you need help with a substance abuse problem you can use our Substance Abuse Treatment Facility Locator at http://findtreatment.samhsa.gov.

There are many other places where you can turn for guidance and support in dealing with the financial problems affecting you or someone you care about. These resources exist at the federal, state and community level and can be found through many sources such as the following:

- Federal and state government
- Civic associations
- Spiritual groups
- Other sources such as the government services section of a phone book

Suicide Warning Signs

Unemployment and other kinds of financial distress do not cause suicide directly, but they can be factors that interact dynamically within individuals and affect their risk for suicide. These financial factors can cause strong feelings such as humiliation and despair, which can precipitate suicidal thoughts or actions among those who may already be vulnerable to having these feelings because of life experiences or underlying mental or emotional conditions (e.g., depression, bipolar disorder) that place them at greater risk of suicide.

These are some of the signs you may want to be aware of in trying to determine whether you or someone you care about could be at risk for suicide:

- Threatening to hurt or kill oneself or talking about wanting to hurt or kill oneself
- Looking for ways to kill oneself
- Thinking or fantasizing about suicide
- Acting recklessly
- Seeing no reason for living or having no sense of purpose in life

If you or someone you care about are having suicidal thoughts or showing these symptoms, seek immediate help. Contact your health-care provider, mental health crisis center, hospital emergency room, or the National Suicide Prevention Lifeline at 800-273-TALK (273-8255) for help.

Chapter 56

Dealing with the Effects of Trauma

This is a serious issue. This text is just an introduction—a starting point that may give you the courage to take action. It is not meant to be a treatment program. The ideas and strategies are not intended to replace treatment you are currently receiving.

You may have had one or many very upsetting, frightening, or traumatic things happen to you in your life, or that threatened or hurt something you love—even your community. When these kinds of things happen, you may not get over them quickly. In fact, you may feel the effects of these traumas for many years, even for the rest of your life. Sometimes you don't even notice effects right after the trauma happens. Years later you may begin having thoughts, nightmares, and other disturbing symptoms. You may develop these symptoms and not even remember the traumatic thing or things that once happened to you.

For many years, the traumatic things that happened to people were overlooked as a possible cause of frightening, distressing, and sometimes disabling emotional symptoms such as depression, anxiety, phobias, delusions, flashbacks, and being out of touch with reality. In recent years, many researchers and health care providers have become convinced of the connection between trauma and these symptoms. They are developing new treatment programs and revising old ones to better meet the needs of people who have had traumatic experiences.

Excerpted from "Dealing with the Effects of Trauma: A Self-Help Guide," by the Substance Abuse and Mental Health Services Administration (SAMHSA, www.samhsa.gov), part of the U.S. Department of Health and Human Services, November 2002. Reviewed by David A. Cooke, MD, FACP, November 23, 2011.

This text can help you to know if traumatic experiences in your life may be causing some or all of the difficult symptoms you are experiencing. It may give you some guidance in working to relieve these symptoms and share with you some simple and safe things you can do to help yourself heal from the effects of trauma.

Some examples of traumatic experiences that may be causing your symptoms include the following:

- Physical, emotional, or sexual abuse
- Neglect
- War experiences
- Outbursts of temper and rage
- Alcoholism (your own or in your family)
- Physical illnesses, surgeries, and disabilities
- Sickness in your family
- Loss of close family members and friends
- Natural disasters
- Accidents

Some things that may be very traumatic to one person hardly seem to bother another person. If something bothers you a lot and it doesn't bother someone else, it doesn't mean there is something wrong with you. People respond to experiences differently.

Do you feel that traumatic things that happened to you may be causing some or all of your distressing and disabling emotional symptoms? Examples of symptoms that may be caused by trauma include the following:

- Anxiety
- Insomnia
- Agitation
- Irritability or rage
- Flashbacks or intrusive memories
- Feeling disconnected from the world
- Unrest in certain situations
- Being shut down
- Being very passive

- Feeling depressed
- Eating problems
- Needing to do certain things over and over
- Unusual fears
- Impatience
- Always having to have things a certain way
- Doing strange or risky things
- Having a hard time concentrating
- Wanting to hurt yourself
- Being unable to trust anyone
- Feeling unlikable
- Feeling unsafe
- Using harmful substances
- Keeping to yourself
- Overworking

Perhaps you have been told that you have a psychiatric or mental illness like depression, bipolar disorder or manic depression, schizophrenia, borderline personality disorder, obsessive-compulsive disorder, dissociative disorder, an eating disorder, or an anxiety disorder. The ways you can help yourself handle these symptoms and the things your health care providers suggest as treatment may be helpful whether your symptoms are caused by trauma or by a psychiatric illness.

Help from Health Care Providers, Counselors, and Groups

You may decide to reach out to health care providers for assistance in relieving the effects of trauma. This is a good idea. The effects of trauma, even trauma that happened many years ago, can affect your health. You may have an illness that needs treatment. In addition, your health care provider may suggest that you take medications or certain food supplements to relieve your symptoms. Many people find that getting this kind of health care support gives them the relief and energy they need to work on other aspects of healing. To find health care providers in your community who have expertise in addressing issues related to trauma, contact your local mental health agency, hospital, or crisis service.

If you possibly can, work with a counselor or in a special program designed for people who have been traumatized. A counselor or people leading the program may refer you to a group. These groups can be very helpful. However, keep in mind that you need to decide for yourself what you are going to do, and how and when you are going to do it. You must be in charge of your recovery in every way.

Wherever you go for help, the program or treatment should include the following:

- **Empowerment:** You must be in charge of your healing in every way to counteract the effects of the trauma where all control was taken away from you.

- **Validation:** You need others to listen to you, to validate the importance of what happened to you, to bear witness, and to understand the role of this trauma in your life.

- **Connection:** Trauma makes you feel very alone. As part of your healing, you need to reconnect with others. This connection may be part of your treatment.

If you feel the cause of your symptoms is related to trauma in your life, you will want to be careful about your treatment and in making decisions about other areas of your life. The following guidelines will help you decide how to help yourself feel better.

Have hope. It is important that you know that you can and will feel better. In the past you may have thought you would never feel better—that the horrible symptoms you experience would go on for the rest of your life. Many people who have experienced the same symptoms that you are experiencing are now feeling much better. They have gone on to make their lives the way they want them to be and to do the things they want to do.

Take personal responsibility. When you have been traumatized, you lose control of your life. You may feel as though you still don't have any control over your life. You begin to take back that control by being in charge of every aspect of your life. Others, including your spouse, family members, friends, and health care professionals will try to tell you what to do. Before you do what they suggest, think about it carefully. Do you feel that it is the best thing for you to do right now? If not, do not do it. You can follow others' advice, but be aware that you are choosing to do so. It is important that you make decisions about your own life. You are responsible for your own behavior. Being traumatized is not an acceptable excuse for behavior that hurts you or hurts others.

Talk to one or more people about what happened to you. Telling others about the trauma is an important part of healing the effects of trauma. Make sure the person or people you decide to tell are safe people, people who would not hurt you, and who understand that what happened to you is serious. They should know, or you could tell them, that describing what happened to you over and over is an important part of the healing process. Don't tell a person who responds with statements that invalidate your experience, like "That wasn't so bad." "You should just forget about it," "Forgive and forget," or "You think that's bad, let me tell you what happened to me." They don't understand. In connecting with others, avoid spending all your time talking about your traumatic experiences. Spend time listening to others and sharing positive life experiences, like going to movies or watching a ball game together. You will know when you have described your trauma enough, because you won't feel like doing it anymore.

Develop a close relationship with another person. You may not feel close to or trust anyone. This may be a result of your traumatic experiences. Part of healing means trusting people again. Think about the person in your life that you like best. Invite them to do something fun with you. If that feels good, make a plan to do something else together at another time—maybe the following week. Keep doing this until you feel close to this person. Then, without giving up on that person, start developing a close relationship with another person. Keep doing this until you have close relationships with at least five people. Support groups and peer support centers are good places to meet people.

Things You Can Do Every Day to Help Yourself Feel Better

There are many things that happen every day that can cause you to feel ill, uncomfortable, upset, anxious, or irritated. You will want to do things to help yourself feel better as quickly as possible, without doing anything that has negative consequences, for example, drinking, committing crimes, hurting yourself, risking your life, or eating lots of junk food.

Read through the following list. Check off the ideas that appeal to you and give each of them a try when you need to help yourself feel better. Make a list of the ones you find to be most useful, along with those you have successfully used in the past, and hang the list in a prominent place—like on your refrigerator door-as a reminder at times when you need to comfort yourself. Use these techniques whenever you are having a hard time or as a special treat to yourself.

- Do something fun or creative, something you really enjoy, like crafts, needlework, painting, drawing, woodworking, making a sculpture, reading fiction, comics, mystery novels, or inspirational writings, doing crossword or jigsaw puzzles, playing a game, taking some photographs, going fishing, going to a movie or other community event, or gardening.

- Get some exercise. Exercise is a great way to help yourself feel better while improving your overall stamina and health. The right exercise can even be fun.

- Write something. Writing can help you feel better. You can keep lists, record dreams, respond to questions, and explore your feelings. All ways are correct. Don't worry about how well you write. It's not important. It is only for you. Writing about the trauma or traumatic events also helps a lot. It allows you to safely process the emotions you are experiencing. It tells your mind that you are taking care of the situation and helps to relieve the difficult symptoms you may be experiencing. Keep your writings in a safe place where others cannot read them. Share them only with people you feel comfortable with. You may even want to write a letter to the person or people who have treated you badly, telling them how it affected you, and not send the letter.

- Use your spiritual resources. Spiritual resources and making use of these resources varies from person to person. For some people it means praying, going to church, or reaching out to a member of the clergy. For others it is meditating or reading affirmations and other kinds of inspirational materials. It may include rituals and ceremonies—whatever feels right to you. Spiritual work does not necessarily occur within the bounds of an organized religion. Remember, you can be spiritual without being religious.

- Do something routine. When you don't feel well, it helps to do something "normal"—the kind of thing you do every day or often, things that are part of your routine like taking a shower, washing your hair, making yourself a sandwich, calling a friend or family member, making your bed, walking the dog, or getting gas in the car.

- Wear something that makes you feel good. Everybody has certain clothes or jewelry that they enjoy wearing. These are the things to wear when you need to comfort yourself.

- Get some little things done. It always helps you feel better if you accomplish something, even if it is a very small thing. Think of some easy things to do that don't take much time. Then do them. Here are some ideas: clean out one drawer, put five pictures in a photo album, dust a book case, read a page in a favorite book, do a load of laundry, cook yourself something healthful, send someone a card.

- Learn something new. Think about a topic that you are interested in but have never explored. Find some information on it in the library. Check it out on the Internet. Go to a class. Look at something in a new way. Read a favorite saying, poem, or piece of scripture, and see if you can find new meaning in it.

- Do a reality check. Checking in on what is really going on rather than responding to your initial "gut reaction" can be very helpful. For instance, if you come in the house and loud music is playing, it may trigger the thinking that someone is playing the music just to annoy you. The initial reaction is to get really angry with them. That would make both of you feel awful. A reality check gives the person playing the loud music a chance to look at what is really going on. Perhaps the person playing the music thought you wouldn't be in until later and took advantage of the opportunity to play loud music. If you would call upstairs and ask him to turn down the music so you could rest, he probably would say, "Sure!" It helps if you can stop yourself from jumping to conclusions before you check the facts.

- Be present in the moment. This is often referred to as mindfulness. Many of us spend so much time focusing on the future or thinking about the past that we miss out on fully experiencing what is going on in the present. Making a conscious effort to focus your attention on what you are doing right now and what is happening around you can help you feel better. Look around at nature. Feel the weather. Look at the sky when it is filled with stars.

- Stare at something pretty or something that has special meaning for you. Stop what you are doing and take a long, close look at a flower, a leaf, a plant, the sky, a work of art, a souvenir from an adventure, a picture of a loved one, or a picture of yourself. Notice how much better you feel after doing this.

- Play with children in your family or with a pet. Romping in the grass with a dog, petting a kitten, reading a story to a child, rocking a baby, and similar activities have a calming effect which translates into feeling better.

- Do a relaxation exercise. There are many good books available that describe relaxation exercises. Try them to discover which ones you prefer. Practice them daily. Use them whenever you need to help yourself feel better. Relaxation tapes which feature relaxing music or nature sounds are available. Just listening for 10 minutes can help you feel better.

- Take a warm bath. This may sound simplistic, but it helps. If you are lucky enough to have access to a Jacuzzi or hot tub, it's even better. Warm water is relaxing and healing.

- Expose yourself to something that smells good to you. Many people have discovered fragrances that help them feel good. Sometimes a bouquet of fragrant flowers or the smell of fresh baked bread will help you feel better.

- Listen to music. Pay attention to your sense of hearing by pampering yourself with delightful music you really enjoy. Libraries often have records and tapes available for loan. If you enjoy music, make it an essential part of every day.

- Make music. Making music is also a good way to help yourself feel better. Drums and other kinds of musical instruments are popular ways of relieving tension and increasing well-being. Perhaps you have an instrument that you enjoy playing, like a harmonica, kazoo, penny whistle, or guitar.

- Sing. Singing helps. It fills your lungs with fresh air and makes you feel better. Sing to yourself. Sing at the top of your lungs. Sing when you are driving your car. Sing when you are in the shower. Sing for the fun of it. Sing along with favorite records, tapes, compact discs, or the radio. Sing the favorite songs you remember from your childhood.

Perhaps you can think of some other things you could do that would help you feel better.

Chapter 57

Grief, Bereavement, and Coping with Loss

People cope with the loss of a loved one in different ways. Most people who experience grief will cope well. Others will have severe grief and may need treatment. There are many things that can affect the grief process of someone who has lost a loved one. They include the following:

- The personality of the person who is grieving

- The relationship with the person who died

- The loved one's cancer experience and the way the disease progressed

- The grieving person's coping skills and mental health history

- The amount of support the grieving person has

- The grieving person's cultural and religious background

- The grieving person's social and financial position

Bereavement and Grief

Bereavement is the period of sadness after losing a loved one through death.

PDQ® Cancer Information Summary. National Cancer Institute; Bethesda, MD. Grief, Bereavement, and Coping with Loss (PDQ®): Patient Version. Updated 08/2010. Available at http://www.cancer.gov. Accessed September 9, 2011.

Grief and mourning occur during the period of bereavement. Grief and mourning are closely related. Mourning is the way we show grief in public. The way people mourn is affected by beliefs, religious practices, and cultural customs. People who are grieving are sometimes described as bereaved.

Grief is the normal process of reacting to the loss.

Grief is the emotional response to the loss of a loved one. Common grief reactions include the following:

- Feeling emotionally numb

- Feeling unable to believe the loss occurred

- Feeling anxiety from the distress of being separated from the loved one

- Mourning along with depression

- A feeling of acceptance

Types of Grief Reactions

Anticipatory Grief

Anticipatory grief occurs when a death is expected, but before it happens. It may be felt by the families of people who are dying and by the person dying. Anticipatory grief helps family members get ready emotionally for the loss. It can be a time to take care of unfinished business with the dying person, such as saying "I love you" or "I forgive you."

Like grief that occurs after the death of a loved one, anticipatory grief involves mental, emotional, cultural, and social responses. However, anticipatory grief is different from grief that occurs after the death. Symptoms of anticipatory grief include the following:

- Depression

- Feeling a greater than usual concern for the dying person

- Imagining what the loved one's death will be like

- Getting ready emotionally for what will happen after the death

Anticipatory grief helps family members cope with what is to come. For the patient who is dying, anticipatory grief may be too much to handle and may cause him or her to withdraw from others.

Anticipatory grief does not always occur. Some researchers report that anticipatory grief is rare. Studies showed that periods of acceptance and recovery usually seen during grief are not common before the patient's actual death. The bereaved may feel that trying to accept the loss of a loved one before death occurs may make it seem that the dying patient has been abandoned.

Also, grief felt before the death will not decrease the grief felt afterward or make it last a shorter time.

Normal Grief

Normal or common grief begins soon after a loss and symptoms go away over time. During normal grief, the bereaved person moves toward accepting the loss and is able to continue normal day-to-day life even though it is hard to do. Common grief reactions include the following:

- **Emotional numbness, shock, disbelief, or denial:** These often occur right after the death, especially if the death was not expected.

- **Anxiety over being separated from the loved one:** The bereaved may wish to bring the person back and become lost in thoughts of the deceased. Images of death may occur often in the person's everyday thoughts.

- **Distress** that leads to crying; sighing; having dreams, illusions, and hallucinations of the deceased; and looking for places or things that were shared with the deceased

- **Anger**

- **Periods of sadness, loss of sleep, loss of appetite, extreme tiredness, guilt, and loss of interest in life:** Day-to-day living may be affected.

In normal grief, symptoms will occur less often and will feel less severe as time passes. Recovery does not happen in a set period of time. For most bereaved people having normal grief, symptoms lessen between six months and two years after the loss.

Many bereaved people will have grief bursts or pangs. Grief bursts or pangs are short periods (20–30 minutes) of very intense distress. Sometimes these bursts are caused by reminders of the deceased person. At other times they seem to happen for no reason.

Grief is sometimes described as a process that has stages. There are several theories about how the normal grief process works. Experts have described different types and numbers of stages that people go through as they cope with loss. At this time, there is not enough information to prove that one of these theories is more correct than the others.

Although many bereaved people have similar responses as they cope with their losses, there is no typical grief response. The grief process is personal.

Complicated Grief

There is no right or wrong way to grieve, but studies have shown that there are patterns of grief that are different from the most common. This has been called complicated grief.

Complicated grief reactions that have been seen in studies include the following:

- **Minimal grief reaction:** A grief pattern in which the person has no, or only a few, signs of distress or problems that occur with other types of grief.

- **Chronic grief:** A grief pattern in which the symptoms of common grief last for a much longer time than usual. These symptoms are a lot like ones that occur with major depression, anxiety, or posttraumatic stress.

Factors That Affect Complicated Grief

Researchers study grief reactions to try to find out what might increase the chance that complicated grief will occur.

Studies have looked at how the following factors affect the grief response:

- **Whether the death is expected or unexpected:** It may seem that any sudden, unexpected loss might lead to more difficult grief. However, studies have found that bereaved people with high self-esteem and/or a feeling that they have control over life are likely to have a normal grief reaction even after an unexpected loss. Bereaved people with low self-esteem and/or a sense that life cannot be controlled are more likely to have complicated grief after an unexpected loss. This includes more depression and physical problems.

- **The personality of the bereaved:** Studies have found that people with certain personality traits are more likely to have long-lasting depression after a loss. These include people who are very dependent on the loved one (such as a spouse), and people who deal with distress by thinking about it all the time.

- **The religious beliefs of the bereaved:** Some studies have shown that religion helps people cope better with grief. Other studies have shown it does not help or causes more distress. Religion seems to help people who go to church often. The positive effect on grief may be because church-goers have more social support.

- **Whether the bereaved is male or female:** In general, men have more problems than women do after a spouse's death. Men tend to have worse depression and more health problems than women do after the loss. Some researchers think this may be because men have less social support after a loss.

- **The age of the bereaved:** In general, younger bereaved people have more problems after a loss than older bereaved people do. They have more severe health problems, grief symptoms, and other mental and physical symptoms. Younger bereaved people, however, may recover more quickly than older bereaved people do, because they have more resources and social support.

- **The amount of social support the bereaved has:** Lack of social support increases the chance of having problems coping with a loss. Social support includes the person's family, friends, neighbors, and community members who can give psychological, physical, and financial help. After the death of a close family member, many people have a number of related losses. The death of a spouse, for example, may cause a loss of income and changes in lifestyle and day-to-day living. These are all related to social support.

Treatment of Grief

Normal grief may not need to be treated. Most bereaved people work through grief and recover within the first six months to two years. Researchers are studying whether bereaved people experiencing normal grief would be helped by formal treatment. They are also studying whether treatment might prevent complicated grief in people who are likely to have it.

For people who have serious grief reactions or symptoms of distress, treatment may be helpful. Complicated grief may be treated with different types of psychotherapy (talk therapy).

Researchers are studying the treatment of mental, emotional, social, and behavioral symptoms of grief. Treatment methods include discussion, listening, and counseling.

Complicated grief treatment (CGT) is a type of grief therapy that was helpful in a clinical trial. Complicated grief treatment (CGT) has three phases:

- The first phase includes talking about the loss and setting goals toward recovery. The bereaved are taught to work on these two things.

- The second phase includes coping with the loss by retelling the story of the death. This helps bereaved people who try not to think about their loss.

- The last phase looks at progress that has been made toward recovery and helps the bereaved make future plans. The bereaved's feelings about ending the sessions are also discussed.

In a clinical trial of patients with complicated grief, CGT was compared to interpersonal psychotherapy (IPT). IPT is a type of psychotherapy that focuses on the person's relationships with others and is helpful in treating depression. In patients with complicated grief, the CGT was more helpful than IPT.

Cognitive behavioral therapy (CBT) for complicated grief was helpful in a clinical trial. Cognitive behavioral therapy (CBT) works with the way a person's thoughts and behaviors are connected. CBT helps the patient learn skills that change attitudes and behaviors by replacing negative thoughts and changing the rewards of certain behaviors.

A clinical trial compared CBT to counseling for complicated grief. Results showed that patients treated with CBT had more improvement in symptoms and general mental distress than those in the counseling group.

Depression related to grief is sometimes treated with drugs. There is no standard drug therapy for depression that occurs with grief. Some health care professionals think depression is a normal part of grief and doesn't need to be treated. Whether to treat grief-related depression with drugs is up to the patient and the health care professional to decide.

Clinical trials of antidepressants for depression related to grief have found that the drugs can help relieve depression. However, they give less relief and take longer to work than they do when used for depression that is not related to grief.

Chapter 58

Coping with the Holidays and Family Celebrations

It's supposed to be the most wonderful time of the year—but not if negative emotions take hold of your holidays. So let's be honest. The holidays are packed with stress, and therefore provoke tons of depression and anxiety. But there is hope. Whether I'm fretting about something as trite as stocking stuffers or as complicated as managing difficult family relationships, I apply a few rules that I've learned over the years. These nine rules help me put the joy back into the festivities—or at least keep me from hurling a mistletoe at Santa and landing myself on the "naughty" list.

1. Expect the Worst

Now that's a cheery thought for this jolly season. What I'm trying to say is that you have to predict bad behavior before it happens so that you can catch it in your holiday mitt and toss it back, instead of having it knock you to the floor. It's simple math, really. If every year for the last decade, Uncle Ted has given you a bottle of Merlot, knowing full well that you are a recovering alcoholic and have been sober for more years than his kids have been out of diapers, you can safely assume he will do this again. So what do you do? Catch it in your "slightly-annoyed" mitt. (And maybe reciprocate by giving him a cheese basket for his high cholesterol.)

559

2. Remember to "SEE"

No, I don't mean for you to schedule an appointment with an ophthalmologist. SEE stands for sleeping regularly, eating well, and exercising. Without these three basics, you can forget about an enjoyable (or even tolerable) holiday. Get your 7 to 9 hours of sleep and practice good sleep hygiene: Go to bed at the same time every night, and wake up in the same nightgown with the same man at the same time in the same house every morning.

Eating well and exercise are codependent, at least in my body, because my biggest motivator for exercising is the reduction in guilt I feel about splurging on dessert. Large quantities of sugar or high fructose corn syrup can poison your brain. If you know your weak spot—the end of the table where Aunt Judy places her homemade hazelnut holiday balls—then swim, walk, or jog 10 extra minutes to compensate for your well-deserved treat. Another acronym to remember during the holidays is HALT: Don't get too hungry, angry, lonely, or tired.

3. Beef up Your Support

If you attend Al-Anon once a week, go twice a week during the holidays. If you attend a yoga class twice a week, try to fit in another. Schedule an extra therapy session as insurance against the potential meltdowns ahead of you. Pad yourself with extra layers of emotional resilience by discussing in advance specific concerns you have about X, Y, and Z with a counselor, minister, or friend (preferably one who doesn't gossip).

In my life with two young kids, this means getting extra babysitters so that if I have a meltdown in Starbucks like I did two years ago—before I knew the mall was menacing to my inner peace—I will have an extra 10 minutes to record in my journal what I learned from that experience.

4. Avoid Toxic People

This one's difficult if the toxic people happen to be hosting Christmas dinner. But in general, just try your best to avoid pernicious humans in December. And if you absolutely must see such folks, then allow only enough time for digestion and gift-giving. Drink no more than one glass of wine in order to preserve your ability to think rationally. You don't want to get confused and decide you really do love these people, only to hear them say something horribly offensive two minutes later, causing you to storm off all aggravated and hurt. (This would also be a good time to remember Rule #1.)

5. Know Thyself

In other words, identify your triggers. As a highly sensitive person (as described in Elaine Aron's book, *The Highly Sensitive Person*), I know that my triggers exist in a petri dish of bacteria known as the Westfield Annapolis Mall. Between Halloween and New Year's, I won't go near that place because Santa is there and he scares me with his long beard, which holds in its cute white curls every virus of every local preschool. Before you make too many plans this holiday season, list your triggers—people, places, and things that tend to trigger your fears and bring out your worst traits.

6. Travel with Polyester, Not Linen

By this, I do not mean sporting the polyester skirt with the red sequinned reindeer. I'm saying that you should lower your standards and make traveling as easy as possible, both literally and figuratively. Do you really want to be looking for an iron for that beautiful linen or cotton dress when you arrive at your destination? I didn't think so—life's too short for travel irons. I used to be adamantly opposed to using a portable DVD player in the car to entertain the kids because I thought it would create two spoiled monsters whose imaginations had rotted courtesy of Disney. One nine-hour car trip home to Ohio for Christmas, I cried uncle after six hours of constant squabbling and screaming coming from the back seat. Now David and Katherine only fight over which movie they get to watch first. If you have a no-food rule policy for the car, I'd amend that one during the holidays as well.

7. Make Your Own Traditions

Of course, you don't need the "polyester" rule if you ban holiday travel altogether. That's what I did this year. As the daughter/sister who abandoned her family in Ohio by moving out east, it has always been my responsibility to travel during the holidays. But my kids are now four and six. I can't continue to haul the family to the Midwest every year. We are our own family. So I said this to my mom a few weeks ago: "It's very important that I spend time with you, but I'd like to do it as a less stressful time, like the summer, when traveling is easier." She wasn't thrilled, but she understood.

Making your own tradition might mean Christmas Eve is reserved for your family and the extended family is invited over for brunch on Christmas Day. Or vice versa. Basically, it's laying down some rules so that you have better control over the situation. As a people-pleaser who hates to cook, I make a better guest than host, but sometimes serenity comes in taking the driver's seat, and telling the passengers to fasten their seatbelts and be quiet.

8. Get out of Yourself

According to Gandhi, the best way to find yourself is to lose yourself in service to others. But that doesn't necessarily mean holding a soup ladle. Since my name and the word "kitchen" have filed a restraining order on each other, I like to think there are a variety of ways you can serve others. Matthew 6:21 says "for where your treasure is, there your heart will be also." In other words, start with the things you like to do. For me, that is saying a rosary for a depressed Beyond Blue reader, or visiting a priest-friend who needs encouragement and support in order to continue his ministry, or helping talented writer friends get published. I'd like to think this is service, too, because if those people are empowered by my actions, then I've contributed to a better world just as much as if I had dished out mashed potatoes to a homeless person at a shelter.

9. Exercise Your Funny Bone

"Time spent laughing is time spent with the gods," says a Japanese proverb. So, if you're with someone who thinks he's God, the natural response would be to laugh! But seriously folks, research shows that laughing is good for your health. And, unlike exercise, it's always enjoyable. The funniest people in my life are those who have been to hell and back, bought the t-shirt, and then accidentally shrunk it in the wash. Humor kept them alive—physically, emotionally, and spiritually. Remember, with a funny bone in place—even if it's in a cast—everything is tolerable.

Chapter 59

Mental Health Support Groups

There has been an increasing awareness of the role that mental health support and self-help groups play in recovery from mental illnesses. Mental health support and self-help groups, historically considered as an alternative to traditional mental health treatment, are now recognized as partners in the continuum of mental health care. The National Survey on Drug Use and Health (NSDUH) gathers information that can help provide a better understanding of the extent to which these groups are used, the characteristics of the people who use them, and the relationship between the more traditional modes of mental health treatment and mental health support or self-help groups.

This text examines the characteristics of adults (i.e., persons aged 18 or older) who received treatment, counseling, or support for emotions, nerves, or mental health in the past year from an in-person support or a self-help group (support and self-help groups hereafter are referred to collectively as self-help groups). All findings presented in this report are annual averages based on combined 2005 to 2008 NSDUH data.

Mental Health Self-Help Groups

An annual average of 2.4 million adults aged 18 or older (1.1 percent of the population in that age group) received support from a mental

Excerpted from "Mental Health Support and Self-Help Groups," a National Survey on Drug Use and Health (NSDUH) Report, by the Substance Abuse and Mental Health Services Administration (SAMHSA, www.oas.samhsa.gov), October 8, 2009.

health self-help group in the past year. The majority were female (61.2 percent)—a proportion higher than expected based on the proportion of females in the total population.

Of the adults who received support from a mental health self-help group, 10.6 percent were aged 18 to 25, 55.3 percent were aged 26 to 49, and 34.1 percent were aged 50 or older. The proportion of adults aged 26 to 49 was higher among persons using mental health self-help groups than among the general adult population. Three fourths (75.2 percent) of those who received support from a mental health self-help group were white, and fewer than half (46.8 percent) were employed full time; these proportions also differed from the expected proportions.

Traditional Mental Health Treatment and Mental Health Self-Help Groups

An average of 28.8 million adults received traditional types of mental health treatment (i.e., inpatient care, outpatient care, or prescription medication) in the past year. Of the 2.4 million adults who received support from a mental health self-help group in the past year, 1.6 million, or 65.6 percent, also received traditional mental health treatment. This number includes 186,000 (7.7 percent of self-help group users) who also received inpatient care, 1.2 million (51.0 percent) who also received outpatient care, and 1.3 million (53.2 percent) who also received prescription medication. An estimated 829,000 users of self-help groups (34.4 percent) did not receive traditional mental health treatment in the past year.

Mental Health Self-Help Group Use among Recipients of Traditional Treatment

About 5.5 percent of adults who received any traditional type of mental health treatment in the past year also received support from a mental health self-help group in that time period.

Use of self-help groups was reported by 9.8 percent of those who received inpatient mental health care in the past year, 8.2 percent of those who got outpatient care, and 5.3 percent of those treated with prescription medications. The proportion using self-help groups was 8.8 percent among adults who received two or more of these traditional types of mental health care and 14.2 percent among those who received all three types.

Demographic Differences in Use of Self-Help Groups among Treatment Recipients

Among adults who received any traditional type of mental health treatment, those aged 26 to 49 were more likely than those aged 18 to 25 or 50 or older to have also received support from a mental health self-help group. Receipt of support from a mental health self-help group by those who received past year traditional mental health treatment ranged from a low of 3.8 percent among Asians to a high of 8.1 percent among blacks or African Americans. Among persons who received traditional mental health treatment in the past year, similar percentages of females and males also received support from a mental health self-help group (5.2 and 6.1 percent, respectively).

Discussion

A continuum of services and supports is important for recovery from mental health problems. For many people, mental health support and self-help groups complement treatment in the traditional mental health sector; two thirds (65.6 percent) of the people who received support for mental health problems from self-help groups also received traditional mental health services (inpatient care, outpatient care, and prescription medication). What was once viewed as an alternative can now be considered an element of mainstream services and supports, especially as even newer "alternatives" to traditional treatment emerge through such avenues as consumer-operated services providing a range of community-based services, wellness programs, peer-provided Medicaid-reimbursable services, Internet support groups, and peer-run crisis alternatives.

Chapter 60

Helping a Family Member or Friend with Depression

Mental illness is a health condition that causes changes in a person's thinking, mood, and behavior.

Mental illness is very common. Mental health and mental illness can be pictured as two points on a continuum with a range of conditions in between. When these conditions are more serious, they are referred to as mental illnesses and include depression, schizophrenia, anxiety, and others that may require treatment and support. They are also widely misunderstood.

Arm yourself with the facts, then use your knowledge to educate others and reach out to those around you with mental illness. Understanding and support are powerful, and they can make a real difference in the life of a person who needs them.

- Among 18- to 25-year-olds, the prevalence of serious mental health conditions is high, yet this age group shows the lowest rate of help-seeking behaviors.

- Those with mental health conditions in this age group have a high potential to minimize future disability if social acceptance is broadened and they receive the right support.

- People with mental illness need to be treated with respect, compassion, and empathy, just as anyone with any other serious but

Excerpted from "What a Difference a Friend Makes," by the Substance Abuse and Mental Health Services Administration (SAMHSA, www.whatadifference.samhsa .gov), part of the U.S. Department of Health and Human Services, 2007.

treatable condition. People with mental illnesses are often stigmatized by others who think it's an uncommon condition. The truth is, mental illness can happen to anybody regardless of age, culture, race, gender, ethnicity, economic status, or location.

One of the most important factors in recovery is the understanding and acceptance of friends. Friends can make a difference by offering reassurance, companionship, and emotional strength.

Recovery

One of the most important things to remember about mental illness is this: People can and do recover. If you have a friend with mental illness, or if you have a mental illness yourself, remember that recovery is possible. Reach out to those around you with compassion, empathy, and understanding.

Here are more things to keep in mind: Mental illness can affect anybody regardless of race, ethnicity, gender, age, or background. You probably know somebody with mental illness. And mental illnesses are not caused by poor decisions or bad habits. They affect a person's physical, mental, and emotional wellbeing, much like heart disease or diabetes.

The stigma associated with mental illness is a big barrier to recovery. If we want to be a truly healthy society, we need to break down the stigma and treat mental illness like any other healthcare condition. It starts with you.

People with mental illness can recover or manage their conditions and go on to lead happy, healthy, productive lives. They contribute to society and make the world a better place. People can often benefit from medication, rehabilitation, psychotherapy, group therapy, self-help, or a combination of these. One of the most important factors in recovery is the understanding and acceptance of friends.

Support

How to Help

If somebody told you he had diabetes, how would you react? If you're like most people, you'd express sympathy and concern, offer your support and reassurance, and feel confident that your friend's condition would improve with treatment. Now, if that same friend told you he had a mental illness, what would you do?

Too many people respond negatively when confronted with a friend's mental illness, and this only fuels the stigma surrounding the diagnosis. The reality is, mental illness is no different from physical illness. Conditions like depression, schizophrenia, and anxiety disorders affect a person's health. The emotional and psychological aspects of mental illness make supportive friends and family even more important to a person's recovery.

So, now you know you can help just by being there and offering your reassurance, companionship, emotional strength, and acceptance. You can make a difference just by understanding and helping your friend throughout the course of his or her illness and beyond.

Respond

Imagine that you've just been diagnosed with a serious but treatable physical condition. You're scared and confused, so you tell a friend. How would you feel if your friend laughed, called you names, made rude gestures, and told you to just snap out of it? People with mental illness face these reactions every day.

We all know better than to hurt people—especially when they're already hurting. Mental illness causes physical, mental, and emotional symptoms that make an added stigma even harder to bear. So put aside any preconceived notions you might have about mental illness and embrace a more helpful way of relating to people.

Instead of blowing off a person's worries, express your interest and concern. Don't change the subject when a mental illness diagnosis comes up—ask questions, listen to ideas, and be responsive. Ask what you can do to help. If other people make insensitive remarks, don't ignore them—educate people so that they understand the facts about mental illness. If someone you work with or go to school with has a mental illness, don't discriminate. Treat people with mental illness just as you would those with any other serious but treatable condition—with respect, compassion, and empathy.

Help a Friend

If your friend tells you he or she has a mental illness, read the tips below for what you might say or how you might respond:

- Express your concern and sympathy.

- Ask for more details about how he or she is managing. Really listen to the answers and continue the conversation. Make sure your friend understands that you honestly care.

- Ask what you can do to help. You can leave this open-ended, or you can suggest specific tasks that might help your friend in his or her specific situation. Rides to medical appointments (or keeping the person company in the waiting room) can ease some of the anxiety and reluctance that people feel when faced with a life-changing diagnosis.

- You might also offer to help your friend with errands, but be careful not to patronize or make the person feel disempowered.

- Reassure your friend that you still care about him or her, and be sure to include him or her in your everyday plans—going out to lunch, catching a movie, taking a jog. If your friend resists these overtures, reassure and reinvite without being overbearing.

- Remind your friend that mental illness is treatable. Find out if the friend is getting the care the friend needs and wants. If not, offer your help in identifying and getting the right kind of care.

- If a friend needs immediate help for mental illness, ask him or her what kind of help is needed and respond immediately. It is important to give him or her hope and encourage them to seek support, including calling a crisis line, or the National Suicide Prevention Line at 800-273-TALK (273-8255).

- Encourage your friend to seek immediate medical attention if your friend is weak or ill from an eating disorder.

Part Eight

Suicide

Chapter 61

Suicide in the United States

Suicide is a major, preventable public health problem. In 2007, it was the 10th leading cause of death in the United States, accounting for 34,598 deaths. The overall rate was 11.3 suicide deaths per 100,000 people. An estimated 11 attempted suicides occur per every suicide death.

Suicidal behavior is complex. Some risk factors vary with age, gender, or ethnic group and may occur in combination or change over time.

What are the risk factors for suicide?

Research shows that risk factors for suicide include the following:

- Depression and other mental disorders or a substance-abuse disorder, often in combination with other mental disorders (More than 90 percent of people who die by suicide have these risk factors.)

- Prior suicide attempt

- Family history of mental disorder or substance abuse

- Family history of suicide

- Family violence, including physical or sexual abuse

- Firearms in the home, the method used in more than half of suicides

From "Suicide in the U.S.: Statistics and Prevention," by the National Institute of Mental Health (NIMH, www.nimh.nih.gov), part of the National Institutes of Health, September 27, 2010.

- Incarceration

- Exposure to the suicidal behavior of others, such as family members, peers, or media figures

However, suicide and suicidal behavior are not normal responses to stress; many people have these risk factors, but are not suicidal. Research also shows that the risk for suicide is associated with changes in brain chemicals called neurotransmitters, including serotonin. Decreased levels of serotonin have been found in people with depression, impulsive disorders, and a history of suicide attempts, and in the brains of suicide victims.

Are women or men at higher risk?

- Suicide was the seventh leading cause of death for males and the 15th leading cause of death for females in 2007.

- Almost four times as many males as females die by suicide.

- Firearms, suffocation, and poison are by far the most common methods of suicide, overall. However, men and women differ in the method used, as shown in Table 61.1.

Table 61.1. Most Common Methods of Suicide

Suicide by	Males (%)	Females (%)
Firearms	56	30
Suffocation	24	21
Poisoning	13	40

Is suicide common among children and young people?

In 2007, suicide was the third leading cause of death for young people ages 15 to 24. Of every 100,000 young people in each age group, the following number died by suicide:

- Children ages 10 to 14—0.9 per 100,000

- Adolescents ages 15 to 19—6.9 per 100,000

- Young adults ages 20 to 24—12.7 per 100,000

As in the general population, young people were much more likely to use firearms, suffocation, and poisoning than other methods of suicide, overall. However, while adolescents and young adults were more likely to use firearms than suffocation, children were dramatically more likely to use suffocation.

There were also gender differences in suicide among young people, as follows:

- Nearly five times as many males as females ages 15 to 19 died by suicide.

- Just under six times as many males as females ages 20 to 24 died by suicide.

Are older adults at risk?

Older Americans are disproportionately likely to die by suicide.

- Of every 100,000 people ages 65 and older, 14.3 died by suicide in 2007. This figure is higher than the national average of 11.3 suicides per 100,000 people in the general population.

- Non-Hispanic white men age 85 or older had an even higher rate, with 47 suicide deaths per 100,000.

Are some ethnic groups or races at higher risk?

Of every 100,000 people in each of the following ethnic/racial groups, the following number died by suicide in 2007. Highest rates:

- American Indian and Alaska Natives—14.3 per 100,000
- Non-Hispanic Whites—13.5 per 100,000

Lowest rates:

- Hispanics—6.0 per 100,000
- Non-Hispanic Blacks—5.1 per 100,000
- Asian and Pacific Islanders—6.2 per 100,000

What are some risk factors for nonfatal suicide attempts?

- As noted, an estimated 11 nonfatal suicide attempts occur per every suicide death. Men and the elderly are more likely to have fatal attempts than are women and youth.

- Risk factors for nonfatal suicide attempts by adults include depression and other mental disorders, alcohol and other substance abuse, and separation or divorce.

- Risk factors for attempted suicide by youth include depression, alcohol or other drug-use disorder, physical or sexual abuse, and disruptive behavior.

- Most suicide attempts are expressions of extreme distress, not harmless bids for attention. A person who appears suicidal should not be left alone and needs immediate mental-health treatment.

What can be done to prevent suicide?

Research helps determine which factors can be modified to help prevent suicide and which interventions are appropriate for specific groups of people. Before being put into practice, prevention programs should be tested through research to determine their safety and effectiveness. For example, because research has shown that mental and substance-abuse disorders are major risk factors for suicide, many programs also focus on treating these disorders as well as addressing suicide risk directly.

Studies showed that a type of psychotherapy called cognitive therapy reduced the rate of repeated suicide attempts by 50 percent during a year of follow-up. A previous suicide attempt is among the strongest predictors of subsequent suicide, and cognitive therapy helps suicide attempters consider alternative actions when thoughts of self-harm arise.

Specific kinds of psychotherapy may be helpful for specific groups of people. For example, a treatment called dialectical behavior therapy reduced suicide attempts by half, compared with other kinds of therapy, in people with borderline personality disorder (a serious disorder of emotion regulation).

The medication clozapine is approved by the Food and Drug Administration for suicide prevention in people with schizophrenia. Other promising medications and psychosocial treatments for suicidal people are being tested.

Since research shows that older adults and women who die by suicide are likely to have seen a primary care provider in the year before death, improving primary-care providers' ability to recognize and treat risk factors may help prevent suicide among these groups. Improving outreach to men at risk is a major challenge in need of investigation.

What should I do if I think someone is suicidal?

If you think someone is suicidal, do not leave him or her alone. Try to get the person to seek immediate help from his or her doctor or the nearest hospital emergency room, or call 911. Eliminate access to firearms or other potential tools for suicide, including unsupervised access to medications.

If you are in a crisis and need help right away, call this toll-free number, available 24 hours a day, every day: 800-273-TALK (273-8255). You will reach the National Suicide Prevention Lifeline, a service available to anyone. You may call for yourself or for someone you care about. All calls are confidential.

Chapter 62

Suicide in Children, Teens, and Young Adults

Chapter Contents

Section 62.1

Suicide in Children and Teens

From "Suicide: A Major, Preventable Mental Health Problem," by the National Institute of Mental Health (NIMH, www.nimh.nih .gov), part of the National Institutes of Health, June 2011.

How common is suicide in children and teens?

In 2007, suicide was the third leading cause of death for young people ages 15–24. Suicide accounted for 4,140 deaths (12%) of the total 34,598 suicide deaths in 2007. While these numbers may make suicide seem common, it is important to realize that suicide and suicidal behavior are not healthy or typical responses to stress.

What are some of the risk factors for suicide?

Risk factors vary with age, gender, or ethnic group. They may occur in combination or change over time. Some important risk factors are the following:

- Depression and other mental disorders, including substance abuse disorder (often in combination with other mental disorders)

- Prior suicide attempt

- Family history of suicide

- Family violence including physical or sexual abuse

- Firearms in the home

- Incarceration

- Exposure to suicidal behavior of others, such as family members or peers

However, it is important to note that many people who have these risk factors, are not suicidal.

What are signs to look for?

The following are some of the signs you might notice in yourself or a friend that may be reason for concern.

- Feelings of hopelessness or worthlessness, depressed mood, poor self-esteem, or guilt

- Not wanting to participate in family or social activities

- Changes in sleeping and eating patterns—eating or sleeping too much or too little

- Feelings of anger, rage, or the need for revenge

- Feeling exhausted most of the time

- Trouble with concentration and problems academically or socially in school

- Feeling listless or irritable

- Regular and frequent crying

- Not taking care of yourself

- Reckless, impulsive behaviors

- Frequent physical symptoms such as headaches or stomachaches

Seeking help is a sign of strength; if you are concerned, go with your instincts and get help.

What can I do for myself or someone else?

If you are concerned, immediate action is very important. Suicide can be prevented and most people who feel suicidal demonstrate warning signs. Recognizing some of these warning signs is the first step in helping yourself or someone you care about.

If you are in crisis and need help: Call this toll-free number, available 24 hours a day, every day—800-273-TALK (8255) or go to www.suicidepreventionlifeline.org. You will reach the National Suicide Prevention Lifeline, a service available to anyone. You may call for yourself or for someone you care about and all calls are confidential.

Section 62.2

Suicide on College Campuses

From "Preventing Suicide on College Campuses," in the *SAMHSA News*, by the Substance Abuse and Mental Health Services Administration (SAMHSA, www.samhsa.gov), part of the U.S. Department of Health and Human Services, March/April 2011.

College can be a stressful time, and the numbers bear that out. The American College Health Association's 2006 National College Health Assessment found that 94 percent of the college and university students surveyed reported that they felt overwhelmed by everything they had to do. Forty-four percent confessed that they had felt so depressed it was difficult to function. And 18 percent had a depressive disorder.

According to SAMHSA's National Survey on Drug Use and Health, in 2008, young adults age 18 to 25 were more likely than adults age 26 to 49 to have had serious thoughts of suicide (6.7 percent vs. 3.9 percent).

These statistics underscore why prevention of substance abuse and mental illness—including suicide prevention—is the first of eight strategic initiatives that will guide SAMHSA's work through 2014.

"Suicide is a preventable tragedy for college students, their families, and our communities," said SAMHSA Administrator Pamela S. Hyde, JD, noting the importance of education about depression, substance abuse, and other suicide risk factors, as well as resources such as SAMHSA's National Suicide Prevention Lifeline. "By working on suicide prevention on campuses and elsewhere, we can save thousands of lives."

For college students, they need all the support they can get. The bad economy is adding to students' stress about debt and job prospects once they graduate. A 2010 Higher Education Research Institute study of more than 200,000 freshmen entering four-year colleges found that their emotional health had declined to the lowest level since the annual survey began 25 years ago.

Chapter 63

Suicidal Thoughts and Behaviors among Adults

Suicidality is a major public health problem that affects many Americans and their families every year. Suicidality ranges from suicide ideation (i.e., thoughts of suicide and making suicide plans) to suicide attempts to completed suicide. Over 32,000 adults committed suicide in 2006; however, these represent only a fraction of the individuals who consider or attempt suicide.

Gaining a better understanding of suicidal thoughts and behaviors among adults may help to identify individuals at risk for suicide, to inform the development of screening tools, and to inform mental health and general practitioners on treatment planning.

Responding to a need for national data on the prevalence of suicidality, a brief series of questions on suicidal thoughts and behaviors was added to the National Survey on Drug Use and Health (NSDUH) questionnaire in 2008. In previous NSDUHs, suicidality questions were asked in the module on major depressive episode (MDE), and suicidality estimates could be generated only for persons who met the criteria for MDE. The new 2008 questions ask all adult respondents aged 18 or older if they had serious thoughts of suicide in the past year. If they had serious thoughts of suicide, respondents were asked if they made plans to commit suicide and if they attempted suicide in the past year. If they reported having made a suicide attempt,

Excerpted from "Suicidal Thoughts and Behaviors among Adults," a National Survey on Drug Use and Health report by the Substance Abuse and Mental Health Services Administration (SAMHSA, www.samhsa.gov), part of the U.S. Department of Health and Human Services, September 17, 2009.

respondents were asked if they received medical attention for their suicide attempt; if they received medical attention, they were asked if they stayed in a hospital overnight or longer for their suicide attempt.

This text examines suicidal thoughts and behaviors among adults aged 18 or older; data are presented by age group, gender, and past year substance use disorder. All findings in the text are based on 2008 data.

Suicidal Thoughts and Behaviors

An estimated 8.3 million adults (3.7 percent of the adult population) had serious thoughts of suicide in the past year, 2.3 million (1.0 percent) made a suicide plan in the past year, and 1.1 million (0.5 percent) attempted suicide in the past year. Table 63.1 displays the numbers of adults who made suicide plans and attempted suicide among those who had serious thoughts of suicide; not all persons who attempted suicide had made a suicide plan. Among the adults who had serious thoughts of suicide, most (5.8 million) had not made a suicide plan or suicide attempt. Approximately 1.4 million adults had serious thoughts of suicide and made a suicide plan, but had not made a suicide attempt; 0.2 million had serious thoughts of suicide and made a suicide attempt, but made no suicide plan. An estimated 0.9 million had serious thoughts of suicide, made a suicide plan, and actually attempted suicide.

Table 63.1. Suicidal Thoughts and Behaviors in the Past Year among Adults: 2008

Suicidal Thoughts and Behavior	Number (in Millions)
Serious Thoughts of Suicide	8.3
Made Suicide Plan	2.3
Made Suicide Plan and Made Suicide Attempt	0.9
Made Suicide Plan But Did Not Make Suicide Attempt	1.4
Did Not Make Suicide Plan	6.0
Did Not Make Suicide Plan but Made Suicide Attempt	0.2
Did Not Make Suicide Plan and Did Not Make Suicide Attempt	5.8

Source: 2008 SAMHSA National Survey on Drug Use and Health (NSDUH).

Suicidal Thoughts and Behaviors, by Demographic and Other Characteristics

Rates of serious thinking about suicide, making plans for suicide, and attempting suicide were higher among young adults aged 18 to 25 than among adults aged 26 to 49 and those aged 50 or older. For example, 6.7 percent of adults aged 18 to 25 had serious thoughts of suicide in the past year compared with 3.9 percent of adults aged 26 to 49 and 2.3 percent of adults aged 50 or older. There was little difference in the rates of suicidal thoughts, plans, and attempts between females and males.

Rates of serious thoughts of suicide, making plans for suicide, and attempting suicide were higher among adults with a past year substance use disorder than among those without a substance use disorder. For example, 11.0 percent of adults with a past-year substance use disorder had serious thoughts of suicide compared with 3.0 percent of those with no past year substance use disorder.

Medical Attention for Suicide Attempts

Of the adults who attempted suicide in the past year, 62.3 percent (678,000 persons) received medical attention for their suicide attempts, and 46.0 percent (500,000 persons) stayed overnight or longer in a hospital for their suicide attempts.

Discussion

A large number of Americans think about, plan for, and attempt suicide every year. In 2008, an estimated 8.3 million adults had serious thoughts of suicide in the past year, 2.3 million made a suicide plan, and 1.1 million attempted suicide. Rates of suicidal behaviors varied by age, with young adults aged 18 to 25 displaying higher rates than older adults. Rates of suicidal behaviors were also significantly higher among those with a past year substance use disorder than among those without a substance use disorder. About six in 10 of the adults who attempted suicide received medical attention for their suicide attempt.

Preventing suicide and addressing the health care needs of persons at risk for suicidal behavior require public health information-sharing efforts that not only highlight the fact that effective preventive interventions exist, but also attempt to reduce the stigma associated with mental and emotional problems and mental health treatment. Further research on additional factors associated with suicidal behaviors (i.e., race/ethnicity, employment and occupation, and mental health and substance abuse problems), as well as on suicidal behaviors among specific subpopulations (i.e., young adults, veterans, and parenting adults), is needed to help guide the development of screening tools and prevention and treatment programs.

Chapter 64

Older Adults: Depression and Suicide Facts

How common is suicide among older adults?

Older Americans are disproportionately likely to die by suicide.

- Although they comprise only 12 percent of the U.S. population, people age 65 and older accounted for 16 percent of suicide deaths in 2004.

- 14.3 of every 100,000 people age 65 and older died by suicide in 2004, higher than the rate of about 11 per 100,000 in the general population.

- Non-Hispanic white men age 85 and older were most likely to die by suicide. They had a rate of 49.8 suicide deaths per 100,000 persons in that age group.

What role does depression play?

Depression, one of the conditions most commonly associated with suicide in older adults, is a widely under-recognized and undertreated medical illness. Studies show that many older adults who die by suicide—up to 75 percent—visited a physician within a month before death. These findings point to the urgency of improving detection and treatment of depression to reduce suicide risk among older adults.

From "Older Adults: Depression and Suicide Facts," a fact sheet by the National Institute of Mental Health (NIMH, www.nimh.nih.gov), part of the National Institutes of Health, September 27, 2010.

The risk of depression in the elderly increases with other illnesses and when ability to function becomes limited. Estimates of major depression in older people living in the community range from less than 1 percent to about 5 percent, but rises to 13.5 percent in those who require home healthcare and to 11.5 percent in elderly hospital patients.

An estimated 5 million have subsyndromal depression, symptoms that fall short of meeting the full diagnostic criteria for a disorder. Subsyndromal depression is especially common among older persons and is associated with an increased risk of developing major depression.

Isn't depression just part of aging?

Depressive disorder is not a normal part of aging. Emotional experiences of sadness, grief, response to loss, and temporary blue moods are normal. Persistent depression that interferes significantly with ability to function is not.

Health professionals may mistakenly think that persistent depression is an acceptable response to other serious illnesses and the social and financial hardships that often accompany aging—an attitude often shared by older people themselves. This contributes to low rates of diagnosis and treatment in older adults.

Depression can and should be treated when it occurs at the same time as other medical illnesses. Untreated depression can delay recovery or worsen the outcome of these other illnesses.

What are the treatments for depression in older adults?

Antidepressant medications or psychotherapy, or a combination of the two, can be effective treatments for late-life depression.

Medications: Antidepressant medications affect brain chemicals called neurotransmitters. For example, medications called SSRIs (selective serotonin reuptake inhibitors) affect the neurotransmitter serotonin. Different medications may affect different neurotransmitters.

Some older adults may find that newer antidepressant medications, including SSRIs, have fewer side effects than older medications, which include tricyclic antidepressants and monoamine oxidase inhibitors (MAOIs). However, others may find that these older medications work well for them.

It's important to be aware that there are several medications for depression, that different medications work for different people, and that it takes 4 to 8 weeks for the medications to work. If one medication doesn't help, research shows that a different antidepressant might.

Also, older adults experiencing depression for the first time should talk to their doctors about continuing medication even if their symptoms have disappeared with treatment. Studies showed that patients age 70 and older who became symptom-free and continued to take their medication for two more years were 60 percent less likely to relapse than those who discontinued their medications.

Psychotherapy: In psychotherapy, people interact with a specially trained health professional to deal with depression, thoughts of suicide, and other problems. Research shows that certain types of psychotherapy are effective treatments for late-life depression.

For many older adults, especially those who are in good physical health, combining psychotherapy with antidepressant medication appears to provide the most benefit. A study showed that about 80 percent of older adults with depression recovered with this kind of combined treatment and had lower recurrence rates than with psychotherapy or medication alone.

Another study of depressed older adults with physical illnesses and problems with memory and thinking showed that combined treatment was no more effective than medication alone. Research can help further determine which older adults appear to be most likely to benefit from a combination of medication and psychotherapy or from either treatment alone.

Are some ethnic/racial groups at higher risk of suicide?

For every 100,000 people age 65 and older in each of the ethnic/racial groups below, the following number died by suicide in 2004:

- Non-Hispanic Whites—15.8 per 100,000
- Asian and Pacific Islanders—10.6 per 100,000
- Hispanics—7.9 per 100,000
- Non-Hispanic Blacks—5.0 per 100,000

Chapter 65

Warning Signs of Suicide and How to Help

Warning Signs of Suicide

Everyone feels sad, depressed, or angry sometimes—especially when the pressures of school, friends, and family become too much to handle. Other times, though, feelings of sadness or hopelessness just won't go away.

These feelings may begin to affect many areas of a person's life and outlook. Someone who experiences very intense feelings of depression or irritability may begin to think about suicide.

You may have heard that people who talk about suicide won't actually go through with it. That's not true. People who talk about suicide may be likely to try it.

Other warning signs that someone may be thinking of suicide include:

- talking about suicide or death in general;

- talking about "going away";

- talking about feeling hopeless or feeling guilty;

- pulling away from friends or family and losing the desire to go out;

"My Friend Is Talking About Suicide. What Should I Do?" June 2008, reprinted with permission from www.kidshealth.org. Copyright © 2008 The Nemours Foundation. This information was provided by KidsHealth, one of the largest resources online for medically reviewed health information written for parents, kids, and teens. For more articles like this one, visit www.KidsHealth.org, or www.Teens Health.org.

- having no desire to take part in favorite activities;
- having trouble concentrating or thinking clearly;
- experiencing changes in eating or sleeping habits;
- engaging in self-destructive behavior (drinking alcohol, taking drugs, or driving too fast, for example).

As a friend, you may also know if the person is going through some tough times. Sometimes, a specific event, stress, or crisis—like a relationship breaking up or a death in the family—can trigger suicidal behavior in someone who is already feeling depressed and showing the warning signs listed in the preceding text.

What You Can Do

Ask

If you have a friend who is talking about suicide or showing other warning signs, don't wait to see if he or she starts to feel better. Talk about it. Most of the time, people who are considering suicide are willing to discuss it if someone asks them out of concern and care.

Some people (both teens and adults) are reluctant to ask teens if they have been thinking about suicide or hurting themselves. That's because they're afraid that, by asking, they may plant the idea of suicide. This is not true. It is always a good thing to ask.

Starting the conversation with someone you think may be considering suicide helps in many ways. First, it allows you to get help for the person. Second, just talking about it may help the person to feel less alone, less isolated, and more cared about and understood—the opposite of the feelings that may have led to suicidal thinking to begin with. Third, talking may provide a chance to consider that there may be another solution.

Asking someone if he or she is having thoughts about suicide can be difficult. Sometimes it helps to let your friend know why you are asking. For instance, you might say, "I've noticed that you've been talking a lot about wanting to be dead. Have you been having thoughts about trying to kill yourself?"

Listen

Listen to your friend without judging and offer reassurance that you're there and you care. If you think your friend is in immediate danger, stay close—make sure he or she isn't left alone.

Tell

Even if you're sworn to secrecy and you feel like you'll be betraying your friend if you tell, you should still seek help. Share your concerns with an adult you trust as soon as possible. If necessary, you can also call a local emergency number (911) or the toll-free number for a suicide crisis line (you can find local suicide crisis numbers listed in your phone book).

The important thing is to notify a responsible adult. Although it may be tempting to try to help your friend on your own, it's always safest to get help.

After Suicide

Sometimes even if you get help and adults intervene, a friend or classmate may attempt or die by suicide. When this happens, it's common to have many different emotions. Some teens say they feel guilty—especially if they felt they could have interpreted their friend's actions and words better. Others say they feel angry with the person for doing something so selfish. Still others say they feel nothing at all—they are too filled with grief.

When someone attempts suicide, those who know that person may feel afraid or uncomfortable about talking to him or her. Try to overcome these feelings of discomfort—this is a time when someone absolutely needs to feel connected to others.

If you are having difficulty dealing with a friend or classmate's suicide, it's best to talk to an adult you trust. Feeling grief after a friend dies by suicide is normal. But if that sadness begins to interfere with your everyday life, it's a sign that you may need to speak with someone about your feelings.

Chapter 66

Coping after Someone You Love Has Attempted Suicide

Suicidal thoughts and actions generate conflicting feelings in family members who love the person who wishes to take his or her own life. This text will give you some important points on how to take care of yourself and your family member following a suicide attempt.

What Happens in the Emergency Department

Goal

The goal of an emergency department visit is to get the best outcome for the person at a time of crisis—resolving the crisis, stabilizing the patient medically and emotionally, and making recommendations and referrals for followup care or treatment. There are several steps in the process, and they all take time.

When someone is admitted to an emergency department for a suicide attempt, a doctor will evaluate the person's physical and mental health.

Emergency department staff should look for underlying physical problems that may have contributed to the suicidal behavior, such as side effects from medications, untreated medical conditions, or the presence of street drugs that can cause emotional distress. While emergency department staff prefer to assess people who are sober, they

From "After an Attempt," by the Substance Abuse and Mental Health Services Administration (SAMHSA, www.samhsa.gov), part of the U.S. Department of Health and Human Services, 2006. Reviewed by David A. Cooke, MD, FACP, November 19, 2011.

should not dismiss things people say or do when intoxicated, especially comments about how they might harm themselves or others.

Assessment

After emergency department staff evaluate your family member's physical health, a mental health assessment should be performed, and the physician doing the exam should put your relative's suicidal behavior into context. The assessment will generally focus on three areas:

1. What psychiatric or medical conditions are present? Are they being or have they been treated? Are the suicidal thoughts and behavior a result of a recent change, or are they a longstanding condition?

2. What did the person do to harm himself or herself? Have there been previous attempts? Why did the person act, and why now? What current stressors, including financial or relationship losses, may have contributed to this decision? Does the person regret surviving the suicide attempt? Is the person angry with someone? Is the person trying to reunite with someone who has died? What is the person's perspective on death?

3. What support systems are there? Who is providing treatment? What treatment programs are a good match for the person? What does the individual and the family feel comfortable with? Finally, a doctor may assess in more detail the actual suicide attempt that brought your relative into the emergency department. Information that the treatment team should look for includes the presence of a suicide note, the seriousness of the attempt, or a history of previous suicide attempts. Inform the emergency department personnel if your relative has the following:

    - Access to a gun, lethal doses of medications, or other means of suicide

    - Stopped taking prescribed medicines

    - Stopped seeing a mental health provider or physician

    - Written a suicide note or will

    - Given possessions away

    - Been in or is currently in an abusive relationship

    - An upcoming anniversary of a loss

    - Started abusing alcohol or drugs

- Recovered well from a previous suicidal crisis following a certain type of intervention

What the Emergency Department Needs to Know: How You Can Help

Confidentiality and Information Sharing

Family members are a source of history and are often key to the discharge plan. Provide as much information as possible to the emergency department staff. Even if confidentiality laws prevent the medical staff from giving you information about your relative, you can always give them information. Find out who is doing the evaluation and talk with that person. You can offer information that may influence the decisions made for your relative.

If you ever again have to accompany your relative to the emergency department after an attempt, remember to bring all medications, suspected causes of overdose, and any names and phone numbers of providers who may have information.

Emergency department personnel should try to contact the medical professionals who know the situation best before making decisions. Other important information about your relative's history to share with the emergency department staff include the following:

- A family history of actual suicide: Mental health professionals are taught to pay attention to this because there is an increased risk in families with a history of suicide.

- Details about your relative's treatment team: A recent change in medication, the therapist is on vacation, etc. This information is relevant for emergency department staff because if they do not feel hospitalization is best, they need to discharge your family member to a professional's care.

- If the person has an advance directive, review this with the emergency department treatment team. If you have a guardianship, let them know that as well.

You may want to get permission from the staff and your relative to sit in on your relative's evaluation in the emergency department to listen and add information as needed. Your role is to balance the emergency department staff's training and the interview of the patient with your perspective. The best emergency department decisions are made with all the relevant information.

Next Steps After the Emergency Department

After your relative's physical and mental health are thoroughly examined, the emergency department personnel will decide if your relative needs to be hospitalized—either voluntarily or by a commitment. If hospitalization is necessary, you can begin to work with the receiving hospital to offer information and support and to develop a plan for the next steps in your relative's care. If involuntary hospitalization is necessary, the hospital staff should explain this legal procedure to your relative and you so that you both have a clear understanding of what will take place over the next 3–10 days, while a court decides on the next steps for treatment.

If your relative has a hearing impairment or does not speak English, he or she may have to wait for someone who knows American Sign Language or an interpreter. It is generally not a good idea to use a family member to interpret in a medical situation.

If the emergency department's treatment team, the patient, and you do not feel hospitalization is necessary, then you should all be a part of developing a followup treatment plan. In developing a plan, consider the following questions:

Questions Family and Friends Should Ask about the Followup Treatment Plan

It is important to be honest and direct with your questions and concerns. Ask your family member:

- Do you feel safe to leave the hospital, and are you comfortable with the discharge plan?

- How is your relationship with your doctor, and when is your next appointment?

- What has changed since your suicidal feelings or actions began?

- What else can I/we do to help you after you leave the emergency department?

- Will you agree to talk with me/us if your suicidal feelings return? If not, is there someone else you can talk to?

Ask the treatment team (This includes the doctor, therapist, nurse, social worker, etc.):

- Do you believe professionally that my family member is ready to leave the hospital?

- Why did you make the decision(s) that you did about my family member's care or treatment?

- Is there a followup appointment scheduled? Can it be moved to an earlier date?

- What is my role as a family member in the safety plan?

- What should we look for and when should we seek more help, such as returning to the emergency department or contacting other local resources and providers?

Remember: It is critical for the patient to schedule a followup appointment as soon as possible after discharge from the emergency department.

What You Need to Know

Make safety a priority for your relative recovering from a suicide attempt.

Research has shown that a person who has attempted to end his or her life has a much higher risk of later dying by suicide.

Safety is ultimately an individual's responsibility, but often a person who feels suicidal has a difficult time making good choices. As a family member, you can help your loved one make a better choice while reducing the risk.

Reduce the Risk at Home

To help reduce the risk of self-harm or suicide at home, here are some things to consider:

- Guns are high risk and the leading means of death for suicidal people—they should be taken out of the home and secured.

- Overdoses are common and can be lethal—if it is necessary to keep pain relievers such as aspirin, Advil, and Tylenol in the home, only keep small quantities or consider keeping medications in a locked container.

- Remove unused or expired medicine from the home.

- Alcohol use or abuse can decrease inhibitions and cause people to act more freely on their feelings. As with pain relievers, keep only small quantities of alcohol in the home, or none at all.

Create a Safety Plan

Following a suicide attempt, a safety plan should be created to help prevent another attempt. The plan should be a joint effort between your relative and his or her doctor, therapist, or the emergency department staff, and you. As a family member, you should know your relative's safety plan and understand your role in it, including the following:

- Knowing your family member's "triggers," such as an anniversary of a loss, alcohol, or stress from relationships

- Building supports for your family member with mental health professionals, family, friends, and community resources

- Working with your family member's strengths to promote his or her safety

- Promoting communication and honesty in your relationship with your family member

Remember that safety cannot be guaranteed by anyone—the goal is to reduce the risks and build supports for everyone in the family. However, it is important for you to believe that the safety plan can help keep your relative safe. If you do not feel that it can, let the emergency department staff know before you leave.

Maintain Hope and Self-Care

Families commonly provide a safety net and a vision of hope for their suicidal relative, and that can be emotionally exhausting. Never try to handle this situation alone—get support from friends, relatives, and organizations such as the National Alliance on Mental Illness (NAMI), and get professional input whenever possible. Use the Internet, family, and friends to help you create a support network. You do not have to travel this road alone.

Moving Forward

Emergency department care is by nature short-term and crisis oriented, but some longer-term interventions have been shown to help reduce suicidal behavior and thoughts. You and your relative can talk to the doctor about various treatments for mental illnesses that may help to reduce the risk of suicide for people diagnosed with illnesses such as schizophrenia, bipolar disorder, or depression. Often, these illnesses require multiple types of interventions, and your relative may benefit from a second opinion from a specialist.

If your relative abuses alcohol or other drugs, it is also important to seek help for this problem along with the suicidal behavior. Seek out a substance abuse specialist. Contact your local substance abuse treatment provider by calling 800-662-4357 or visiting www.findtreat ment.samhsa.gov, or contact groups like Alcoholics Anonymous (AA) or Narcotics Anonymous (NA) to help your loved one; Al-Anon may be a good resource for you as a family member. If it is available in your area, an integrated treatment program like Assertive Community Treatment (ACT) may provide better outcomes than traditional care for some severely ill individuals.

Ultimately, please reach out for help in supporting your family member and yourself through this crisis. See the list below of hotlines, information, and support organizations to help you and your family member move forward with your lives.

Remember that the emergency department is open 24 hours a day, 365 days a year to treat your family member, if the problem continues and if your family member's medical team is unavailable to provide the needed care.

Part Nine

Additional Help and Information

Chapter 67

Glossary of Terms Related to Depression

antidepressants: A name for a category of medications used to treat depression.[1]

anxiety disorder: Serious medical illness that fills people's lives with anxiety and fear. Some anxiety disorders include panic disorder, obsessive-compulsive disorder, posttraumatic stress disorder, social phobia (or social anxiety disorder), specific phobias, and generalized anxiety disorder.[1]

behavioral therapy: Behavioral therapy focuses on a person's actions and aims to change unhealthy behavior patterns.[2]

bipolar disorder: Medical illness that causes unusual shifts in mood, energy, and activity levels. It is also known as manic-depressive illness. A person with bipolar disorder may switch from feeling extremely joyful or excited to feeling extremely sad and hopeless very quickly.[1]

cognitive behavioral therapy: This therapy helps a person focus on his or her current problems and how to solve them. Both patient and therapist need to be actively involved in this process. The therapist

---

Definitions in this chapter were compiled from documents published by several public domain sources. Terms marked 1 are from publications by the Office on Women's Health (www.womenshealth.gov); terms marked 2 are from the National Institute of Mental Health (www.nimh.nih.gov); terms marked 3 are from the Substance Abuse and Mental Health Services Administration (www.samhsa .gov); and terms marked 4 are from the Centers for Disease Control and Prevention (CDC).

helps the patient learn how to identify distorted or unhelpful thinking patterns, recognize and change inaccurate beliefs, relate to others in more positive ways, and change behaviors accordingly.[2]

cognitive therapy: Cognitive therapy focuses on a person's thoughts and beliefs, and how they influence a person's mood and actions, and aims to change a person's thinking to be more adaptive and healthy.[2]

depression: Used to describe an emotional state involving sadness, lack of energy, and low self-esteem.[1]

dysthymia: Also called dysthymic disorder. This kind of depression lasts for a long time (2 years or longer). The symptoms are less severe than major depression but can prevent one from living normally or feeling well.[1]

eating disorder: Eating disorders, such as anorexia nervosa, bulimia nervosa, and binge-eating disorder, involve serious problems with eating. This could include an extreme decrease of food or severe overeating, as well as feelings of distress and concern about body shape or weight.[1]

electroconvulsive therapy (ECT): Treatment for depression. This option may be particularly useful for individuals whose depression is severe or life threatening, or who cannot take antidepressant medication. Before treatment, which is done under brief anesthesia, patients are given a muscle relaxant. Electrodes are placed at precise locations on the head to deliver electrical impulses. The stimulation causes a brief (about 30 seconds) generalized seizure within the brain, which is necessary for therapeutic efficacy. A typical course of ECT requires 6 to 12 treatments.[2]

family-focused therapy: Therapy that includes family members in sessions to improve family relationships, which may support better treatment results.[2]

gene: The functional and physical unit of heredity made up of deoxyribonucleic acid (DNA), which has a specific function and is passed from parent to offspring.[1]

interpersonal therapy: This therapy is based on the idea that improving communication patterns and the ways people relate to others will effectively treat depression. IPT helps identify how a person interacts with other people. When a behavior is causing problems, IPT guides the person to change the behavior.[2]

light therapy: Light therapy is used to treat seasonal affective disorder (SAD), a form of depression that usually occurs during the autumn and winter months, when the amount of natural sunlight decreases.

During light therapy, a person sits in front of a "light box" for periods of time, usually in the morning. The box emits a full spectrum light, and sitting in front of it appears to help reset the body's daily rhythms.[2]

major depressive disorder: Also called major depression, this is a combination of symptoms that interfere with a person's ability to work, sleep, study, eat, and enjoy once-pleasurable activities.[1]

postpartum depression (PPD): A serious condition that requires treatment from a health care provider. With this condition, feelings of the baby blues (feeling sad, anxious, afraid, or confused after having a baby) do not go away or get worse.[1]

posttraumatic stress disorder (PTSD): An anxiety disorder that can occur after you have been through a traumatic event.[1]

premenstrual dysphoric disorder (PMDD): A severe form of premenstrual syndrome, which causes feelings of sadness or despair, or even thoughts of suicide, feelings of tension or anxiety, panic attacks, mood swings or frequent crying, and other severe symptoms.[1]

psychiatrist: A doctor (MD) who treats mental illness. Psychiatrists must receive additional training and serve a supervised residency in their specialty. They can prescribe medications.[1]

psychologist: A clinical psychologist is a professional who treats mental illness, emotional disturbance, and behavior problems. They use talk therapy as treatment, and cannot prescribe medication. A clinical psychologist will have a master's degree (MA) or doctorate (PhD) in psychology, and possibly more training in a specific type of therapy.[1]

psychotherapy: Counseling or talk therapy with a qualified practitioner in which a person can explore difficult, and often painful, emotions and experiences, such as feelings of anxiety, depression, or trauma. It is a process that aims to help the patient become better at making positive choices in his or her life, and to become more self-sufficient. Psychotherapy can be given for an individual or in a group setting.[1]

psychotic depression: A mental health disorder that occurs when a severe depressive illness is accompanied by some form of psychosis, such as a break with reality, hallucinations, and delusions.[1]

resilience: The ability of an individual, family, organization, or community to cope with adversity and adapt to challenges or change. Resilience implies that after an event, a person or community may not only be able to cope and recover, but also change to reflect different priorities arising from the experience and prepare for the next stressful situation.[3]

schizophrenia: A brain disease that can cause loss of personality, agitation, catatonia (being in a statue-like state), confusion, psychosis (a disorder in which a person is not in touch with reality), unusual behavior, and withdrawal. The illness usually begins in early adulthood.[1]

seasonal affective disorder (SAD): A depression during the winter months, when there is less natural sunlight.[1]

selective serotonin reuptake inhibitors (SSRIs): A kind of antidepressant for treating depression and anxiety disorders. SSRI medications are considered an improvement over older antidepressant medications because they have fewer side effects and are less likely to be harmful if taken in an overdose, which is an issue for patients with depression already at risk for suicide.[2]

self-esteem: How a person feels about himself or herself. When a person does not think too highly of themselves, he or she is said to have low self-esteem.[1]

serotonin syndrome: Serotonin syndrome usually occurs when older antidepressants are combined with selective serotonin reuptake inhibitors. A person with serotonin syndrome may be agitated, have hallucinations (see or hear things that are not real), have a high temperature, or have unusual blood pressure changes.[2]

social worker: A licensed clinical social worker (LCSW) is trained in psychotherapy and helps people with many different mental health and daily living problems to improve overall functioning. Usually has a master's degree in social work (MSW).[1]

St. John's wort: St. John's wort is a plant with yellow flowers that has been used for centuries for health purposes, including depression and anxiety.[1]

suicidal ideation: Thinking about, considering, or planning for suicide.[4]

suicide attempt: A non-fatal self-directed potentially injurious behavior with any intent to die as a result of the behavior. A suicide attempt may or may not result in injury.[4]

suicide: Death caused by self-directed injurious behavior with any intent to die as a result of the behavior.[4]

Chapter 68

Directory of Organizations That Help People with Depression and Suicidal Thoughts

Government Agencies That Provide Information about Depression

Agency for Healthcare Research and Quality (AHRQ)
Office of Communications and Knowledge Transfer
540 Gaither Road, Suite 2000
Rockville, MD 20850
Phone: 301-427-1104
Website: www.ahrq.gov

Centers for Disease Control and Prevention (CDC)
1600 Clifton Road
Atlanta, GA 30333
Toll-Free: 800-CDC-INFO
(800-232-4636)
Toll-Free TTY: 888-232-6348
Phone: 404-639-3311
Website: www.cdc.gov
E-mail: cdcinfo@cdc.gov

Healthfinder®
National Health Information Center
P.O. Box 1133
Washington, DC 20013-1133
Toll-Free: 800-336-4797
Phone: 301-565-4167
Fax: 301-984-4256
Website: www.healthfinder.gov
E-mail: healthfinder@nhic.org

Resources in this chapter were compiled from several sources deemed reliable; all contact information was verified and updated in October 2011.

National Cancer Institute (NCI)
NCI Office of Communications and Education
Public Inquiries Office
6116 Executive Boulevard
Suite 300
Bethesda, MD 20892-8322
Toll-Free: 800-4-CANCER
(800-422-6237)
Toll-Free TTY: 800-332-8615
Website: www.cancer.gov
E-mail: cancergovstaff@mail.nih.gov

National Center for Complementary and Alternative Medicine (NCCAM)
National Institutes of Health
NCCAM Clearinghouse
P.O. 7923
Gaithersburg, MD 20898-7923
Toll-Free: 888-644-6226
Toll-Free TTY: 866-464-3615
Toll-Free Fax: 866-464-3616
Website: www.nccam.nih.gov
E-mail: info@nccam.nih.gov

National Center for Health Statistics (NCHS)
3311 Toledo Road
Hyattsville, MD 20782
Toll-Free: 800-CDC-INFO
(800-232-4636)
Website: www.cdc.gov/nchs
E-mail: cdcinfo@cdc.gov

National Center for Posttraumatic Stress Disorder (NCPTSD)
U.S. Department of Veterans Affairs (VA)
810 Vermont Avenue, NW
Washington, DC 20420
Toll-Free: 800-827-1000
Website: www.va.gov

National Institute of Mental Health (NIMH)
Science Writing, Press, and Dissemination Branch
6001 Executive Boulevard
Room 8184, MSC 9663
Bethesda, MD 20892-9663
Toll-Free: 866-615-6464
Toll-Free TTY: 866-415-8051
Phone: 301-443-4513
TTY: 301-443-8431
Fax: 301-443-4279
Website: www.nimh.nih.gov
E-mail: nimhinfo@nih.gov

National Institute on Aging (NIA)
Building 31, Room 5C27
31 Center Drive, MSC 2292
Bethesda, MD 20892
Phone: 301-496-1752
Toll-Free: 800-222-2225
Toll-Free TTY: 800-222-4225
Fax: 301-496-1072
Website: www.nia.nih.gov
E-mail: nianews3@mail.nih.gov

National Institutes of Health (NIH)
9000 Rockville Pike
Bethesda, Maryland 20892
Phone: 301-496-4000
TTY: 301-402-9612
Website: www.nih.gov
E-mail: NIHinfo@od.nih.gov

National Women's Health Information Center (NWHIC)
Office on Women's Health
200 Independence Avenue, SW
Room 712E
Washington DC 20201
Toll-Free: 800-994-9662
Toll-Free TDD: 888-220-5446
Phone: 202-690-7650
Fax: 202-205-2631
Website: www.womenshealth.gov

Office of Disability Employment Policy (ODEP)
U.S. Department of Labor
200 Constitution Avenue, NW
Washington, DC 20210
Toll-Free: 866-ODEP-DOL
(866-633-7365)
Toll-Free TTY: 877-889-5627
Website: www.dol.gov/odep

Office of Minority Health (OMH)
Resource Center
P.O. Box 37337
Washington, DC 20013-7337
Toll-Free: 800-444-6472
Phone: 240-453-2882
TDD: 301-251-1432
Fax: 301-251-2160
Fax: 240-453-2883
Website: minorityhealth.hhs.gov
E-mail: info@minorityhealth
.hhs.gov

Substance Abuse and Mental Health Services Administration (SAMHSA)
1 Choke Cherry Road
Rockville, MD 20857
Toll-Free: 877-SAMHSA-7
(877-726-4727)
Fax: 240-221-4295
Website:
mentalhealth.samhsa.gov
Mental Health Services Locator:
mentalhealth.samhsa.gov/
databases

U.S. Department of Education (ED)
Information Resource Center
400 Maryland Avenue, SW
Washington, DC 20202
Toll-Free: 800-USA-LEARN
(800-872-5327)
Toll-Free TTY: 800-437-0833
Phone: 202-401-2000
Website: www.ed.gov

U.S. Department of Health and Human Services (HHS)
200 Independence Avenue, SW
Washington, DC 20201
Toll-Free: 877-696-6775
Website: www.hhs.gov

U.S. Food and Drug Administration (FDA)
10903 New Hampshire Avenue
Silver Spring, MD 20993
Toll-Free: 888-INFO-FDA
(888-463-6332)
Website: www.fda.gov

U.S. National Library of Medicine (NLM)
8600 Rockville Pike
Bethesda, MD 20894
Toll-Free: 888-FIND-NLM
(888-346-3656)
Toll-Free TDD: 800-735-2258
Phone: 301-594-5983
Fax: 301-402-1384
Website: www.nlm.nih.gov
E-mail: custserv@nlm.nih.gov

Private Agencies That Provide Information about Depression

AIDS InfoNet
P.O. Box 810
Arroyo Seco, NM 87514
Website: www.aidsinfonet.org
E-mail:
AIDSInfoNet@taosnet.com

Alzheimer's Association
225 North Michigan Avenue
Floor 17
Chicago, IL 60601-7633
Toll-Free: 800-272-3900
Toll-Free TDD: 866-403-3073
Phone: 312-335-8700
TDD: 312-335-5886
Toll-Free Fax: 866-699-1246
Website: www.alz.org
E-mail: info@alz.org

American Academy of Child and Adolescent Psychiatry
3615 Wisconsin Avenue, NW
Washington, DC 20016-3007
Phone: 202-966-7300
Fax: 202-966-2891
Website: www.aacap.org

American Academy of Family Physicians
P.O. Box 11210
Shawnee Mission, KS 66207-1210
Toll-Free: 800-274-2237
Phone: 913-906-6000
Fax: 913-906-6075
Website: www.aafp.org
E-mail: contactcenter@aafp.org

American Academy of Pediatrics
141 Northwest Point Boulevard
Elk Grove Village, IL 60007-1098
Phone: 847-434-4000
Fax: 847-434-8000
Website: www.aap.org
E-mail: kidsdocs@aap.org

American Art Therapy Association
225 North Fairfax Street
Alexandria, VA 22314
Toll-Free: 888-290-0878
Phone: 703-548-5860
Fax: 703-783-8468
Website: www.arttherapy.org
E-mail: info@arttherapy.org

American Association for Geriatric Psychiatry
7910 Woodmont Avenue
Suite 1050
Bethesda, MD 20814-3004
Phone: 301-654-7850
Fax: 301-654-4137
Website: www.aagponline.org
E-mail: main@aagponline.org

American Association for Marriage and Family Therapy
112 South Alfred Street
Alexandria, VA 22314-3061
Phone: 703-838-9808
Fax: 703-838-9805
Website: www.aamft.org
E-mail: central@aamft.org

American Counseling Association
5999 Stevenson Avenue
Alexandria, VA 22304
Toll-Free: 800-347-6647
TDD: 703-823-6862
Toll-Free Fax: 800-473-2329
Fax: 703-823-0252
Website: www.counseling.org
E-mail: webmaster@counseling.org

American Medical Association
515 North State Street
Chicago, IL 60654
Toll-Free: 800-621-8335
Website: www.ama-assn.org

American Psychiatric Association
1000 Wilson Boulevard
Suite 1825
Arlington, VA 22209-3901
Toll-Free: 888-35-PSYCH
(888-357-7924)
Phone: 703-907-7300
Website: www.psych.org
E-mail: apa@psych.org

American Psychological Association
750 First Street, NE
Washington, DC 20002-4242
Toll-Free: 800-374-2721
Phone: 202-336-5500
TDD/TTY: 202-336-6123
Website: www.apa.org
E-mail: public.affairs@apa.org

American Psychotherapy Association
2750 East Sunshine Street
Springfield, MO 65804
Toll-Free: 800-205-9165
Phone: 417-823-0173
Fax: 417-823-9959
Website: www
.americanpsychotherapy.com

Anxiety Disorders Association of America
8730 Georgia Avenue
Silver Spring, MD 20910
Phone: 240-485-1001
Fax: 240-485-1035
Website: www.adaa.org

Arthritis Foundation
P.O. Box 7669
Atlanta, GA 30357-0669
Toll-Free: 800-283-7800
Website: www.arthritis.org

Association for Behavioral and Cognitive Therapies
305 7th Avenue, 16th Floor
New York, NY 10001
Phone: 212-647-1890
Fax: 212-647-1865
Website: www.abct.org

The Balanced Mind Foundation
820 Davis Street, Suite 520
Evanston, IL 60201
Phone: 847-492-8510
Fax: 847-492-8520
Website:
www.thebalancedmind.org
E-mail:
info@thebalancedmind.org

Brain and Behavior Research Foundation
60 Cutter Mill Road, Suite 404
Great Neck, NY 11021
Toll-Free: 800-829-8289
Phone: 516-829-0091
Fax: 516-487-6930
Website: www.bbrfoundation.org
E-mail: info@bbrfoundation.org

Brain Injury Association of America
1608 Spring Hill Road, Suite 110
Vienna, VA 22182
Toll-Free: 800-444-6443
Phone: 703-761-0750
Fax: 703-761-0755
Website: www.biausa.org
E-mail:
braininjuryinfo@biausa.org

Canadian Mental Health Association
Phenix Professional Building
595 Montreal Road, Suite 303
Ottawa ON K1K 4L2
Fax: 613-745-5522
Website: www.cmha.ca

Canadian Psychological Association
141 Laurier Avenue West
Suite 702
Ottawa, ON K1P 5J3
Toll-Free: 888-472-0657
Phone: 613-237-2144
Fax: 613-237-1674
Website: www.cpa.ca
E-mail: cpa@cpa.ca

Caring.com
2600 South El Camino Real
Suite 300
San Mateo, CA 94403
Website: www.caring.com

Cleveland Clinic
9500 Euclid Avenue
Cleveland, OH 44195
Toll-Free: 800-223-2273
Toll-Free: 866-588-2264 (Info Line)
Phone: 216-636-5860 (Info Line)
TTY: 216-444-0261
Website: my.clevelandclinic.org

The Dana Foundation
505 Fifth Avenue, 6th Floor
New York, NY 10017
Phone: 212-223-4040
Fax: 212-317-8721
Website: www.dana.org
E-mail: danainfo@dana.org

Depressed Anonymous
P.O. Box 17414
Louisville, KY 40217
Phone: 502-569-1989
Website:
www.depressedanon.com
E-mail: info@depressedanon.com

Depression and Bipolar Support Alliance
730 North Franklin Street
Suite 501
Chicago, IL 60654-7225
Toll-Free: 800-826-3632
Fax: 312-642-7243
Website: www.dbsalliance.org
E-mail: info@dbsalliance.org

Eating Disorder Referral and Information Center
Website: www.edreferral.com

Family Caregiver Alliance
180 Montgomery Street
Suite 900
San Francisco, CA 94104
Toll-Free: 800-445-8106
Phone: 415-434-3388
Website: www.caregiver.org
E-mail: info@caregiver.org

Geriatric Mental Health Foundation
7910 Woodmont Avenue
Suite 1050
Bethesda, MD 20814
Phone: 301-654-7850
Fax: 301-654-4137
Website: www.gmhfonline.org
E-mail: web@GMHFonline.org

International Foundation for Research and Education on Depression
P.O. Box 17598
Baltimore, MD 21297-1598
Fax: 443-782-0739
Website: www.ifred.org
E-mail: info@ifred.org

International OCD Foundation
P.O. Box 961029
Boston, MA 02196
Phone: 617-973-5801
Fax: 617-973-5803
Website: www.ocfoundation.org
E-mail: info@ocfoundation.org

Mental Health America
2000 North Beauregard Street
6th Floor
Alexandria, VA 22311
Toll-Free: 800-969-6642
Toll-Free Crisis Line:
800-273-TALK (800-273-8255)
Phone: 703-684-7722
Fax: 703-684-5968
Website: www.nmha.org
E-mail: webmaster
@mentalhealthamerica.net

Mind
15-19 Broadway
Stratford, London, UK E15 4BQ
Phone: +44 208-519-2122
Fax: +44 208-522-1725
Website: www.mind.org.uk
E-mail: contact@mind.org.uk

**Multiple Sclerosis
Association of America**
706 Haddonfield Road
Cherry Hill, NJ 08002
Toll-Free: 800-532-7667
Phone: 856-488-4500
Fax: 856-661-9797
Website: www.msassociation.org
E-mail: MSquestions
@msassociation.org

**National Alliance on
Mental Illness**
3803 North Fairfax Drive
Suite 100
Arlington, VA 22203
Toll-Free:
800-950-NAMI (800-950-6264)
Phone: 703-524-7600
Fax: 703-524-9094
Website: www.nami.org

**National Association of
Anorexia Nervosa and
Associated Disorders**
P.O. Box 640
Naperville, IL 60566
Phone: 630-577-1333
Phone: 630-577-1330 (Helpline)
Fax: 630-577-1323
Website: www.anad.org
E-mail: anadhelp@anad.org

**National Association of
School Psychologists**
4340 East West Highway
Suite 402
Bethesda, MD 20814
Toll-Free: 866-331-NASP
(866-331-6277)
Phone: 301-657-0270
TTY: 301-657-4155
Fax: 301-657-0275
Website: www.nasponline.org
E-mail: center@naspweb.org

**National Eating Disorders
Association**
165 West 46th Street
New York, NY 10036
Toll-Free: 800-931-2237
Phone: 212-575-6200
Fax: 212-575-1650
Website:
www.nationaleatingdisorders.org
E-mail:
info@NationalEatingDisorders.org

National Federation of Families for Children's Mental Health
9605 Medical Center Drive
Suite 280
Rockville, MD 20850
Phone: 240-403-1901
Fax: 240-403-1909
Website: www.ffcmh.org
E-mail: ffcmh@ffcmh.org

Nemours Foundation Center for Children's Health Media
1600 Rockland Road
Wilmington, DE 19803
Phone: 302-651-4000
Website: www.kidshealth.org
E-mail: info@kidshealth.org

Parkinson's Disease Foundation
1359 Broadway, Suite 1509
New York, NY 10018
Toll-Free: 800-457-6676
Phone: 212-923-4700
Fax: 212-923-4778
Website: www.pdf.org
E-mail: info@pdf.org

Postpartum Support International
6706 SW 54th Avenue
Portland, OR 97219
Toll-Free: 800-944-4PPD
(800-944-4773)
Phone: 503-894-9453
Fax: 503-894-9452
Website: www.postpartum.net
E-mail: support@postpartum.net

Psych Central
55 Pleasant Street, Suite 207
Newburyport, MA 01950
Phone: 978-992-0008
Website: www.psychcentral.com
E-mail:
talkback@psychcentral.com

Psychology Today
115 East 23rd Street, 9th Floor
New York, NY 10010
Phone: 212-260-7210
Website:
www.psychologytoday.com

Suicide and Suicide Prevention Resources

National Suicide Prevention Lifeline
Toll-free: 800-273-TALK (800-273-8255)
Website:
www.suicidepreventionlifeline.org

American Association of Suicidology
5221 Wisconsin Avenue, NW
Washington, DC 20015
Phone: 202-237-2280
Fax: 202-237-2282
Website: www.suicidology.org

American Foundation for Suicide Prevention
120 Wall Street, 29th Floor
New York, NY 10005
Toll-Free: 888-333-AFSP
(888-333-2377)
Phone: 212-363-3500
Fax: 212-363-6237
Website: www.afsp.org
E-mail: inquiry@afsp.org

Kristin Brooks Hope Center
1250 24th Street, NW, Suite 300
Washington, DC 20037
Toll-Free: 800-442-HOPE
(800-442-4673)
Toll-Free Helpline:
800-SUICIDE (800-784-2433)
Toll-Free for Veterans:
877-VET-2-VET (877-838-2838)
Phone: 202-536-3200
Fax: 202-536-3206
Website: www.hopeline.com
Website: www.hopeline.com/
gethelpnow.html
E-mail: reese@hopeline.com

Suicide Awareness Voices of Education
8120 Penn Avenue South
Suite 470
Bloomington, MN 55431
Phone: 952-946-7998
Website: www.save.org

Suicide Prevention Resource Center
Education Development
Center, Inc.
55 Chapel Street
Newton, MA 02458-1060
Toll-Free: 877-GET-SPRC
(877-438-7772)
TTY: 617-964-5448
Fax: 617-969-9186
Website: www.sprc.org
E-mail: info@sprc.org

Index

Index

Page numbers followed by 'n' indicate a footnote. Page numbers in *italics* indicate a table or illustration.

V

vagus nerve stimulation (VNS)
 depression 28
 described 481–82
"Valerian" (NCCAM) 430n
valerian, described 450–51
Valium (diazepam),
 approved age *408*
valproic acid
 approved age 404n
 bipolar disorder 80
 side effects 406–7
Vanscoy, Holly 116n
varenicline 423–24
venlafaxine
 Alzheimer disease 333
 anxiety disorders 408
 approved age *400*
 depression 25, 54
 substance abuse 467–68
violence
 mental health problems 197–98
 mental illness 16
Vivactil (protriptyline)
 approved age *400*
 depression 55
Vyvanse (lisdexamfetamine
 dimesylate), approved age *411*

W

warning labels
 anticonvulsant medications 81
 antidepressant medications 123,
  403, 406, 413, 465
warning signs
 depression 541–42
 mental illness 5–6
 suicide 591–93
Weissenburger, J.E. 347n
Weissman, Myrna 116
Wellbutrin (bupropion)
 Alzheimer disease 332
 anxiety disorders 408
 approved age *400*
 bipolar disorder 82
 depression 54
 dysthymia 64
 side effects 59–60

"What a Difference a Friend
 Makes" (SAMHSA) 567n
"What Causes Depression?"
 (Centre for Clinical
 Interventions) 204n
"What to Do When Someone
 Experiences Depression After a
 Stroke" (Caring, Inc.) 338n
Whipple, Beverly 497
Widom, Cathy 229
women
 caregivers 183
 depression 22–23
 depression overview 125–30
 stress 213
 suicide statistics 574
"Women and Depression:
 Discovering Hope" (NIMH) 125n
workplace, depression coping
 strategies 537–40
 see also employment;
  occupations

X

Xanax (alprazolam)
 anxiety disorders 409
 approved age *408*

Y

yoga, overview 451–54
"Yoga for Health: An Introduction"
 (NCCAM) 451n

Z

Zarate, Carlos 422
ziprasidone
 approved age *396*
 bipolar disorder 405
 schizophrenia 395
Zoloft (sertraline)
 Alzheimer disease 333
 anxiety disorders 408
 approved age *400*
 bipolar disorder 82
 depression 25, 54
 described 399
 dysthymia 64

Health Reference Series